ESSENTIALS OF
Psychiatric nursing

ESSENTIALS OF
Psychiatric nursing

DOROTHY MERENESS
R.N., Ed.D.

*Dean, School of Nursing, University of Pennsylvania,
Philadelphia, Pa.; formerly Director of the
Psychiatric-Mental Health Nursing Program,
School of Education,
New York University, New York, N. Y.*

EIGHTH EDITION

With 20 illustrations

Saint Louis
THE C. V. MOSBY COMPANY
1970

EIGHTH EDITION

Copyright © 1970 by

THE C. V. MOSBY COMPANY

Sixth printing

*All rights reserved. No part of this book may be
reproduced in any manner without written permission
of the publisher.*

Previous editions copyrighted 1940, 1944, 1949, 1953, 1958, 1962, 1966

Printed in the United States of America

Standard Book Number 8016-3397-4

Library of Congress Catalog Card Number 70-119365

Distributed in Great Britain by Henry Kimpton, London

To

FRANCES PAYNE BOLTON

*Patron of the nursing arts and tireless
champion of higher standards in nursing education*

Preface to eighth edition

Like all other areas of human knowledge, psychiatric nursing is constantly changing. Each year more information is added to the essential knowledge required of those who are focusing their attention upon this aspect of nursing. In keeping with the need for nurses to have more knowledge about human behavior, the eighth edition of this text has provided a chapter on understanding children and adolescents who are emotionally ill. In addition, a discussion that focuses on understanding individuals with faulty intellectual development has also been included.

For twenty-five years the number of children and adolescents who have required psychiatric help has steadily increased. Because caring for very young patients has now been included among the psychiatric nurse's responsibilities, I concluded that a chapter on children and adolescents should become a part of the eighth edition. This was a difficult decision because understanding and providing care for mentally ill children and adolescents is a highly specialized activity and should have an enlarged treatment if it is to be adequate. Likewise, understanding and providing care for individuals with faulty intellectual development requires a greatly enlarged treatment if it is to be completely adequate. This chapter was included because of the nurse's need for information about individuals with faulty intellectual development whose numbers in psychiatric situations appear to be increasing rapidly.

Community psychiatry, a new concept that has gained popularity within the last few years, has been included. In addition,

emphasis has been placed on the nurse's role with groups of patients. The inclusion of these four new chapters makes it possible for the eighth edition of *Essentials of Psychiatric Nursing* to provide the student with a complete survey of the entire field of psychiatric nursing. Of course, a single text cannot provide all the information needed for students to gain an in-depth understanding of the topic being studied; thus a bibliography of readily available articles has been provided at the end of each chapter. The sequence of chapters has been rearranged for a more logical organization of the material presented, and new illustrations of psychiatric nurses in action have been added throughout the book.

The eighth revision has been accomplished in the hope of providing the students of psychiatric nursing with a more effective study tool that will assist in making this most interesting aspect of nursing more meaningful and more significant to the user.

No one ever revises a text without becoming indebted to many persons who have assisted by making suggestions, giving encouragement, or having contributed in other ways.

I am especially grateful to one of my former graduate students, Mrs. Cecelia Monat Taylor, now Educational Director at Brooklyn Downstate Medical Center, who made many valuable suggestions for revising some of the content and rearranging the sequence of chapters.

I am grateful to Mr. William Sippel, one of my former graduate students who is currently an administrative officer at Philadelphia Community College, for making suggestions for revision of some of the content.

Special gratitude is due the nursing staff and affiliating students at Cleveland Psychiatric Institute for providing some of the illustrations that were used in the books. Some of those who provided leadership in the photographic project were Mrs. Helen Kreigh, former Director of Nursing, Miss Janice Somppi, formerly Director of Nursing Education and currently Director of Nursing, and Mrs. May Wykle, Instructor in Nursing.

Gratitude is also due Dr. F. A. Lingl, Superintendent of Cleveland Psychiatric Institute, for making it possible for photographs of the nursing staff to be taken at Cleveland Psychiatric Institute.

Dorothy Mereness

Preface to seventh edition

We have developed this textbook in the hope of assisting students of nursing to gain a beginning understanding of the causes, prevention, and treatment of mental illness and the potential therapeutic role of the psychiatric nurse. Because the role of the psychiatric nurse is constantly developing and ever expanding, an attempt has been made to identify principles and concepts that will provide a sound basis upon which to build an understanding of human behavior and to perfect the skills required in psychiatric nursing.

To achieve these goals we have devoted the first section of the text to the nurse as an individual and have entitled it The Nurse Focuses upon Herself and Her Role. Since many authorities believe that self-understanding is an important beginning in the development of an understanding of others, one of the first chapters focuses upon the early reactions of the student to psychiatric nursing. This emphasis upon the student as an individual was a deliberate attempt to encourage self-examination and reflection upon personal feelings and the relationships developed with patients.

The most profitable time for study and discussion of this portion of the text would be before the student actually embarks upon the psychiatric nursing experience or during the first week of the experience.

Although the work roles of the psychiatric nurse almost never occur singly, they have been discussed individually in order to assist the student in identifying and understanding them. Likewise, separate chapters have been devoted to the nursing skills that have been found to be most useful in the psychiatric situation. Thus it is hoped that the student of nursing will become more consciously aware of the potentially therapeutic skills at her command and will work toward perfecting skill in communicating with patients and co-workers, skill in using self therapeutically, skill in developing therapeutic potentials of the environment, and skill in contributing to the therapeutic aspects of specific therapies that are provided for patients.

The second section of the text, entitled The Nurse Focuses upon Understanding Her Patients, is devoted to the patient and to understanding abnormal behaviors that are expressions of unmet human needs. Short patient histories are included, followed by a discussion of the probable dynamics underlying the behavior which is described. Such explanations and analyses of patient behavior provide a basis for understanding the abnormal expression of human needs and for developing insights into possible useful nursing interventions.

The third section includes discussions of essential topics that contribute to the development of a broad understanding of the field of psychiatric nursing. These topics include a discussion of psychophysiological disorders, a historical review of psychiatry, psychiatry and the law, and mental hygiene.

The appendix provides a quick and easy reference to some of the more common psychiatric terms, some of the necessary information about the more common and generic forms of the ataractic agents (tranquilizers) the nurse will administer to patients, and the most recent diagnostic classification of mental illnesses currently in use by psychiatrists.

Although this text was written specifically for students of nursing who are having initial experience with psychiatrically ill patients, it is recognized that all nurses require these skills and understandings if they are to function in a therapeutic role with any group of human beings. Thus a chapter is devoted to understanding patients who are hospitalized in settings other than psychiatric ones.

In keeping with the belief that nurses themselves can best understand and describe the work of the nurse meaningfully, the references included at the end of each chapter are primarily the works of other psychiatric nurses. References from medical authorities serve to help the nurse develop some basic concepts concerning the cause and development of the illnesses discussed in this text.

This book cannot include all of the information a student must have if a breadth of understanding of the field of psychiatric nursing is to be developed. However, it does seek to initiate the nurse into this field of nursing, to interest the nurse so that she will continue to work toward developing an understanding of self and patients throughout her professional career, and to motivate her to read more widely in the available literature.

Teachers who use this text are encouraged to begin the study of psychiatric nursing with Section Two, The Nurse Focuses upon Understanding Her Patients, if this approach seems more appropriate to the situation. Hopefully, Section One, The Nurse Focuses upon Herself and Her Role, will be studied before the student embarks upon the psychiatric nursing experience or in the very early days of the experience.

We hope that students who use this book will be encouraged to elect psychiatric nursing as the area of their specialized nursing interest when they are ready to embark upon a professional career.

Dorothy Mereness
Philadelphia, Pennsylvania

Louis J. Karnosh
Cleveland, Ohio

Contents

xi

Contents

SECTION THREE

The nurse focuses on understanding her patients

Contents

Contents

Contents

SECTION FOUR

The nurse focuses upon psychiatric nursing in relation to its history, to the law, and to future trends

Contents

Appendixes

SECTION ONE
The nurse focuses on understanding self and others

CHAPTER ONE

Introduction—the nature of psychiatric nursing

This text has been written specifically for the student of nursing who is beginning the study of psychiatric nursing and who is being initiated into an experience in a clinical setting where care is given to mentally ill patients. We believe that such a nurse will welcome some guidance in accepting and understanding the situation and in studying her role in the care of these patients.

The student nurse's previous professional experience probably has been limited to situations in which attention was focused upon the physical needs of patients. In spite of the fact that the nurse's initial professional education may have emphasized the relationship between the emotional and physical aspects of sickness and health, the student nurse may be surprised and a little confused by the approach that is made to the care of patients in psychiatric settings. She may raise many questions and may feel that much she has learned previously is of little help to her in this new situation. Many of the attitudes and approaches used in the psychiatric setting may be unfamiliar. The student may notice that few nurses are involved in measuring and recording the temperature, pulse, and respirations of the patients. She may observe that nurses are required to take very few blood pressure readings. She may wonder if there is enough concern on the part of the doctors and nurses for the physical welfare of these patients.

Vital statistics show that the physical health of patients in psychiatric hospitals is slightly above the average of the physical health of a comparable group of people in the community outside the hospital. This is probably because of the relatively safe environment in which the patients live. Although psychiatric hospitals do not have the physical health of patients as their primary concern, nurses and doctors are constantly aware of the importance of safeguarding and maintaining the physical health of mentally ill patients. They are also aware of the significant interrelationship between physical and emotional health.

In addition to wondering if there is enough professional concern about the physical welfare of mentally ill patients, the student nurse may wonder about many other activities in which she observes the nurses participating. She may be surprised at the amount of time that hospital personnel spend talking to patients and engaging in recreational activities with them. She may wonder how some of these recreational activities can be classified as nursing.

She may question the wisdom of allowing patients to spend a good deal of time away from the hospital on weekends and during the evening. She may question the importance of hospitalization for patients who seem not to require the services of the hospital staff for many of the highly technical procedures employed in other areas of the hospital.

It is not surprising or difficult to understand that during the first day in psychiatric nursing the student nurse may believe that she is going to have a few weeks of comparative inactivity as far as nursing is concerned.

WHAT IS PSYCHIATRIC NURSING?

It may be helpful to consider broadly the meaning of the concept that is expressed by the words nursing care. Unfortunately, there was a time in the development of the nursing profession when nursing care was thought to be limited to the performance of comfort measures and restorative techniques. Under this somewhat limited view, nursing care focused upon giving the bath, making the patient comfortable, and administering restorative treatments and medicines. Although comfort measures and restorative techniques are still essential elements in the total nursing care of physically ill patients, the nursing profession has broadened its concept of the role of the nurse. Today, in addition to her traditional role, the nurse is expected to be a teacher of positive health, to participate in activities that are designed to prevent illness, to understand emotional aspects of health and disease, to recognize emotional needs, and to give understanding, support, and guidance to persons in trouble. Helping the patient to resume his role as an independent, self-directing, functioning individual is also part of the nurse's professional responsibility.

Nursing care may consist of any therapeutic activity within the professional competence of the nurse and under the direction of the physician that is designed to assist the patient to resume, within the limitations of his capabilities, the role of a functioning, self-directing individual or that will help him live out the remainder of his life as comfortably and happily as possible. The nurse may perform intimate, personal services for a patient while he is experiencing a physical illness and until he is able to function as an independent, self-directing individual.

A mentally ill patient may require help in coping with the everyday problems of life. This assistance may involve the physical functions of his body, but it is more likely to involve his feelings about himself and other people, his social relationships, and his response to his environment.

Helping patients to accept themselves, to improve their relationships with other people, and to function independently are probably the most fundamental goals in psychiatric nursing. Because helping patients to improve their interpersonal relationships is one of the therapeutic goals of psychiatric nursing, the nurse needs to be prepared to make positive use of her own personality. Some essential abilities that are involved in using oneself therapeutically include the following: the acceptance of patients as unique, important human beings, the acceptance of all human behavior as being meaningful and having developed in response to a need, and the ability to convey to the patient a feeling of acceptance, warmth, and genuine interest in him. All patients, whether they are mentally or physically ill, deserve a nurse who is capable of using self therapeutically. Many nurses successfully achieve this ability without actually recognizing it or being able to analyze how success was accomplished. Psychiatric nurses cannot trust to luck in the hope of developing the attitudes that are fundamental in becoming a therapeutic person. The nurse who works with mentally ill patients needs to learn to know herself, to analyze her relationships with others, and to work constantly to improve her understanding of human behavior and her approach to patients. Psychiatric nursing probably does not require unique personality attributes or attitudes, but it does require an interest in developing a therapeutic approach to patients and consistent, thoughtful effort directed toward developing understanding of self and others.

Because the psychiatric nurse is the professional person who is with the patient the greatest length of time, she has a unique opportunity to influence his hospital experience in the direction of positive therapeutic results. The therapeutic role of the psychiatric nurse involves creating a daily, 24-hour environment that will provide opportunities for patients to establish positive relationships with individuals and groups in anticipation of eventually returning to the community as contributing, self-directing members. In light of the psychiatric nurse's opportunity to make hospitalization a therapeutic experience for patients, each daily activity in which patients participate needs to be examined from the standpoint of its therapeutic potential. It is obvious that the therapeutic role of the psychiatric nurse cannot be described in terms of routines and procedures but must be discussed in terms of attitudes, feelings, relationships, and understandings.

THE PSYCHIATRIC NURSE'S NEED TO UNDERSTAND HERSELF

All nurses need to develop self-awareness in order to understand how they respond to patients and how patients respond to them. It is also necessary for nurses to be able to identify emotional needs of patients and to understand ways in which these emotional needs can be met. This is an essential aspect of the professional nurse's role because emotional needs of human beings can be met only by other human beings. It is reasonable to believe that the nurse will identify emotional needs more accurately and will meet them more effectively if she has some awareness of herself as a person and the role that she can play in the emotional lives of patients.

When a nurse cares for any patient some kind of reciprocal relationship develops. This relationship has unlimited therapeutic possibilities. It may develop into something extremely positive and may be an important factor in the eventual recovery of the patient. It may develop many unhealthy features and may actually affect the hospital experience of the patient negatively. It is possible that the relationship between nurse and patient may develop both positive and negative aspects. Whatever relationship develops, the nurse should have some understanding of the relationship and her role in it.

Many nurses are only partially aware of how they affect the outcome of the patient's hospital experience. It is not uncommon for nurses who deal primarily with the physical aspects of illness to function intuitively when dealing in the area of emotions. This method of dealing with the emotional problems of illness may result in acceptable outcomes with patients who are not mentally ill. However, because psychiatric nurses strive to deal therapeutically with emotional problems, it is important for them to develop an understanding of self and others that goes beyond the intuitive level.

All psychiatric nurses will not be able to have professional help in understanding the reciprocal relationship that develops between themselves and patients and co-workers. However, it is possible for all

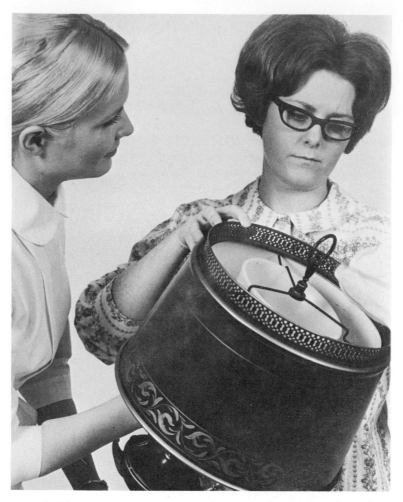

FIG. 1. *The nurse strives to meet the patient's emotional needs.*

nurses to develop an interest in learning to understand themselves. They can consider their own responses, and they can develop the habit of studying responses they evoke from others. Nurses can develop the practice of recognizing and admitting their feelings and examining them in group discussions with other professional people who are also striving to develop and improve awareness of self. Nurses can learn a great deal by studying their own behavior and the behavior of others and by asking themselves such questions as these: "Why did I do what I did?" What do I do that makes the other individual respond as he does?" How can I alter my behavior in order to achieve more positive responses on the part of the other person?"

ADJUSTING TO THE PSYCHIATRIC SITUATION

Among many adjustments the student nurse will find she has to make in the psychiatric situation, there are a few that seem to require particular attention. They include the problem of fear of people who are mentally ill, adjustment to the slower pace of the psychiatric hospital, handling the guilt feelings that sometimes arise when student nurses are not required to expend a great deal of energy in giving physical care to patients, and the continuous adjustment and readjustment of attitudes and feelings as they relate to the needs and the behavior of patients. These aspects of adjustment to the psychiatric situation are discussed more completely in chapters that follow.

In many ways mentally ill patients are the most challenging group of individuals with whom the nurse has had an opportunity to work. In a very real sense, the relationship the nurse and the patient develop can be one of the most important factors in the patient's therapeutic experience. Whether the nurse can be a force for developing a truly therapeutic situation for the patient depends on her ability to give the patient new and more positive experiences in living with other people. To accomplish this the nurse must continuously strive to understand the patient's behavior and the emotional needs expressed by the behavior. She must seek to understand herself and the role into which she is cast in the emotional lives of the patients with whom she relates. She must constantly adjust and readjust her approaches, her attitudes, and her feelings. To do this the nurse must give much thought and consideration to her own behavior as it influences the behavior of others. It is helpful to reflect upon the activities of the day, to reconstruct conversations and experiences in written form, and to share these with other students in a small discussion group. In reliving these experiences by sharing them, the student can see more clearly their meaning and the role that she was cast in or assumed. With the help of a teacher and other students, such discussions can provide an opportunity for learning for all members of a student group.

IMPORTANT CONCEPTS

1. Helping patients to accept themselves, to improve their relationships with other people, and to function independently are probably the most fundamental goals in psychiatric nursing.
2. Effective performance in psychiatric nursing does not require unique personality attributes or abilities, but it does demand that emphasis be placed upon accepting and understanding oneself and others and the ability to relate positively to others.
3. One of the most important responsibilities of the psychiatric nurse is to create an environment that will provide opportunities for patients to establish positive relationships with individuals and groups.
4. The nurse will identify emotional needs more accurately and will meet them more effectively if she has some awareness of herself as a person and of her role in the reciprocal relationship between herself and patients.
5. The nurse can be one of the most significant therapeutic influences in a patient's hospital experience because she spends more time with the patient than does any other professional worker.

7

CHAPTER TWO

Personality—its structure, development, and mechanisms of defense

Understanding human behavior and the many adjustment problems that arise in the lives of people depends to a large extent on understanding the process through which the personality develops. It is also important to recognize the relationship between the early interpersonal experiences that human beings undergo and the development of the personality.

Much of the information that we have today about the evolution of personality has been derived from psychological theories and not from scientific research. Actually, much of our current knowledge is based upon theories proposed by Sigmund Freud, who lived from 1856 to 1939. He did much of his important work in Vienna around the turn of the century. During and after the time when Freud was formulating his theories, other men contributed important ideas to the total understanding of human behavior. Many of these contributors were Freud's students. However, Freud deserves most of the credit for developing the foundational theories. It was Freud's writing that first stressed the crucial importance of early childhood experiences in the development of human personality and the relationship between some of the emotional problems in adult life and the negative influences that sometimes occur during the early years.

The psychiatric theories currently in use in the United States are sometimes called *eclectic*. That is, concepts from more than one school of thought have been used in developing a usable theory of personality development.

Before a discussion of personality development can become meaningful, it is essential to understand the definition of personality used by students of human behavior. Unfortunately, this word has been used to convey many different meanings and ideas. In ordinary conversation it usually refers to the personal response that the individual evokes from others. It is not unusual for someone to comment that an individual has a pleasing personality or that a certain person has a poor personality. When used technically, the word personality refers to the aggregate of the physical and mental qualities, as these interact in characteristic fashion with the individual's environment. Thus it can be seen that personality is expressed through behavior. The characteristic combinations of behavior distinguish one individual from another and endow individuals with their own unique identity.

This definition of personality includes the individual's biological and intellectual endowment, the attributes that have been acquired through experience, and his conscious and unconscious reactions and feelings. Personality development is a complex and dynamic process that is constantly evolving from what it was to something different, yet it always retains a certain identifiable consistency. It is important to remember that from birth to death personality is ever changing and ever developing. This fact makes it possible for individuals of all ages to profit from corrective experiences and to modify behavior in a positive direction. This is the rationale underlying all psychotherapeutic endeavors on the behalf of patients.

TOPOGRAPHICAL DESCRIPTION OF THE PSYCHE

It is important for the student of human behavior to understand Freud's theoretical delineation of the mind or psyche. These concepts are used almost universally in this country and contribute much to understanding the accepted theories concerning personality development.

Levels of consciousness

One way in which Freud described the mind topographically was from the standpoint of levels of consciousness. These levels are referred to as the conscious, the preconscious, and the unconscious parts of the mind.

The *conscious* part of the mind is aware of the here and now as it relates to the individual and his environment. It functions only when the individual is awake. The conscious mind is concerned with thoughts, feelings, and sensations. It directs the individual as he behaves in a rational, thoughtful way.

The *preconscious* or *subconscious,* as it has been described by some psychologists, is that part of the mind in which ideas and reactions are stored and partially forgotten. It also acts as a watchman, since it prevents certain unacceptable, disturbing unconscious memories from reaching the conscious mind. Material relegated to this handy storehouse usually can be brought into conscious awareness if the individual concentrates on recall. Because it is not economical for human beings to burden the conscious mind with a multitude of facts that are infrequently used and currently not in demand, the preconscious is an extremely valuable device.

The unconscious is by far the largest part of the mind and is sometimes compared to the large hidden part of an iceberg that floats under the water. In this comparison the small part of the iceberg that appears above the water represents the conscious mind. The unconscious is the storehouse for all the memories, feelings, and responses experienced by the individual during his entire life. It is one of Freud's most important concepts. Authorities believe that the human mind never actually forgets any experience but stores all knowledge, information, and feeling about all experiences in the unconscious. These memories cannot be recalled at will by the individual. He is rarely aware of the unconscious mind, except as it demonstrates its presence through dreams, slips of the tongue, unexplained behavioral responses, jokes, and lapses of memory. Psychotic symptoms are expressions of unconscious thoughts or feelings. Material stored in the unconscious has a powerful influence upon behavior because the accompanying feelings continue to act as motivating, dynamic forces. The individual is unaware of the ideas themselves, but he may continue to experience an emotional reaction as if the material were in the conscious mind.

Structure of the personality

The second topographical description developed by Freud is frequently referred to as the structure of the personality. This structure includes the concepts of the id, the ego, and the superego.

The *id* is part of and derived from the unconscious. It is unlearned, primitive, selfish, and the source of all energy. It contains the instinctual drives, which are said to be the drive for self-preservation, the drive to reproduce, and the drive for group association. The id is without a sense of right and wrong and ruthlessly insists upon the satisfaction of its impulses and desires.

When the new individual is born he is said to be a bundle of id, seeking only to satisfy his needs and to find release for physiological tensions. By crying, the infant insists upon receiving attention when tensions build up. He disregards all other factors in his environment as he demands that his needs be met.

During the individual's entire life the id persists in pushing the organism toward the achievement of its primitive, instinctual goals. It is described as operating on the bass of the *pleasure principle*. That is to say, the id presses for avoidance of pain at all costs and seeks to maintain pleasure. Pleasure in this sense refers to release of tension and the establishment of emotional and physiological equilibrium. Pain refers to tensions that are present when the infant is cold, hungry, frightened, or anxious. As the child matures, the concept of pain encompasses additional aspects of body equilibrium, including sexual tension, tensions that result from cultural pressures, and tension from physiological needs. Throughout the individual's entire life the id insists that the individual seek release of tension regardless of the social outcome. It is the duty of other parts of the personality to censor the id and to keep it under control.

The *ego* is that part of the personality that represents the self or the "I" and gives the individual identity. The development of the ego is a result of the individual's interaction with the environment. It is initiated when the infant recognizes the breast or the bottle as part of the environment rather than as part of his own body.

The ego promotes the individual's satisfactory adjustment in relation to his environment. Its main function is to effect an acceptable compromise between the crude pleasure-seeking strivings of the id and the excessive inhibitions of the superego. The ego deals with the demands of reality as it strives to control and derive satisfaction from the environment. Thus, as the individual matures the ego becomes the rational, reasonable, conscious part of the personality and strives to integrate the total personality into a smoothly functioning unified, coherent whole.

Chronologically the *superego* develops last. Its development is partially a result of the socialization process that the child undergoes. The superego encorporates the taboos, prohibitions, ideals, and standards of the parents and the other significant adults with whom the child associates. It operates mostly at unconscious levels and at this level is an inhibitor of the id. At the conscious levels it may be regarded as the voice of conscience or the phase of personality that is keenly sensitive to the demands of strict convention. The term superego refers to the blindly rigid, strict moralistic part of the mind, which can be as unrelenting and ruthless as the id. One aspect of the *superego* is the *ego ideal*, which directs behavior to simulate that of individuals the person admires and wishes to emulate.

If the individual does not develop an ego that is strong enough to arbitrate effectively between the id and the superego, he will surely develop interpersonal and intrapersonal conflicts. When the id is not controlled effectively, the individual functions in antisocial, lawless ways because his primitive impulses are expressed freely. When individuals suffer from emotional illness they are frequently suffering from a conflict between the ego and the id. If the superego is so strong that the individual's life is dominated by its restrictions on behavior, he is likely to be inhibited, repressed, unhappy, and guilt ridden. Thus development of a mature, effective, stable adult life is dependent on a powerful ego and a strong superego.

DEVELOPMENT OF THE PERSONALITY

It has been said that the first six years in a child's life contribute the most to personality development. When one considers that these years provide the foundation for future patterns of behavior, this statement appears to be true. For the sake of convenience the early developmental years have been divided into periods or stages. The boundaries of these periods are not rigidly fixed, and each period overlaps with the period that follows. The stages of personality development, as described by Freud, are differentiated by the changing focus of the child's libidinal energies as he matures emotionally, socially, and physically. Freud theorized that development of the personality was intimately involved with the maturation of the libidinal drives or love energies as they focused first upon the self and later upon other appropriate persons in the environment. This interrelationship is referred to as *psychosexual* development and has proved to be an essentially useful concept.

At first the infant directs his libidinal drives toward himself. This process is technically referred to as *primary narcissim*, which means self-love. It seems logical that the infant needs to focus upon

himself in his initial struggle to survive. As he develops, his initial self-love is slowly directed toward others, beginning with the mother and finally including the other significant members of his immediate environment. According to Freud's theories, the individual achieves psychosexual maturity after successfully advancing through several stages of development. The behavior of the mature individual is characterized by the direction of his libidinal drives, which are focused upon a member of the opposite sex for whom he has tender, protective feelings and with whom he hopes to establish a home and nurture a family. At the same time he retains enough self-love to seek satisfaction for his own needs without being destructive to others. In addition, he is able to direct positive feelings toward other people in his environment, to work effectively and to achieve creatively, and to fully utilize the capacities with which he has been endowed without being hampered by crippling anxieties. The ability to achieve these mature capabilities depends to a large extent on the child's heredity and constitutional endowment. However, psychosexual development is powerfully influenced by the responses that the child receives from the significant people in his environment during his early formative years and by other crucial events that occur as he grows.

Infancy

The period of infancy roughly extends over the first year and a half of life and is sometimes referred to as the *oral period*. This descriptive title is applied to it because the child's whole being is focused upon the mouth and its functions. In the first weeks of life most of the infant's satisfactions come from the sensation of sucking or swallowing. At this stage in the infant's life he is unable to differentiate between himself and his environment. His awareness of himself is in terms of comfort or discomfort. His total being is focused upon fulfilling the demands of the id, which insists on relief from hunger, cold, or tension. As far as the infant is concerned his environment exists to satisfy his needs for oral satisfaction. At this period the infant is said to be in the early or passive oral stage of development. Tensions are relieved by breast-feeding, nursing a bottle, or sucking a thumb. In the infant's feelings food intake becomes closely identified with the tender, comforting care given by the mother, who becomes the most important single source of satisfaction for him. If the mother is a giving, comforting parent, the child will probably develop a general feeling of security and an expectant attitude regarding the meeting of his needs. If she is a withholding mother, he may develop anxious, insecure feelings.

The lips, mouth, tongue, and skin are the areas of an infant's body from which he receives pleasure. As he learns to achieve pleasurable reactions from parts of his own body he begins to separate himself from his mother. Thus the infant begins to develop narcissistic behavior or self-love. In this way the ego or the recognition of the self or the "me" as opposed to the "not me" begins to develop.

When weaning is initiated the infant begins to receive fewer oral satisfactions from his environment. When the cup and solid food are substituted for the breast or bottle, the infant feels frustrated. With the adoption of more rigid schedules the infant is denied the complete attention of the mother. He may react to these frustrations orally in an aggressive, sometimes destructive way and may begin to bite and may seek symbolic oral gratification by sucking other objects. This behavior is characteristic of the agressive oral phase of this period.

Significance of the oral phase. The child's future attitude toward life may be powerfully conditioned by his feeding experiences. If his great need for love and attention has been met unconditionally by a giving, loving mother he will begin to develop a general attitude toward life that will have been conditioned in the direction of optimism.

Because food and love are given simultaneously during the oral period, oral needs become synonymous with protective love and security. These needs are universal and continue throughout life in one form or another. In adult life release of tension through oral gratification is achieved through chewing gum, smoking, eating, and drinking. These activities are residuals of the oral phase of development.

More incapacitating residuals of the oral phase can be observed in the extremely dependent individual or the person who eats compulsively in an attempt to relieve anxiety and to satisfy an insatiable need for love and security. Likewise, excessive drinking of alcohol may be an attempt to relieve anxiety and to return emotionally to a period when love was given unconditionally without concomitant demands being made. By observing some alcoholics it is strikingly obvious that they have substituted the whiskey bottle for the pleasures of the nursing bottle.

Early childhood

The period of early childhood is a phase of personality development that occurs between the ages of 1½ and 3 years. It is sometimes described as the anal or habit-training period. This descriptive terminology focuses upon the tasks to be achieved in the child's maturation during these years. In our culture this is the period when the mother insists that the infant achieve sphincter control and begin to communicate through the use of language.

In the early part of this period, the child freely gratifies his love of self with the pleasurable sensations involved in evacuating the bladder and bowels naturally and without restriction. Although the mouth remains an important zone of pleasure, the infant derives much pleasure from the anus and the urethra during these early years.

Ego development continues in this period as the child constantly develops a better defined concept of self. Superego development is initiated as the mother begins to insist that the child accept certain restrictions and controls regarding toileting. It is at this point that the child experiences the first major frustration of his id drives. He is forced to come to terms with the reality of the situation. To retain his mother's love the child must learn to postpone the immediate pleasure of urinating or evacuating until the appropriate time and place. The necessity

for making an adaptation to the mother's wishes regarding toileting places the infant and the mother in conflict. This stage of psychosexual development is sometimes called the late anal aggressive phase. As the mother withholds love in an attempt to force the child to accept her standards in relation to toileting, the child develops ambivalent feelings toward her. If the mother is too forceful or too harsh in enforcing rigid toileting schedules the child may express anal aggression in the form of retention of feces, soiling, scattering, and other hostile behavior directed toward parents and other adults.

If the mother-child relationship during the first year was developed out of the provision of adequate love and security, the conflict between them will be resolved without too much difficulty. Eventually the child accepts and internalizes the inhibitions and standards of the mother.

This is frequently the period in a child's life when a new baby arrives and replaces him as the focus for all his mother's attention. When the child is struggling to master sphincter control, the birth of a sibling may cause him to regress to the earlier and more dependent behavior that was satisfying during the oral period. Essentially he is competing for his mother's attention in the best way he knows. This rivalrous situation in which the child vies with a brother or sister for the love and attention of the parents is referred to as *sibling rivalry.*

Significance of the habit-training period. The habit-training period is an extremely important period because patterns of behavior involving self-control are initiated. The child-mother conflict may also initiate a pattern of interaction that may persist into adult life.

Some of the residuals of this period may dominate adult behavior. If great stress is placed upon the child in relation to remaining clean during this period he may grow up to be compulsively clean and meticulous. Other adult attitudes thought to be traceable to rigid toilet training include stubbornness, hoarding and collecting, excessive concern with bowel function, and sadistic or masochistic tendencies.

Later childhood

The period of later childhood is a phase of psychosexual development that includes the years of age from 3 to 6. It has been variously described as the phallic period or the period of the family triangle. These descriptive terms refer to the fact that the focus of pleasurable sensations has shifted from the mouth and the excretory organs to the genitalia and that the child begins to identify with the parent of the same sex and to unconsciously wish to replace that parent in the family situation. Thus it is not uncommon to hear a girl in this age group speak of "marrying Daddy" or a little boy say "Go away, Daddy, I will take care of Mommie."

Between the ages of 3 and 6 years children begin to examine their own bodies. They discover that pleasurable sensations can be aroused from manipulation of the penis or the clitoris. They also become aware of the difference between the sexual structure of men and women and wonder about the girl's lack of a sexual organ. Children of this age may conclude that the penis can be lost in some way, since some people whose bodies they have observed have apparently lost this organ. Anxiety about the loss of the sex organ may develop among children in this age group. Fears may be expressed by a little boy concerning the loss of his penis through punishment or an accident. These fears are referred to as *castration fears.* Unfortunately, some parents reinforce these fears by threatening to cut off the penis if the child is observed fondling it. A little girl notices that she has no penis and may conclude that she lost it or that it has been taken away. She naturally wants what she observes some other children possess. This attitude on the part of a little girl is called *penis envy.* It is sometimes basic to the problem of *sibling rivalry.*

Some people ridicule these concepts and deny that normal children are concerned about loss of the penis. However, evidence that these ideas are frequently found among young children can be gathered by observing children in any permissive nursery school. One little 4-year-old girl was observed to hold up a lump of clay she had fashioned and call to her nursery school group, "See my penis!" Parents do not always observe these attitudes because children learn even before they begin to talk that parents react as if there were something shameful about the genitalia. Thus some children avoid telling their parents about their sexual phantasies or asking questions about sex.

During this period the little boy who has always had a great deal of attention and love from his mother begins to feel very possessive toward her. He wants her for himself, and he resents the close tie that he feels exists between his mother and father. He develops rivalrous feelings toward his father and tries to compete with him for his mother's love. The father is such a large and formidable opponent that the little boy develops a good deal of resentment and fear of him. This situation is referred to as the *Oedipus complex* or *situation*. It may precipitate *castration fears* because the little boy may begin to fear that the father will punish him for his resentment toward him and his attempt to replace him in his mother's life. Eventually the little boy concludes that being like his father is a more effective way of achieving his mother's love and attention. Thus he begins to take on the masculine behavior of the father. This is referred to as *identification*. In this way the little boy begins to learn the role of the male in our culture. The initiation of *role identification* is probably the most significant psychosexual task of this period.

Similarly, during this period the little girl begins to identify with the feminine role. The process through which the girl passes in identifying with the parent of the same sex is not as clearly understood as is the process for little boys. The girl feels that somehow her mother is responsible for the fact that she does not have a penis. She also notices that she does not have breasts as her mother does. She may blame her mother for not having provided her with a complete body and may display a good deal of hostility and antagonism toward her. The little girl turns to her father for love and affection and frequently competes openly with the mother for his attention. She begins to imitate her mother because she feels that in this way she may be able to please her father. This is a difficult period for the little girl who must keep her mother's love and approval because she is still dependent upon her. It is essential that the child maintain a positive relationship with her mother if she is to accomplish the task of identifying with the feminine role.

Sibling rivalry presents a particularly difficult adjustment problem for both boys and girls during this period when they are struggling to resolve the *oedipal situation*. The arrival of a new baby in the family at this time presents children with a situation in which they feel that they must compete for the parents' love. They are particularly in need of the mother's love during this phase and may develop tremendous resentment of the newcomer.

Significance of later childhood. Later childhood is a crucial time in the life of both the boy and the girl because the basic life pattern for future relationships with men and women is initiated during this period. If for many reasons the parents are people with whom the children cannot identify, their future sexual adjustment may be seriously jeopardized. If the father is cruel or overly harsh, the boy may reject the father and emulate the mother. This may begin a life pattern of identification with the female instead of the male role. The girl may carry hostility and resentment of her mother into her adult life and may fail to develop positive working relationships with female peers. On the other hand, if the girl cannot identify with her mother's role she may emulate her father and may be handicapped in adult life by a confused role identification.

Latency

The period of latency falls roughly between the ages of 6 and 12 years. By the beginning of this period most children have resolved the oedipal conflict, at least temporarily. During this period the child represses sexual thoughts and channels his libidinal energies into the pursuit of intellectual interests. The term latency is used to describe this period because sexual interests are repressed and lie more or less dormant until the advent of puberty. The child begins the process of emancipating himself from the family by seeking security and companionship from peer groups of the same sex. This is the period of gang formation and fierce gang loyalties. The gang requires strict adherence to the rules of the group and the child slavishly complies with them. During this period the child tries to find his place among his peers. His major character patterns are formed at this time, and he begins to conform to some of the norms of the culture into which he was born.

This period is sometimes referred to as the *normal homosexual* period because groups of boys cling together and shun girls. On the other hand, groups of girls band together and declare that they despise boys. Although children of this age have an active phantasy life that sometimes is concerned with the opposite sex, they disregard the opposite sex as much as possible at school and at play. Up to this time the child's love has been *narcissistic* or has been directed primarily toward himself. Now he seeks a companion or chum with whom he can share some of his self-love. It is easier to love someone like himself so he seeks someone of the same sex. Thus love for another person, the most important task in preparation for a normal love relationship with someone of the opposite sex, is initiated in this stage of psychosexual development.

Every person normally passes through this phase of development.

The *superego* that was initiated in an earlier period functions actively during this period. It is strict and demanding and forces the child to resort to both magic and compulsive behavior to conform to its demands.

Significance of period of latency. The term latency is somewhat misleading when applied to this period. The child at this age is constantly finding it necessary to reorganize his thinking and behavior and thus he is frequently in a state of emotional conflict. During this period the child becomes somewhat emancipated from his family and finds a place for himself among his peer group. At school and on the playground he develops skills that help him to compete, cooperate, and get along successfully with others. He also begins to develop a deep personal concern for at least one other person who is not a member of his immediate family—a chum. This initiates the capacity for loving another person.

One of the dangers of this period is that the youngster may become fixated at this level and may not be able to move forward emotionally in developing the capacity to focus his love upon a member of the opposite sex in order to achieve the more mature relationship of the next or heterosexual phase of psychosexual development.

Concept of self as a reflection of the environment

It cannot be stressed too emphatically that awareness of self, which is learned early in the life of every individual, develops from responses to the individual by significant adults in the environment. The earliest and probably the most important and lasting influences are from the mothering adult. As has been stated earlier in this chapter, the child's reactions toward life in general are powerfully influenced by the attitudes encountered during feeding and toileting experiences.

The cultural expectations of an individual are usually conveyed through the attitudes and reactions of adults in the child's environment. In this way the child learns what behavior is expected from one of his sex, what behavior is valued and what is not tolerated, which roles he is expected to assume and which are taboo for him, and which activities he may aspire to engage in and which ones will bring disapproval.

Although the individual is endowed with unique characteristics and abilities, the direction of his growth and development and the personality characteristics that will emerge as he becomes a part of his environment will depend upon the significant adults with whom he is intimately involved.

The school plays an important role in the development of the child's personality. It is at school that children meet significant adults who greatly influence the development of their self-concepts. In this culture, success at school is rewarded with much approval, whereas lack of success often begins a series of defeats that carries over into adult life. The self-concept of children who do poorly in school may be irreparably damaged by the reactions of teachers, the significant adults in that

important environment. On the other hand, understanding, helpful teachers may provide the child with a positive basis for self-evaluation and, in some instances, may constitute an opportunity for corrective interpersonal experiences with adults. Teachers are of tremendous importance in the lives of children. They need to become more aware of their potential for providing therapeutic experiences in their day-to-day contacts with children.

Puberty and adolescence

The period of puberty and adolescence covers the years from age 12 to approximately age 18. It is difficult to make a definite statement concerning the span of years included in adolescence because individuals mature at different rates. This period is initiated by the active functioning of the sexual glands and continues until the individual is socially, psychologically, and emotionally mature. Part of emotional maturity is developing a stable love relationship with someone of the opposite sex. Because the chief task of this period is to develop a love relationship with the opposite sex, it has been called the heterosexual period of psychosexual adjustment.

Adolescence may be an extremely stormy and precarious period. Every aspect of life is apt to be characterized by turmoil as the young individual attempts to become completely emancipated from his family. Because of conflict over dependent-independent needs, the adolescent may be hostile toward adults, particularly his parents, and rebellious toward authority. His life is apt to be in a state of disequilibrium. This period may be an anxiety-ridden time of life because many important decisions about life must be made.

Unresolved conflicts and unsolved problems of earlier developmental periods often reappear at this time. The oedipal conflict is frequently reactivated, and conflict over sexual longings and masturbation are particularly troublesome. Adolescents are confusing to themselves as well as to their parents and other adults. They vacillate between behaving in an immature, childlike way and behaving as mature adults.

Relationships with members of the opposite sex are the most troublesome part of this difficult period. It is understandable that many shy, inhibited, insecure adolescents require expert professional help to cope with some of their more serious emotional conflicts.

The best preparation for this period is successful achievement of the developmental tasks of all the preceding periods of psychosexual growth. This requires a stable, loving, home life and wise mature parents who understand the needs of children. Supportive, loving, wise parents are also the best insurance that an adolescent will complete this period successfully.

EARLY ADULTHOOD

Making decisions about significant aspects of life is a continuing task during early adulthood. If the individual has been able to accept the sexual role the culture has assigned, he will be ready to select a mate and establish the marriage relationship. Living as a married person is a unique role and makes different demands upon the individuals involved than does the relationship of dating, which is actually preparation for marriage. In this culture the relationship of marriage is encouraged for the purpose of establishing a family and providing a safe and congenial environment for the growth and development of children who will perpetuate the culture. Thus the major developmental tasks of early adulthood include choosing a mate, establishing a home and a congenial relationship with the mate, and accepting the role of parent and the responsibility for nurturing, safeguarding, and rearing children. Children cannot be effectively nurtured unless the family has a reasonable degree of security. Thus acceptance of family responsibilities requires that the young adult be reasonably effective in performing some aspect of work. In addition, a successful parent must accept the roles of citizen in the community and participating member of a social group.

MIDDLE AGE

As children grow and develop, their needs for parental love and guidance are altered. The role of the parent is an ever changing and evolving one as each child advances from infancy to adolescence. The needs and requirements of marital partners, like those of their children, change as the relationship matures. Thus the maintenance of a happy and successful marriage relationship requires that the partners continuously seek to relate to each other as individuals. The developmental tasks of the mature adult with grown children includes acceptance of physiological changes brought on by middle age, coping with the problems of aging parents, serving the community as a socially responsible adult, and assisting grown children to establish independent lives.

ADJUSTMENT TO THE ROLE
OF AN AGED PERSON

The role of aged individuals who have retired from an active social and economic life is unique in this culture. Unfortunately the wisdom that they have accumulated through the years is not considered to be of value as it is in some cultures. Aging individuals find it necessary to adjust to a reduced income, waning physical strength, and deteriorating health. This may be an anxiety-producing experience, since it represents a loss of power and of independence. Loneliness is another experience with which aged people must cope. Frequently their friends and marital partners pass away, leaving them in the position of being socially isolated. Such lonely individuals who are no longer able to cope efficiently with their own physical requirements need to adjust to the establishment of living arrangements that are acceptable, while at the same time being faced with the need to accept a dependent role. Such aged individuals need to establish social relationships with a group of interested, sympathetic peers. This need leads many aged individuals to seek an affiliation with a "golden age" club or a similar organization.

One authority believes that the developmental task of the aged person is to gradually disengage himself from the social systems to which he belongs so that he initiates a type of social distance. This process carried to its ultimate conclusion suggests that the transition from life to death becomes a logical one.

ANXIETY—ITS RELATIONSHIP TO
DEFENSE MECHANISMS

As will be explained in the following discussion, it is accurate to speak of defense mechanisms of personality because they actually defend the individual's intrapsychic balance against the intolerable pain and unpleasant tensions of anxiety. Anxiety can be produced by any situation that threatens the individual's identity or self-image or causes him to feel helpless, isolated, or insecure. Since anxiety is a basic concept in psychiatry and a key problem in the development of emotional problems, it will be discussed as a separate entity.

Anxiety occurs in degrees and is a reaction to something that is perceived or felt to be a danger. When it is experienced, anxiety is indistinguishable from fear, but unlike fear it does not occur in response to a specific environmental threat. Individuals experiencing anxiety describe it as a vague, uneasy feeling of dread, nervousness, and apprehension. These feelings may cause the individual to become more alert mentally and physically, and through the actions of the autonomic nervous system the body may be made ready for "flight or fight." That is to say that the body may be ready to fly from the danger or to fight the cause of the danger. Therefore a mild degree of anxiety may actually assist the actor to give an excellent performance or the student to write an unusually well-thought-out examination paper by increasing alertness and focusing attention specifically on the task at hand.

When the level of anxiety is extremely high, the individual may be incapable of action or may react with unusual behavior or what appears to be irrational behavior. This irrational behavior is referred to as a panic state. The degree of anxiety expressed and the behavior the individual uses to defend himself depends upon the way the individual perceives the threat to his self-image. It must be remembered that the use of defense mechanisms to defend against these threats takes place well below the level of the individual's conscious awareness.

Some authorities distinguish between normal anxiety and neurotic anxiety. Normal anxiety consists of the feelings of tension, nervousness, and apprehension that accompany a realistic situation. Thus the feelings of fear and tension a bridegroom experiences before a wedding are called normal anxiety and arise out of what he feels to be a threat to his identity as an adequate male.

Anxiety that is aroused by the individual's own unacceptable thoughts, feelings, wishes, or desires and that would cause the loss of approval or love from significant individuals or groups is sometimes termed neurotic anxiety. Individuals who develop overwhelming sexual thoughts and desires that are unacceptable to the social group frequently respond with behavior described as panic. Such an individual might choose unconsciously to utilize one of the defense mechanisms. In such an instance he might blame someone else for planting unacceptable thoughts in his mind.

Children who have been brought up by parents or other significant adults who punish them severely for minor indiscretions or who consistently disapprove of their behavior no matter how hard they try to please may develop persistent severe anxiety that becomes a lifelong problem. Corrective experiences to counteract such a long-standing problem require consistent long-term treatment in depth.

Since defense mechanisms are initiated in a less sophisticated form during the early phases of personality development, they will be discussed from the standpoint of the phase where they may have originated. It should not be forgotten that a defense mechanism may originate in more than one phase of personality development or it may originate in one phase and be reinforced in other phases. Defense mechanisms are not clear-cut and almost never appear as an isolated phenomenon.

DEFENSE MECHANISMS OF PERSONALITY

When the primitive id drives are in serious conflict with the controls imposed by the ego or the superego, the individual suffers from tension and anxiety that cannot be tolerated for long. This uncomfortable situation is reflected in the individual's behavior. Some method of developing a compromise and of relieving the tension and anxiety is essential. The human being usually is able to relieve the conflict by utilizing certain forms of adaptation, that is, *defense mechanisms* or *mental dynamisms*. These methods of thinking and acting are actually patterns of behavior initiated during one of the earlier phases of personality development. They are further developed and elaborated as the individual grows and struggles with problems. Even during their early development they are utilized to protect the individual from threatening aspects of his environment or from his own feelings of tension and anxiety that are unacceptable and upsetting to him. Thus the use of these defense mechanisms is a matter of resorting to earlier patterns of behavior that have already proved helpful in relieving tension and anxiety. Many of these methods of thinking are wholly unconscious while others are partially conscious and partially unconscious.

All persons utilize defense mechanisms to a certain degree to relieve intrapsychic tension. Under abnormal stress the use of the mental mechanisms may become a very prominent characteristic of behavior and may be so bizarre and unusual as to suggest that the individual is mentally ill.

In a sense mental mechanisms are a means of compromising with forbidden desires, feelings of guilt, or an admission that one is inadequate in facing certain problems. They salvage the individual's self-respect, avoid an open admission of failure, and save psychic energy.

Defense mechanisms that may originate in the oral phase

Compensation. Compensation is a pattern of adjustive behavior by which tension or anxiety is relieved as the individual makes up for a personal lack or a feeling of inadequacy by emphasizing some personal or social attribute that overshadows the weakness and gains social approval.

The origins of this device can be seen in the young infant who substitutes a thumb or a toy for the nipple or the bottle in order to relieve tension and make up for some of the pleasurable sensations of sucking that the infant may be lacking in sufficient quantity.

Obviously, compensation is far more complicated in adults than in infants and is usually prompted by feelings of guilt or inferiority. It may explain much of the behavior observed in adults who work zealously to promote philanthropic enterprises. Compensation is operating in the behavior of a man who is very small in physical stature but who is extremely successful in the business world through his aggressive practices. It may also be a part of the adjustive behavior of a young woman who becomes a religious zealot but whose family ran a gambling casino when she was a child. This may be one of the mechanisms operating when a young person who is paralyzed as a result of poliomyelitis is able to achieve many honors for outstanding scholarship in college.

Displacement or substitution. Displacement or substitution refers to the discharge of emotions, feelings, or ideas upon a subject entirely different from the one to which the feelings rightly belong. This is usually a safety operation with the feelings being discharged away from the actual source of the emotion because it is not considered safe to express them directly. Displacement may be used by a teacher who is angry with her immediate supervisor but does not show these feelings in his presence. However, when this same teacher reacts with unreasonable anger when one of her pupils accidentally breaks a window pane on that same day, she may be displacing her feelings by expressing anger toward the student rather than toward the supervisor. Actually she has unconsciously substituted the student for the supervisor and has displaced her feelings accordingly.

An individual with a deep, instinctual conflict may displace the anger arising from unacceptable repressed feelings in the unconscious by soundly beating an opponent in a boxing contest.

Fixation. Fixation refers to the point in the individual's psychosexual development at which certain aspects of the emotional development cease to advance. For reasons that are usually obscure, further development seems to be blocked. This blocking appears to arise from the inability of the individual to solve the problems of the specific phase of development at which the progress ceased. Thus the individual is unable to achieve the developmental tasks of that phase and, since it is not possible to entirely bypass a stage, he is always handicapped in proceeding to the stages that follow. Individuals who have not experienced the love and security required in the oral stage of development may spend the remainder of their lives pursuing this goal or pattern of behavior. Many adults are said to be fixated at the oral-dependent level of development. They seek to find ways of answering this need. Since food and liquid intake are so closely allied to love and security in the unconscious emotional life, some fixated individuals may imbibe huge quantities of alcohol or overeat compulsively.

Defense mechanisms that may originate in the habit-training period

Fixation and substitution are mental mechanisms that may originate in the anal period of psychosexual development, although they more frequently originate in the earlier oral period.

Suppression. Suppression is the conscious and intentional dismissal to the preconscious mind of impulses, feelings, and thoughts that are unpleasant or unacceptable to the individual. Suppressed material is easily recalled and is thus available to the conscious mind.

Sublimation. Sublimation is a mechanism by which the energy involved in primitive impulses and cravings is redirected into socially constructive and acceptable channels. This is one of the chief mechanisms operating when a child learns to redirect the pleasurable sensations involved in expelling excrement at will into the more socially acceptable patterns of toilet training.

Sublimation is one of the more positive mechanisms of adjustment and is at least partially responsible for much of the artistic and cultural achievement of civilized people. It is operating when a women redirects her sexual drives, which might be expected to result in a home and children, into a successful career as a nursery school teacher. It is probably operating when a young man who has lost his lover turns to writing poetry about love.

Reaction formation. Reaction formation occurs when an individual expresses an attitude or act that is directly opposite to his unconscious feelings or wishes. Thus the individual is denying, in a sense of the word, his true feelings or desires. People who are extremely friendly, overly polite, and very socially correct frequently have unconscious feelings of anger and hatred toward many people. These true feelings may be evident in slips of the tongue or in their biting humor.

Reaction formation sometimes develops out of rigid toilet training experiences. One evidence of reaction formation may be observed in adults who are untidy about their homes and their personal hygiene but whose mothers required meticulous conformity to rules of cleanliness and tidiness.

Identification. Identification is a much used and extremely useful mechanism since it plays a large part in the development of a child's personality and in the process of acculturation. Through the process of identification the individual takes on desirable attributes found in the personalities of people in his environment for whom he has admiration and affection. He integrates these personality attributes into his own ego. Thus the little boy takes on masculine attributes that he admires in his father. The student integrates into his personality makeup the attributes he admires in his professor. Another form of identification is observed when one individual develops an unreasoning sympathy for a criminal because of an unconscious sense of guilt.

Introjection. The introjection mechanism is closely related to identification, and the two are difficult to differentiate.

Introjection rests on the psychoanalytical concept of oral receptivity and refers to the phantasied swallowing or incorporation of a loved or hated object or person into the individual's own ego structure. Introjection is operating when the child develops the superego by incorporating the ideals and standards of the parents. When introjection is operating in adults it suggests that the entire personality of a second person has been incorporated and has replaced the original personality. A psychotic patient who claimed to be Moses wore a beard, let his hair grow long, talked in biblical phrases, and acted as Moses might have acted. The personality of Moses had been incorporated by the patient and he had given up his own personality. In contrast, identification is a mechanism by means of which an individual's ego is added to, not replaced. Introjection may operate in a less constructive way than identification, especially when it is observed in adults. For instance, a depressed patient may phantasize that he has incorporated a person within himself and may attempt to commit suicide in order to kill the introjected person whom he unconsciously hates or loves.

Defense mechanisms that may originate in the later period of childhood

Rationalization. Rationalization is a mental mechanism that is almost universally employed. It is an attempt to make one's behavior appear to be the result of logical thinking rather than the result of unconscious desires or cravings. It is used when the individual has a sense of guilt about something he does or believes or when he is uncertain about his behavior. It is a face-saving device that may or may not deal with the actual truth. Rationalization should not be confused with falsehoods or alibis since the latter are conscious avoidance maneuvers. Rationalization is almost totally unconscious and, although it is used to put the individual in the best possible light, does not have the deliberate aspect of other conscious avoidance maneuvers.

The person who does not keep an appointment but says that the appointment slipped his mind is not telling a falsehood, although he may not have wanted to keep the appointment for a very good reason. The following example of rationalization involves a group of persons who decided to write a letter to protest a decision that affected all of them. Two members of the group failed to write the letter. They seemed surprised that they were expected to write and said that they did not remember that any group action had been decided upon. The two who did not write were obviously not in favor of the decision when it was being made but gave the impression that they would go along with the group. Although rationalization relieves anxiety temporarily, it is not an effective mechanism of adjustment because it assists the individual to avoid facing the reality factors in the situation.

Repression. Repression is a widely used and completely unconscious mechanism. Painful experiences, unacceptable thoughts and impulses, and disagreeable memories are forcibly dismissed from consciousness. The psychic energy with which they were invested becomes an active source of anxiety in the unconscious mind. Many painful experiences are repressed during early childhood and become unconscious sources of emotional conflict in later life. The stronger the superego the more material will be repressed. Selfish, hostile feelings and sexual impulses are the most frequently repressed. Such repression always causes internal conflict. This repressed material may find escape through conversion into physical defects, into obsessions, and into morbid anxiety that arises without apparent reason.

Regression. Regression occurs when an individual is faced with a conflict or problem that cannot be solved with the adjustment mechanisms with which he customarily solves problems. In such a situation he may resort to behavior that was successful at an earlier stage in his development but which he had presumably outgrown. Thus regression is a return to patterns of earlier immature behavior. Any retreat into a state of dependency on others to avoid facing acute problems can be called a regressive trait. "Crying on someone's shoulder" is a reenactment of the infant's seeking comfort on the maternal bosom. Although some seeking for a dependency relationship is a benign form of neurotic regression, this dynamism becomes the main element in grave psychoses.

Defense mechanisms that may originate in the latency period

Projection. Projection is a frequently used unconscious mechanism that relieves tension and anxiety by transferring the responsibility for unacceptable ideas, impulses, wishes, or thoughts to another person. The mechanism is used when the individual cannot accept the responsibility for his own hostile, aggressive thoughts. Although all people use this mechanism to some extent, it is not a healthy method of adaptation and is more frequently used by mentally ill persons than by normal individuals. It is observed in psychotic symptoms such as delusions and hallucinations. In the latter the patient hears voices saying things about him that he unconsciously fears are true. The paranoid patient may project his own inner hate of others by saying that a group of persons is plotting to kill him. Less pathological use of projection is evident when a worker blames the boss for his difficulties on the job or when a student blames the teacher for his failure on the final examination. Paranoid patients frequently project their feelings of sexual inadequacy upon others. Thus a common delusion concerns the unfaithful spouse when the actual lack of fidelity is in the mind of the accuser.

Other commonly used defense mechanisms

Symbolization and condensation. A symbol is an idea or object used by the conscious mind in lieu of the actual idea or object.

Instinctual desires may appear through symbols, the meanings of which are not exactly clear to the conscious mind. These symbols are the language of the unconscious. Such symbols appear in dreams or in phantasies and may emerge through various rituals or obsessive behavior.

Symbols may become further merged by condensation to represent a wide range of emotionally painful ideas that thus become lumped together so as to lose their painful significance. When they rise to conscious levels, they take the form of an apparently incoherent jumble of words, the real meaning of which is hidden in the unconscious. Such condensations of thinking are frequently noted in the apparently irrational language of the schizophrenic patient. The condensations have meaning and significance for the patient.

Conversion. Conversion refers to the expression of emotional conflicts through physical symptoms. When disagreeable experiences and unacceptable desires are repressed into the unconscious, they may reappear as physical symptoms without the patient being aware of any connection between the two phenomena. Thus a child who is torn by a conflict arising out of a chronic friction between her parents, both of whom she loves, may find herself suddenly blind. This symptom relieves her of the necessity of looking upon such incompatibility. A young girl who fears that she must account for her misbehavior may suddenly develop a paralysis of her vocal cords. Conversion is not always expressed in such a direct and easily recognized manner. Frequently it is difficult to determine just what conflicts in the repressed unconscious produce a certain physical symptom. The symptom always serves to distract attention from the individual's real problems. Conversion is a dynamism particularly useful to the person who is prone to hysteria. It is entirely unconscious and is not utilized by mature well-adjusted individuals.

IMPORTANT CONCEPTS

1. Much of our current knowledge concerning personality development is based upon the theories proposed by Sigmund Freud, who lived from 1856 to 1939.

2. Personality refers to the aggregate of physical and mental qualities as they interact in characteristic fashion with the individual's environment.

3. The levels of consciousness were described by Freud as the conscious, the preconscious, and the unconscious.

4. The conscious mind is concerned with thoughts, feelings, and sensations and directs the individual in rational, thoughtful behavior.

5. The unconscious mind is the storehouse for all the memories, feelings, and responses that the individual has experienced in his entire life.

6. According to Freud the structure of the personality includes the id, the ego, and the superego.

7. The id is unlearned, primitive, selfish, and the source of all instinctual energy. The ego represents the self or the "I" and is the rational, reasonable, conscious part of the personality. The superego is the voice of conscience and is that part of the personality that is keenly sensitive to the demands of strict convention.

8. The stages of personality development, as described by Freud, are differentiated by the changing focus of the child's libidinal energies as he matures emotionally, socially, and physically.

9. Psychosexual maturity is achieved only after successfully advancing through several stages of development until the libidinal drives are focused upon a member of the opposite sex for whom there are tender, protective feelings and the goal is to establish a home and a family.

10. The phases of psychosexual development include infancy or the oral period; early childhood or the habit-training period; later childhood or the period of family triangle; the period of latency or the normal homosexual period; and the period of puberty and adolescence or the period of heterosexual adjustment.

11. The human being utilizes certain forms of adaptive behavior, called defense mechanisms or mental dynamisms, to relieve the tension that results from a serious conflict between the primitive id drives and the controls imposed by the ego or superego.

12. All people utilize defense mechanisms to a certain degree to relieve intrapsychic tension and anxiety, but if these mechanisms become a very prominent characteristic of behavior or are bizarre and unusual the individual may be mentally ill.

13. Most defense mechanisms are initiated early during the development of the personality. They are not clear-cut and almost never appear as an isolated phenomenon.

14. In a sense, mental mechanisms are a means of compromising with forbidden desires, feelings of guilt, or an admission that one is inadequate in facing certain problems. They salvage self-respect, avoid an open admission of failure, and save psychic energy.

SUGGESTED SOURCES OF ADDITIONAL INFORMATION

Berlien, Ivan C.: Growth as related to mental health, Amer. J. Nurs. **56**:1142-1145, Sept., 1956.

Brill, A. A.: The basic writings of Sigmund Freud, New York, 1938, Modern Library, Inc.

Brill, A. A.: Freud's contribution to psychiatry, New York, 1944, W. W. Norton & Co., Inc.

Committee on Psychiatric Nursing, National League for Nursing Education: Psychological concepts of personality development, Amer. J. Nurs. **50**:122-125, Feb.; 182-184, March; 242-243, April, 1950.

Cumming, Elaine, and Henry, William E.: Growing old; the process of disengagement, New York, 1961, Basic Books, Inc., Publishers.

English, Spurgeon O., and Pearson, G. H. J.: Emotional problems of living, ed. 3, New York, 1963, W. W. Norton & Co., Inc.

Erikson, Erik H.: Childhood in society, New York, 1950, W. W. Norton & Co., Inc., pp. 219-234.

Freud, Sigmund: New introductory lectures on psychoanalysis, New York, 1933, W. W. Norton & Co., Inc.

Freud, Sigmund: A general introduction to psychoanalysis, Garden City, New York, 1943, Doubleday & Co., Inc.

King, Joan M.: Denial, Amer. J. Nurs. **66**:1010-1013, May, 1966.

Lidz, Theodore: The person; his development throughout the life cycle, New York, 1968, Basic Books, Inc., Publishers, pp. 93-263.

Munroe, Ruth L.: Schools of psychoanalytic thought, New York, 1955, The Dryden Press, Inc.

Nehren, Jeanette, and Gilliam, Naomi R.: Separation anxiety, Amer. J. Nurs. **65**:109-112, Jan., 1965.

Sullivan, Harry Stack: The interpersonal theory of psychiatry, New York, 1953, W. W. Norton & Co., Inc.

Thompson, Clare: The different schools of psychoanalysis, Amer. J. Nurs. **57**:1304-1307, Oct., 1957.

CHAPTER THREE

The nurse develops an understanding of self

Nurses strive to be as helpful as possible to patients in whatever situation they find them. One of the ways to develop professional ability is to learn as much as possible about the patient, his illness, the helping role of the nurse, and the way in which this knowledge applies to the total situation. However, in some situations the nurse finds that her own anxieties, fears, and personal concerns are so compelling that it is difficult to focus upon the problems of the patients.

FEARS AND ANXIETIES

One of the most effective tools available to the psychiatric nurse is the therapeutic use of her own personality. However, when the nurse is burdened with personal fears and anxieties, she finds it difficult to focus attention or interest upon the patient and his emotional problems. To overcome this difficulty it is necessary for the nurse to identify the source of her fears and anxiety, to learn to understand these disturbing influences, and to cope with these reactions. Until this goal is accomplished, it is unlikely that the nurse will be able to achieve the knowledge, skills, and attitudes that will assist her in becoming a therapeutic influence in the patient's environment. Some frequent concerns of nurses who are beginning an experience in psychiatric nursing include fear of bodily harm, fear of personal inadequacy, fear of loss of emotional control, fear of rejection by patients, and fear of harming patients psychologically. Each of these fears will be discussed separately in an effort to help the nurse recognize that these feelings are not unusual and that

it is possible to cope with such reactions.

Initially most of these feelings are experienced in varying degrees by almost everyone who works with mentally ill patients. They usually disappear as knowledge and understanding develop. One of the most helpful ways to view such feelings objectively is to share them with other people who are likely to have had similar experiences. When fears are discussed with a sympathetic peer group under the guidance of a wise leader or teacher, one discovers that they are almost universally shared by the others. This knowledge plus the experience of examining these feelings objectively makes them more easily understood and accepted.

Fear of bodily harm

New situations are feared by most people. Some nurses fear the clinical practice of psychiatric nursing not only because it is a new experience but also because of many preconceived ideas about the behavior of mentally ill patients. Nurses may have heard discussions about unusual and frightening behavior of such patients. These discussions often exaggerate the behavior that is being described and tend to arouse fear on the part of the listener.

The nurse with these feelings can cope more readily with the situation by admitting that she has some concerns about her personal safety, by facing the fact frankly, and by examining these fears to discover where they came from and what they involve. As has been suggested, it is usually helpful to discuss such attitudes in situations where students and the teacher can help each other in examining, understanding, and coping with these feelings. This method is particularly effective when the discussion focuses upon the individual patient whose behavior is causing concern.

Much of the fear of mentally ill patients grows out of cultural attitudes and beliefs that are handed down from one generation to another. In spite of attempts to educate the public about mental illness, there are still many persons who believe that all mentally ill patients are dangerous and require drastic measures to control their behavior. The nurse who is being introduced to a psychiatric situation will be surprised at the large number of patients whose behavior is socially acceptable. She will be surprised to find that many psychiatric patients seem content to be inactive. Instead of requiring controls, many patients require stimulation and need to be helped to develop an interest in the available activities.

The nurse will learn that the behavior of mentally ill persons differs only in degree from that of any group of people of similar age, culture, and socioeconomic background. As she learns more about human behavior and mental illness she will realize that all behavior has meaning, that all behavior is in response to a human need, and that abnormal behavior differs from normal behavior in degree but not in kind.

Fear of personal inadequacy

Nurses who are beginning an experience in psychiatric nursing sometimes find that they are filled with sympathy and deep concern for mentally ill patients. At the same time they are likely to feel that they are not skillful enough to offer any significant help to the patient. These feelings present the nurse with an uncomfortable personal dilemma from which she may seek to escape by developing an attitude of indifference. This is unfortunate because indifference is one of the reactions with which most mentally ill patients have already had far too much experience in their relations with family and friends.

It is surprising to find nurses who express more sympathy and concern for mentally ill patients than for patients who are suffering from physical conditions for which little medical help is available. These feelings probably develop from attitudes about mental illness that were learned early in life and persist in spite of scientific information. They suggest that the nurse believes mental illness is even more hopeless than the most baffling of the physical illnesses. Actually, the symptoms of mental illness usually exist because the patient has unconsciously selected them to assist himself in coping with unbearable emotional conflicts or unmet personal needs. Through the use of knowledge, personal warmth, and interpersonal skills the nurse can assist the patient to solve a problem or meet a need. The nurse does not work alone or without direction, but she may be the most significant person with whom the patient has a relationship.

At the beginning of the psychiatric experience the nurse may feel that she is working without tools because she cannot rely upon many of the nursing activities that were so helpful to her in dealing with physically ill patients. In addition, she may not have developed interpersonal skills to a level that helps her to feel adequate in the situation. With guidance, practice, and persistent study of self, the early feelings of inadequacy will be replaced with a developing ability to help patients cope with interpersonal problems.

Fear of loss of emotional control

Mentally ill patients present a young nurse with a unique situation. These patients are rarely in need of bed rest and are usually physically well. They may be the same age as the nurse herself or her parents. In many psychiatric settings the patients wear their own clothing and present a superficial picture of being personally and socially competent. Thus the inexperienced nurse may unconsciously apply to the group of patients with whom she is becoming acquainted the same ready-made set of standards of behavior that she uses for other groups of strangers. Her expectations may include chivalrous behavior toward her from the young men, friendly attitudes of a peer group from the young women, an attitude of motherly helpfulness from the middle-aged woman, and fatherly suggestions from the middle-aged men. She may not be emotionally or intellectually prepared for a profane outburst from a motherly looking patient who may have appeared to be perfectly calm when they were introduced earlier. The nurse may react to such an outburst with horror in the same way she would respond if her mother became profane. The sarcastic remarks of an attractive young male patient are understandably

difficult to accept. The nurse may react with the same angry response that she might use in a social situation. These are examples of initial reactions of a nurse who has not become familiar with the problems or needs of the patients with whom she is becoming acquainted. It is understandable that the nurse may react to unusual behavior of patients with a characteristic response until she has had an opportunity to develop some understanding and insight into the behavior patterns of individual patients and has developed skill in helping these patients.

The nurse will quickly develop the habit of seeking answers to questions such as the following: "Why does this patient need to behave in this way?" "What was there in the situation that precipitated this behavior?" "Where can I find information about this patient that will help me to understand his behavior?" "How can I be of more help to him?"

It is understandable and reasonable for a nurse to react with controlled anger to some kinds of patient behavior. For instance, it is resonable for the nurse to be angry if a patient deliberately trips her. In such a situation the nurse would undoubtedly speak to the patient about the fact that tripping other people is dangerous. It would be reasonable for her to make it clear that she disapproves of such behavior. The thoughtful nurse would wonder what it is about her that precipitated such a hostile reaction on the part of the patient. It would be important to discuss this incident with other workers who are acquainted with the patient in order to discover whether he reacts similarly to all women or if his reaction is unique and directed toward specific workers. Finally, it would be important for the nurse, in cooperation with other members of the professional staff, to make some decisions as to how to help this patient express his hostile feelings in a more appropriate way.

It is helpful for nurses to remember that the reality of the situation is always a good basis upon which to develop an approach to any behavioral problem. In dealing with the incident referred to in the preceding paragraph, the nurse would appropriately place the emphasis upon the dangerous aspects of such behavior as it involves other people rather than upon her personal anger at the patient who would treat her in such a way.

Nurses who work with mentally ill patients are not expected to operate as automatons who do not respond with appropriate feelings. Actually, the nurse who is rigidly controlling her personal behavior and her emotional responses will probably find it difficult to develop a helping relationship with mentally ill patients. Patients need nurses who understand their own emotional reactions and who can analyze situations, determine how their emotions contribute to the situation, and identify that part the patient's feelings are contributing. Patients can accept and learn from the nurse who responds emotionally in a sincere, genuine, and appropriate way.

Fear of rejection by patients

Members of the professional staffs in hospitals want to be liked by patients. A large part of the satisfaction a nurse derives from her work comes from patient approval and gratitude. Physically ill patients are usually ready and willing to accept the nurse. They often bring ready-made attitudes to the hospital that encourage the immediate development of a cooperative, friendly relationship. Such patients often help bridge the gap that sometimes exists between strangers so that a relationship is usually established without too much thought having been given to this aspect of the patient's care.

In contrast, mentally ill patients may be shy, suspicious, withdrawn, and preoccupied with their own thoughts and problems. They may view the nurse as a stranger and observe her cautiously from a distance. By actions or statements some patients may demonstrate what appears to be an obvious dislike for the nurse. This situation is disturbing and confusing, especially to the nurse who has not had previous experience in a psychiatric setting.

As the nurse develops an understanding of mental illness her concern about rejection by patients will become less acute. She will realize that some patients remain aloof, even when they want very much to become acquainted, because they fear that they will not be acceptable. She will soon learn that a patient who appears to be disturbed by her presence may be misidentifying her and that as far as the patient is concerned the nurse is the hated woman who lived across the street. A patient may show dislike for the nurse because he has always had difficulty with his sister; he may be treating the nurse as he would like to treat his sister. The nurse will learn to understand that rejection on the part of the patient is one expression of the mental illness for which he is receiving treatment.

As the nurse learns to know patients as people, as she develops some understanding of their individual needs, and as she develops skill in offering professional help to these people, they will begin to accept her as someone who belongs to the group. The nurse cannot expect to thoroughly like all patients nor can she expect all patients to genuinely like her. She can expect to develop some understanding and appreciation of the problems of all patients.

Fear of injuring patients psychologically

Among the unique and baffling aspects of a psychiatric setting is the unfamiliar terminology used by the professional staff. There are a number of special terms that must be learned before a professional worker is able to communicate with other members of the psychiatric team. Furthermore, it becomes apparent almost immediately that the young nurse lacks much knowledge about the emotional aspects of illness. Nurses sometimes believe that the slightest change in the environment of a mentally ill person will precipitate an untoward emotional response. Because of this attitude nurses may feel that such a patient must be approached with great caution. It is not unusual for a nurse to believe that the mentally ill patient is so emotionally fragile that he can be traumatized by an inexpertly phrased statement. These attitudes may cause some nurses to avoid contact with patients because of a fear that they may actually harm the patient psychologically.

It is well to remember that emotionally ill patients are not defenseless and that they withstand the inappropriate approach of new workers remarkably well. They, like all human beings, are usually able to sense the innate friendliness behind a nurse's approach even if it is not skillfully executed. They likewise are able to sense the negative feelings that sometimes underlie the statements and actions of a few professional workers. The most significant qualities of the nurse's approach to any patient are sincerity, warmth of feeling, and genuine caring.

Patients usually have one avenue of escape available to them when a professional worker is upsetting them. Except in rare instances, they are free to walk away from the worker to another part of the hospital unit. Instead of avoiding patients because of the fear of harming them psychologically, the nurse can help by developing understanding and skill as quickly as possible. Developing skill for working therapeutically with psychiatric patients requires that the nurse initiate a relationship with patients early in her experience, reflect thoughtfully upon the content of the experience, discuss the aspects of the developing relationship with a more skilled and experienced professional person, and return to the patient prepared to proceed with more understanding and in a more helpful way.

EMOTIONAL INVOLVEMENT VERSUS AN OBJECTIVE ATTITUDE

"Maintain an objective attitude" has been the theme of teachers of nursing throughout the years. Although students of nursing have been told to maintain an objective attitude, teachers have not always defined the meaning of these words. Many nurses adopt an aloof, impersonal approach to all patients because they interpret objectivity to mean social and professional distance. When the nurse enters the psychiatric nursing aspect of the curriculum, an even greater emphasis may be placed upon objectivity in nurse-patient relationships. This emphasis grows out of the hope that students will avoid possible pitfalls in the area of interpersonal relations. It is hoped that students will avoid becoming so emotionally related to the patient that problems are viewed through the eyes of the patient instead of through the eyes of a professional person. It is hoped that the nurse will focus upon the patient's needs and not upon her needs. It is hoped that emotional maturity of the patient will be encouraged by making sure that he is free to relate to others. The goals of psychiatric nursing might more realistically be achieved if students are helped to develop a mature professional relationship with patients. Instead of emphasizing objectivity, nurses could more profitably receive help in identifying the patient's needs and the ways in which the patient can be assisted to achieve these needs in a mature way. Instead of emphasizing aloof detachment, the nurse can more profitably use help in becoming aware of her own reactions in relation to the patient.

Today psychiatric nurses are encouraged to become emotionally involved with patients. In fact, many authorities believe that without such involvement the nurse can be of little real therapeutic help. However, it is essential to understand the meaning of involvement. In-volvement implies that the nurse is genuinely and sincerely interested in the patient, that she gives of her time and of herself without expecting anything in return, and that she is warm and helpful in a way that meets the needs of the patient instead of her own. Finally, the nurse who is emotionally involved professionally with a patient can help him to develop meaningful relationships with other appropriate people.

IMPORTANT CONCEPTS

1. Developing the professional skills of a psychiatric nurse is dependent upon learning as much as possible about the patient, his illness, and the helping role of the nurse as it specically applies to the patient.
2. Until the nurse is able to cope with personal fears and anxieties in relation to psychiatric nursing, it is unlikely that she can become a therapeutic influence in the patient's environment.
3. Sharing disturbing feelings about psychiatric nursing with a peer group under the guidance of a wise leader is helpful to the nurse in understanding and dealing with such feelings.
4. The behavior of mentally ill persons differs only in degree from that of any group of people of similar age, culture, and socioeconomic background.
5. The symptoms of mental illness usually exist because the patient has unconsciously selected them as useful methods for relieving tensions derived from emotional problems.
6. Although the nurse does not work

33

alone or without direction, she may be the most significant person with whom the patient has a relationship during his hospital experience.

7. The reality of the situation is always a good basis upon which to develop an approach to any behavioral problem involving a mentally ill patient.

8. Patients need nurses who understand their own emotional reactions and who can analyze the situation, determine how their emotions may contribute to the situation, and identify the contribution made by the patient's feelings.

9. The nurse learns to understand that rejection of other people is one expression of the mental illness from which the patient suffers.

10. The nurse cannot expect to thoroughly like all patients, neither can she expect all patients to genuinely like her. She can expect to develop some understanding and acceptance of all patients.

11. The most significant part of the nurse's approach to any patient is the sincerity, warmth of feeling, and genuine caring that is conveyed to the patient.

12. Many authorities believe that psychiatric nurses can be of little real therapeutic help to mentally ill patients unless they become involved in a mature emotional relationship with them. It is essential for the nurse to have a clear concept of the meaning and significance of a mature emotional involvement.

SUGGESTED SOURCES OF ADDITIONAL INFORMATION

Brill, Norman Q.: The importance of understanding yourself, Amer. J. Nurs. **57**:1325-1326, Oct., 1957.

Frances, Gloria M.: How do I feel about myself? Amer. J. Nurs. **67**:1244-1245, June, 1967.

Goldstein, Joan: Exploring attitudes that affect nursing care, Nurs. Outlook **16**:50-51, June, 1968.

Holmes, Marguerite J.: What's wrong with getting involved? Nurs. Outlook **8**:250-251, May, 1960.

Hyde, R. M., and Coggan, C. M.: When nurses have guilt feelings, Amer. J. Nurs. **58**:233-236, Feb., 1958.

Lewis, Garland K., and Holmes, Marguerite J.: Meddling with emotions, Nurs. Outlook **9**:405-407, July, 1961.

Lewis, John A.: Reflections on self, Amer. J. Nurs. **60**:828-830, June, 1960.

Schwartz, Morris S., and Shockley, Emmy Lanning: The nurse and the mental patient, New York, 1956, Russell Sage Foundation, pp. 21-71.

Stevens, Leonard F.: Understanding ourselves, Amer. J. Nurs. **57**:1022-1023, Aug., 1957.

Tuteur, Werner: As you enter psychiatric nursing, Amer. J. Nurs. **56**:72-74, Jan., 1956.

CHAPTER FOUR

Communication skills—an essential aspect of psychiatric nursing

Communication refers to the reciprocal exchange of information, ideas, beliefs, feelings, and attitudes between at least two persons or among a group of persons. It is basic to all nursing and contributes to the development of all therapeutic relationships. An understanding of the principles of effective communication is important for the nurse because success with mentally ill patients depends upon developing skill in this area.

MODES OF COMMUNICATION

Everyone is familiar with communication through the written word. When written material is read, the reciprocal aspects of communication are limited to the student's ability to understand and react to the ideas and concepts that the authors are attempting to convey. If the reader does not receive the intended message, successful communication has not been achieved.

Another mode of communication with which everyone is familiar is the spoken word. If persons who are speaking together understand the same language, a major reciprocal element is present as they question, challenge, clarify, and enlarge upon statements. Nonverbal communication is closely related to verbal communication and is usually an integral part of it. Nonverbal communication refers to the information revealed by facial expressions, voice quality, physical posture, gestures, and general emotional and intellectual attitudes. Observed behavior conveys a great deal to the observer. Inner feelings are revealed by the manner in which an individual conducts himself in such simple activities as walking down the hall, opening and closing doors, reclining in an easy chair, speaking to other people, and asking questions. The nonverbal aspects of communication sometimes convey general attitudes, feelings, and reactions more clearly and more accurately than do spoken words. An understanding of the implications of nonverbal communication is important for all nurses, especially psychiatric nurses. Mentally ill patients are more aware of the nurse and her verbal and nonverbal behavior than many nurses realize. The nurse who works rapidly, walks down the hall briskly, closes doors emphatically, and answers questions sharply is likely to be seen by the patient as an angry person who is unapproachable. The nurse who smiles as if she were happy, speaks in a warm, friendly manner, and seems to approach her work calmly conveys to the patient an acceptance that may prompt him to turn to her for help.

Mentally ill patients quickly learn to know and to anticipate the behavioral responses of the workers with whom they deal. With the possible exception of patients who are pathologically suspicious of other people, mentally ill patients, like all other patients, usually evaluate the sincerity and kindness of the hospital staff accurately. Thus it has been observed that a worker who is gruff and outspoken with patients may be respected and loved by them if he communicates nonverbally a basic attitude of kindness and a sincere interest in their welfare. A nurse who has adopted an unusually saccharine approach to patients may be deeply resented by them because she conveys nonverbally a feeling of rejection.

It is essential for the nurse to examine

her own feelings toward patients and if possible to focus her activities upon those patients for whom she has genuine feelings of interest and acceptance. If the nurse attempts to work closely with patients about whom she has many negative feelings, she will surely communicate these feelings nonverbally. The nurse needs to recognize the importance of her personal feelings in developing a reciprocal relationship with a patient. It is also essential to recognize the role of nonverbal communication and to understand that it is impossible for every nurse to work therapeutically with every mentally ill patient. Equipped with this knowledge and understanding, the nurse can feel comfortable in admitting that she is not the appropriate person to be assigned to work closely with a specific patient with whom she has not been able to establish a positive relationship.

DEVELOPING A CLIMATE THAT ENCOURAGES COMMUNICATION

Mentally ill patients need the opportunity to communicate with others who are sincerely interested in their problems and who care about them as people. It is important for the nurse to learn to talk with patients so that conversation will become a part of the total therapeutic environment. The ability to talk therapeutically with patients requires that the nurse have an attitude of acceptance, tolerance, and genuine interest in the patient.

A climate of mutual trust and respect must be developed before mentally ill patients can feel safe enough to communicate with a nurse. This is not an easy climate to establish; it requires time, patience, knowledge, and skill. When a patient is helped to converse meaningfully with a professional person, a release of tension may result. Such an opportunity can be an emotionally supportive experience for the patient.

The patient and the nurse are strangers when she first joins the professional staff of a psychiatric unit. They must become acquainted before her work can be meaningful. Most patients approach the nurse cautiously at first, as they approach other strangers. Some shy patients may not approach the nurse at all. A few of the more aggressive ones may insist upon monopolizing her total attention. The wise nurse will utilize some of the same skills in building a relationship with a patient that she has used successfully to build relationships with other strangers.

If the nurse has not already been introduced to the patients on the unit to which she is assigned she will begin by introducing herself. It will be helpful if she explains her status on the unit at the same time. This can be done by saying "I am Miss Jones, a student nurse, and I have been assigned to this unit for four weeks." Or she might say "I am Miss Smith, a graduate nurse, and I have come to work on this unit for a while." If the nurse cannot recall the name of a patient to whom she has introduced herself, she might say "Will you please help me learn your name? I am sorry that I do not know it." With this invitation most patients will introduce themselves. Thus the nurse will begin the necessary task of learning the names, faces, and personalities of the patient population with whom she will be working.

INITIATING A CONVERSATION

A conversation is one of the most common of the shared activities in which people engage. It is the logical beginning for any relationship. Just as the nurse initiates conversational topics with other strangers, she may find it helpful with patients to introduce a neutral conversational topic appropriate for the time and place. If the time of year is right, baseball may be an appropriate topic. If the patient group is interested in baseball the nurse may choose to initiate a conversation with a question about a recent game. For example, she may begin by saying "I did not have a chance to follow the game yesterday. What was the final score?" Other neutral topics that may be used include the headlines in the newspaper, the weather, or an approaching hospital party. If the nurse notices that a patient is holding a newspaper she may begin a conversation by inquiring "What interesting happenings are in the headlines today?"

Having introduced a topic, the sensitive nurse will wait for a response and will not feel compelled to avoid silences by immediately adding her own comments or opinions. After ample opportunity has been given for a response, it is suggested that she introduce a second conversational idea that logically follows the first.

Patients often ask new nurses personal questions such as "Are you married?" or "What nursing school are you from?" or "Where do you live?" The natural curiosity of patients about the personal life of the professional staff is understandable. However, if the conversation is allowed to be focused upon the personal life of the nurse it quickly loses its original goal —to achieve therapeutic communication.

If the nurse wishes to do so, it would seem logical for her to respond to factual questions such as "Are you married?" with a simple "Yes" or "No." If the patient persists with further personal questions directed at the nurse, she might say in a friendly way "Why do you ask?" or comment "I wonder if we could not find a more interesting topic than my personal life to discuss." Personal questions directed to the nurse alert her to the need for focusing future conversation more carefully. It may suggest that the specific patient in question hopes to direct attention away from his own problems or that the patient is somewhat hostile toward nurses.

One of the first steps the nurse can take in creating a permissive environment is to sit near or beside the patient when talking to him. Some nurses hesitate to sit beside patients even when they are trying to converse with them. This hesitancy probably comes from experience in other nursing situations when the nurse was expected to be constantly busy carrying out comfort measures or therapeutic treatment procedures.

When the nurse stands during a conversation she conveys the idea that she is in a hurry, that she expects the conversation to be a short one, and that she is prepared to remain with the patient for only a few minutes. In such a hurried atmosphere no one can expect a patient to feel that there is interest or time enough for him to talk about anything important. It is essential to establish a physical climate in which the patient will feel that the nurse is giving him her interest and her time. The nurse can expect a positive nurse-patient relationship to be initiated when a permissive, accepting climate is established and when she conveys her sincere interest in the patient through the warmth of her voice and her facial expression.

PRACTICAL SUGGESTIONS FOR IMPROVING COMMUNICATION

Some nurses attempt to communicate with patients by doing most of the talking while the patient sits or stands passively nearby. If the patient responds at all in a situation like this it is usually to give a one-word answer. When the nurse communicates in such a way, her comments usually fall into the category of giving advice or persuading the patient to do something that someone believes will benefit him. Neither advice nor persuasion are of much help if the goal is to assist the patient to become a self-directing adult. Giving advice suggests that one person is attempting to impose his values and personal choices upon a second person who is not capable of making such choices. The giver of advice usually begins the conversation by saying "If I were you." The nurse is not the patient and cannot know the choices that are best for him to make in most situations. She does not know all the past experiences that influence the patient's present thinking and feeling and therefore is not qualified to make suggestions about his many problems and concerns. Advice may result in a temporary and positive response because it may relieve the patient from the responsibility of making an immediate decision. In the long run it is likely to encourage the patient to remain dependent upon some other person for decisions.

Giving advice is not always a safe practice. If the advice is accepted and the situation remains unimproved or worsens, the patient is likely to blame the giver of the advice. Advice should be avoided. Instead of offering advice it is more helpful to explore with the patient the positive and negative aspects of the possible decisions that are open to him. Ultimately, the goal of the professional person is to help the patient identify the decision he can feel most comfortable about making.

Nurses make many comments to patients that they hope will give reassurance but fall far short of this goal. Even though the nurse intends to be helpful, it is never helpful to a patient to make comments such as the following: "Don't worry." "Your doctor says this medicine will help you." "There are a great many people who are worse off than you are." "Don't cry; you do not want people to see you crying." Such comments are meaningless and are likely to convince the patient that the nurse is not able to understand his problems. Reassurance is never achieved by using meaningless clichés. Instead, reassurance is more likely to be achieved by spending time with the patient and by listening to his expressions of feelings as long as he seems to need to talk. It is reassuring for the nurse to consider the problem thoughtfully and to ask intelligent, reality-oriented questions about the situation that is upsetting the patient. It is reassuring for the nurse to accept the patient's tears without comment or to assure the patient that crying is a reasonable thing to do under the circumstances, provided, of course, the circumstances do warrant such emotional expression. It is reassuring to listen to the patient's personal problems without showing surprise or disapproval when the patient talks about past social behavior that is unusual or below the standards that the nurse has set for herself. It is reassuring when the nurse agrees that the patient has a problem and works with him in trying to think through solutions to it. It may be reassuring to sit with the patient even when he does not feel like talking. If the nurse can convey to the patient her genuine interest in his problem and acceptance of him, she may be able to reassure the patient in a very real sense by sitting quietly with him.

Persuasion suggests that some pressure is being placed upon the patient to accept a prescribed course of action. This, like advice, is not a practice that is likely to help the patient to move toward more self-reliance.

Suggestion is an aspect of communication that may be helpful to patients. Much can be done to stimulate interest in activities and to help patients alter social attitudes by using skillfully phrased suggestions. For instance, encouraging a patient to participate in the activities offered in the occupational therapy department may be accomplished by telling him about the activities available there and by using suggestions such as "You might enjoy the finger painting class." At another time a second comment about this activity might be "Everybody seems to have an interesting time when they go to the occupational therapy department; I think you might, too." One suggestion is usually not sufficient to alter an attitude or help a patient accept a new idea. Suggestion must be used frequently and skill-fully by persons whose opinion the patient respects.

The patient who has refused to have his hair cut for several weeks may request a visit to the barber shop if several people with whom he is acquainted comment about his attractive appearance when his hair was cut a few weeks before.

EFFECTIVE VERBAL INTERACTIONS

To be effective, verbal interactions must be guided by goals.

Certainly the nurse should avoid approaching any patient with a barrage of words. In their desire to communicate with patients, nurses sometimes resort to asking a series of questions. Unfortunately this is too often the type of conversation that is reported when nurses are asked to tell something of a recent conversation with a patient. "How are you today?" is one of the usual questions with which many nurses begin a conversation. Such an opening sentence usually does little to develop a conversation.

The nurse's therapeutic potential will be greatly increased if a conscious effort is made to establish a goal for each nurse-patient interaction before initiating a conversation. The identified purpose for the interaction will provide a guide as to the appropriate approach and attitude to be used, the approximate length of the conversation, and the manner in which it will be terminated.

Frequently the nurse interacts with the patient for the purpose of giving or getting specific information. Although the attitude toward the patient will be friendly, the nurse will initiate the conversation by explaining the purpose of the questions she will ask. In this instance it is appropriate that the questions will be more direct than those usually employed. Such a conversation would undoubtedly be brief and terminated with a polite expression of thanks.

Direct questions may be perceived by the patient as threatening to personal security. "Why did you come to the hospital"? or "How do you feel about your job"? may touch upon sensitive feelings. Thus direct questions are usually helpful only when specific information must be obtained or when the patient is confused. When a patient is responding to intrapsychic stimulation, it may be necessary to use direct questions to communicate with him.

A second goal for initiating a nurse-patient interaction may be to establish a beginning rapport that can serve as a basis for developing a meaningful future relationship. With such a goal, attention would be focused upon the patient in a friendly, relaxed way in order to convey a willingness to listen. In such a situation, emphasis is upon getting acquainted and establishing a feeling of trust on the part of the patient.

If the purpose of the interaction is to encourage the patient to express his thoughts and feelings, a nondirective approach would undoubtedly achieve the most positive results. In such a situation the patient would be encouraged to initiate the conversation. Responding to the patient's comments by reflecting his thoughts might be helpful in encouraging him to continue expressing his feelings without introducing new or unrelated ideas. For example, if the patient speaks of his unhappy home life, the nurse might respond to the patient, "Your home life is unhappy."

REASONABLE EXPECTATIONS IN DEVELOPING RELATIONSHIPS

It is not possible for a nurse to develop relationships that have the same potential and the same meaning for each individual patient. It is possible, however, for the nurse to learn to know the names and something of the needs of all patients with whom she comes in close contact. With many of these patients the nurse can expect to develop a positive working relationship. With a limited number she will be able to develop a mutual give and take that will have the potential of growing into a therapeutic relationship. Some patients in this last group undoubtedly will seek out the nurse almost daily to talk with her or to ask her to participate in some recreational activity. It is with this group that she will be able to carry on discussions that have therapeutic potential because she will know the patients, will have developed a genuine interest in them as people, and will have been able to talk with the physician about the goals he has established for therapy.

LISTENING AS AN ASPECT OF COMMUNICATION

A general rule to follow when talking with patients is to encourage the patient to take the conversational lead. Although the nurse may initiate communication and may keep the conversation alive, it must focus upon the interests and concerns of the patient if it is to be of value to him.

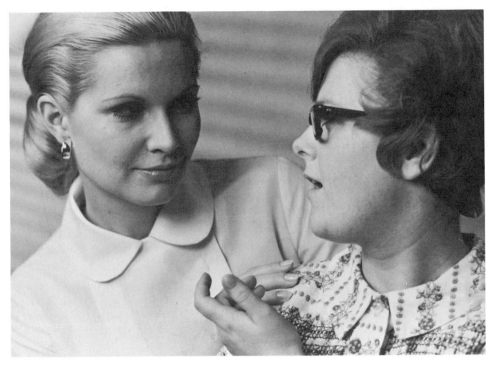

FIG. 2. *The nurse helps the patient by listening.*

Listening implies silence, but it does not imply passivity. The listener can and should be an active, alert, and interested participant even though she may make very few verbal contributions. The nurse gives evidence of interest by actually being genuinely interested in the patient and in what he is saying. This interest cannot be feigned. Evidence of genuine, sincere interest is shown by the expression on the listener's face, by the way the listener looks at the speaker, and by the verbal encouragement that is given to the speaker. Nodding the head to suggest that one understands or agrees is one way of giving encouragement. Comments such as "I can understand that." or "That must have been difficult for you." or "I see. Go on." are encouraging when said at an appropriate time in a friendly, interested tone. If the listener cannot follow the logic of the speaker or the sequence of the related incidents, it is best to ask the speaker to review that part of the story again. The nurse might say "Could you explain that last statement again for me? I do not believe I understood it clearly." Or she might say "I am afraid you lost me there a minute ago. Could you go over that last point again?" If the nurse fails to ask for clarification when it is needed, the patient will soon discover that she has lost the sequence and meaning of the conversation and is trying to act as if she understands when she does not. This is one way of losing the patient's confidence.

When the nurse needs to leave the patient she should break off the conversation in such a way that it can be resumed at another time. Thus she might say "I have been interested in what you have been telling me, and I hope we can continue this discussion later on. Just now I must take care of some other duties that have been assigned to me." Of course, such a

41

statement must be true. If the nurse has no other duties to perform she should mention some other real reason for leaving the patient. If she has promised to talk to the patient at another time she must find a time for taking up the conversation again. She might begin by saying "I have been thinking about our conversation of yesterday. I have some free time right now and I am wondering if we could talk some more about the last point that you were making." The nurse would use this statement only if there were a last point she wished to explore. If such a statement were not apropos, she would choose one appropriate for the conversation.

WHEN PATIENTS REQUEST THAT CONVERSATIONS BE KEPT SECRET

Many mentally ill patients struggle with the problem of not being able to trust other people. One of the ways a nurse can help such a patient is to demonstrate to him that she can be trusted. If a patient can begin to trust one person, it is possible that eventually that trust can be extended to other people. When trying to help a patient learn to trust her, the nurse sometimes finds herself in a dilemma. A patient with whom the nurse is establishing a relationship may confide information that places her in an untenable position. On the one hand she wishes to respect the patient's confidences while at the same time she hopes to carry out her responsibilities as a member of the professional staff. The following situation precipitated such a dilemma.

A patient confided that he was planning to leave the city during the next weekend, at which time he expected to be given permission to visit his family. He told the nurse that he had stolen enough money from his family to purchase a train ticket to a distant city where he was unknown and where he hoped to make a fresh start in the world. The patient cautioned the nurse not to tell anyone about these plans until after he had gone. The nurse was, with reason, concerned about the patient's safety, about keeping the patient's confidences, and about fulfilling her role as a member of the professional staff of the hospital. She was understandably distressed about the situation.

Unfortunately the nurse failed to remind the patient that she was a member of the professional staff and therefore had a responsibility to report his plan to the nurse in charge of the unit and the physician in charge of his therapy. A reasonable guide to follow is that the nurse has a responsibility to tell the patient's physician and the nurse in charge of the unit if the patient tells her of plans that are dangerous to him or others or that interfere with the treatment plan. When the patient begins to confide information to the nurse that should be shared with other members of the professional staff, she has a responsibility to remind him that she must report the conversation to the appropriate people. The nurse might ask the patient, "Are you sure that you want to tell me this? You know it will be necessary for me to share this with the treatment team."

When a patient confides his feelings about an emotionally laden situation to the nurse, she may be presented with a second problem. The information and feelings about which the patient has told her should be handled in the therapeutic session with the physician, but for various reasons the patient may not have been able to share this information with him. The nurse should suggest that she is not the appropriate person with whom he should share this particular information.

When the nurse has established a relationship with the patient that makes it possible for him to express his anxiety to her, she has a responsibility to listen with acceptance and understanding. In addition, she is obligated to encourage the patient to share his feeling with the physician. It is also suggested that the nurse ask the physician for an opportunity to discuss the patient and his problems.

RECORDING PATIENTS' CONVERSATIONS

The professional and nonprofessional staff in a psychiatric setting need to communicate continuously with each other. An effective communication system is one way of improving consistency of patient care and of avoiding many errors that occur when information about the needs and behavior of patients is not shared. Talking together about ward problems and patient care is probably the best method to improve staff communication. The written records that are made by the professional staff are another important way of communicating with one another. Recording done by nurses should give an accurate account of the patient's 24-hour behavior, since the nursing staff has the opportunity of being with the patient continuously. Usually the most meaningful source of recorded material is the patient's verbal communication. The nurse's record

should quote the patient as accurately as possible and should be written in a reasonably short time after the conversation has taken place. The nurse's personal impressions and reactions should be avoided, except in situations where the patient's mood or attitude is being described. Psychiatric terminology and impressions should be omitted. Psychiatric labels and symptomatology contribute little information to the reader and should be avoided. Recording in the nurse's notes should emphasize the patient's conversation and should be written simply, accurately, and straightforwardly. The reader should be free to make his own judgments concerning the meaning of the behavior about which the nurse has written.

IMPORTANT CONCEPTS

1. It is essential for the psychiatric nurse to develop an understanding of the principles of effective communication.
2. Nonverbal communication often conveys general attitudes, feelings, and reactions more clearly and more accurately than do spoken words.
3. The nurse needs to examine her own feelings toward patients because she communicates these feelings nonverbally.
4. The ability to talk therapeutically with patients requires an attitude of acceptance, tolerance, and genuine interest in the patient.
5. The wise nurse will utilize some of the same skills in building a relationship with a patient that she has used successfully with other strangers.
6. Conversation that is focused upon

the personal life of the nurse loses its real goal of achieving therapeutic conversation.

7. The therapeutic potential of the nurse's verbal interaction with the patient will be greatly increased if it is guided by goals established before the conversation is initiated.

8. The nurse works toward creating a climate in which the patient can feel safe enough to converse with her freely.

9. Neither advice nor persuasion is helpful when the therapeutic goal is to help the patient become a self-directing adult.

10. Reassurance can be helpful to patients if the method used is appropriate for the patient and his problem, but statements that represent meaningless clichés are rarely reassuring.

11. Skillfully phrased suggestions are useful in altering social attitudes, in changing ideas, and in stimulating interest in therapeutic activities.

12. Direct questions are rarely helpful in stimulating conversation and may give the effect of probing into the patient's personal life.

13. Patients should be encouraged to take the conversational lead.

14. Patients must be helped to understand that the nurse has a responsibility to share confidences with the physician and the head nurse when confiding behavior that may be dangerous to themselves or others or may interfere with the physician's treatment goals.

15. The nurse's written records of conversations with patients should be accurate and should avoid psychiatric terminology, labels, or impressions.

SUGGESTED SOURCES OF ADDITIONAL INFORMATION

Ball, Geraldine: Speaking without words, Amer. J. Nurs. **60**:692-693, May, 1960.

Davidson, Henry A.: Nonverbal communication in a hospital setting, Perspect. Psychiat. Care **1**: 12-17, 1963.

Davis, Anne J.: The skills of communication, Amer. J. Nurs. **63**:66-70, Jan., 1963.

Eldred, Stanley H.: Improving nurse-patient communication, Amer. J. Nurs. **60**:1600-1603, Nov., 1960.

Hall, Bernard H.: A colleague looks at psychiatric nursing, Nurs. Outlook **2**:66-69, Feb., 1954.

Hewitt, Helon E., and Pesznecker, Betty L.: Blocks to communicating with patients, Amer. J. Nurs. **64**:101-103, July, 1964.

Ingles, Thelma: Understanding the nurse-patient relationship, Nurs. Outlook **9**:698-700, Nov., 1961.

Knowles, Lois N.: How can we reassure patients? Amer. J. Nurs. **59**:834-835, June, 1959.

Lewis, Garland K.: Communication; a factor in meeting emotional crises, Nurs. Outlook **13**: 36-39, Aug., 1965.

Peplau, Hildegard E.: Talking with patients, Amer. J. Nurs. **60**:964-966, July, 1960.

Peplau, Hildegard E.: Interpersonal techniques; the crux of psychiatric nursing, Amer. J. Nurs. **62**:50-54, June, 1962.

Rector, Cynthia: Content in the initial therapist-patient interview, Perspect. Psychiat. Care **3**:33-35, 1965.

Robinson, Alice M.: Communicating with schizophrenic patients, Amer. J. Nurs. **60**:1120-1123, Aug., 1960.

Schwartz, Morris S., and Shockley, Emmy Lanning: The nurse and the mental patient, New York, 1956, Russell Sage Foundation, pp. 218-230, 231-243.

Stoneberg, Carla Johnson: Communication through art on a psychiatric ward, Perspect. Psychiat. Care **2**:12-22, 1964.

Travelbee, Joyce: What do we mean by rapport? Amer. J. Nurs. **63**:70-72, Feb., 1963.

The nurse focuses on developing therapeutic nursing roles

CHAPTER FIVE

Therapeutic roles of the psychiatric nurse

One of the most challenging aspects of the work of the psychiatric nurse is the opportunity to fill a variety of therapeutic roles while participating in patient care. The daily living activities of the patient provide the psychiatric nurse with a unique opportunity to make a distinct therapeutic contribution. Although no other professional group concerns itself solely with this aspect of the patient's hospital experience, it may be the most important single factor that helps to alter the patient's behavior in a positive direction. There are unlimited therapeutic opportunities for the nurse who spends 8 hours a day with patients and really learns to know and understand them.

The psychiatric nurse's role shifts frequently as she strives to develop the hospital environment into a therapeutic situation for mentally ill patients. She fills the role of creator of a therapeutic environment when she provides opportunities for patients to experience acceptance in social relationships. Frequently she fills the role of socializing agent when she helps individuals or groups of patients plan and participate in hospital dances and ward parties. The nurse finds that she must assume the role of counselor when patients need someone to listen with understanding and sympathy while they talk about troublesome problems. The nurse is sometimes a teacher, especially when she helps patients learn to function in more socially acceptable ways. Frequently she fills the role of mother substitute when she gives emotional support and understanding or when she performs a mothering activity such as feeding a patient. Sometimes she functions in the traditional role of nurse as she performs technical nursing duties such as administering medications or treatments. The nurse probably never functions in any single role at any given time; usually she fulfills all or several of these roles at once. For the sake of clarity, however, these roles will be discussed separately.

THE NURSE AS CREATOR OF A THERAPEUTIC ENVIRONMENT

One of the major therapeutic contributions the nurse can make to improving a patient's hospital experience is to develop a warm, accepting atmosphere. Although this atmosphere is related superficially to the physical equipment and decoration of the ward, no amount of decoration can substitute for genuine human warmth, which springs solely from other human beings. If the situation is to be therapeutic for patients, it is essential that the nurses and attendants who are in close daily contact with them be honest, sincere, friendly people who really care about other people. The skill of the psychiatrist cannot be completely effective if the patient is living in a cold, sterile, routinized hospital atmosphere. If the psychiatric nurse is able to establish a warm, accepting atmosphere, the way will have been prepared so that the contributions of the other members of the psychiatric treatment team can be of maximum effectiveness.

When opportunities are provided through ward activities for new and more positive experiences in living and relating to other people, the patient may be helped to behave in more mature ways. Certain ingredients must be present in the emo-

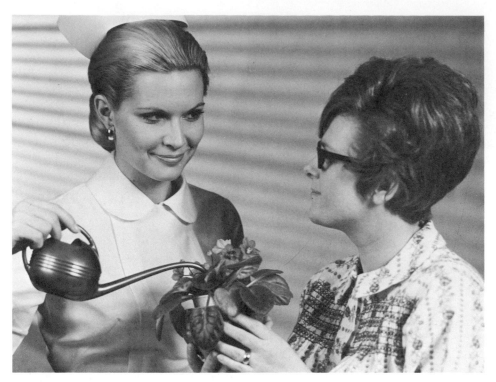

FIG. **3.** *The nurse helps create a homelike atmosphere.*

tional climate before opportunities for developing social confidence and emotional maturity can be provided in a hospital setting. The first of these is a genuine interest in and respect for individual patients on the part of all hospital personnel. When there is real respect for patients as individuals, they are given as much responsibility as possible for making their own decisions, and they are expected to assume some responsibility for their own control.

A feeling of security is a second essential element in developing a therapeutic climate. When patients are provided with an emotionally secure climate, feelings of acceptance, friendliness, warmth, safety, and relaxation are present. Many emotionally sick people enter the hospital because they are fearful, anxiety-ridden, and insecure in their relationships with other people. A therapeutic climate should

make it possible for emotionally sick individuals to behave as they need to behave because of their illness, secure in the knowledge that they will not be rejected and that they do not need to fear retaliation.

A third essential element in creating a therapeutic climate is an attitude that anticipates positive change and growth. If the climate is to be therapeutic, everyone working with patients will project an attitude that encourages improvement and positive change in behavior.

THE NURSE AS A SOCIALIZING AGENT

Another important role is that of socializing agent. In fulfilling this role the nurse helps patients live and participate successfully in group activities. Units for patients in psychiatric facilities are ideal

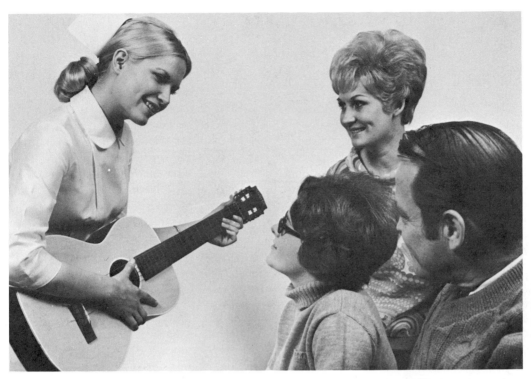

FIG. 4. *The nurse helps patients develop socialization skills.*

settings for organizing and directing group activities. Group activities are particularly needed during that period in the day that comes after the evening meal has been served. Many hospital activities stop before supper, and patients are frequently faced with long, unoccupied, dull evenings. The clever, imaginative nurse who cares for patients during the evening hours has a real opportunity to contribute to the mental health of the patients on the unit where she is assigned. Such a simple activity as an evening snack period can be the focus for group singing, group games, or group conversation. Ward activities, organized by the patients themselves, uncover and utilize hidden talent. In this way the group has an opportunity to recognize and encourage its own members and to contribute to developing the ego strengths of individuals. The dining room situation may lend itself to group

activity if groups of patients eat in individual dining rooms. In such a situation the nurse in charge during mealtime has an opportunity to create a leisurely, happy experience from which a feeling of belonging can develop. Mealtime is too often viewed solely from the standpoint of nutrition. Sometimes patients are hurried so that the ward personnel can get on to some other activity. Sometimes conversation is discouraged because it slows up eating. The nurse or attendant who supervises the dining room may stand about like a policeman and may view the task solely from the standpoint of getting the patients fed as efficiently and quickly as possible.

No one questions the value of an adequate dietary intake. When personnel are in short supply, the only realistic approach to dining room supervision may be a hurried one. But in some hospitals where there are adequate personnel, mealtime is part of a therapeutic approach to patient care. When the supervising nurse adopts a permissive attitude toward activities in the dining room, mealtime recaptures the spirit of a family gathering. When the nurse eats at the table with the patients and assumes the role of hostess, a positive learning situation results.

The nurse makes a contribution to improving the socialization skills of patients by encouraging and developing the healthy aspects of their personalities. Many mentally ill patients have utilized withdrawal because of their extreme sensitivity and anxiety in relation to other people. The hospital provides opportunities for patients to learn to achieve success in social situations by creating opportunities through which patients develop feelings of security with other people. The skillful nurse utilizes ward recreational activities, the dining room situation, and even activities centering around the housekeeping chores in the ward situation to help patients learn to participate successfully in social situations.

THE NURSE AS A COUNSELOR

Sympathetic listening is another important aspect of psychiatric nursing. There is probably no more important task than listening to a patient in a positive, dynamic, sympathetic way without at the same time giving advice, stating opinions, or making suggestions. This type of listening encourages the patient to think through his problems and to arrive at a decision, which is helpful to him. It helps the patient to discharge anxiety and ten-sion. It conveys to the patient the realization that the nurse really cares.

Sympathetic listening demands a great deal from the nurse both in time and in emotional energy. It demands that she be skillful in reflecting the patient's comments to him in such a manner that he will realize that she is interested in the discussion and wants to hear as much as he needs to tell. Some nurses may not understand the vital importance of this kind of listening and may feel that they should stop the patient's outpouring of problems. Unfortunately, this is easily done by a comment such as "You can tell all of that to your doctor tomorrow. He's the one who needs to know these things." The nurse may respond with an even less helpful comment, "Things will be better tomorrow. Just keep a stiff upper lip."

Sometimes patients pour out problems more freely to the nurse than to anyone else. It is unfortunate when the patient feels that he is better able to talk to the nurse than to the psychiatrist about his problem. The role of the psychiatrist is to deal primarily with the problems of the unconscious, whereas the nurse deals with reality-oriented concerns. The nurse seeks to assist the patient to channel those problems that are the legitimate concern of the psychiatrist to him. The nurse and the psychiatrist need to work out together their mutually therapeutic roles with the patient who actively seeks help from both of them.

The role of the nurse is to help the patient with problems of reality that deal with the here and now. There are scores of times when patients discuss problems with the nurse that do deal with the areas that are her special concern, and it is in

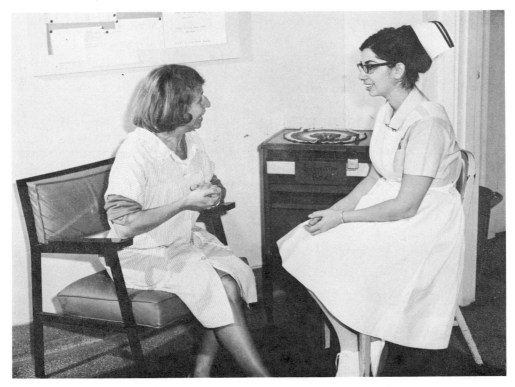

FIG. 5. *Sympathetic listening is an important aspect of psychiatric nursing.*

these situations that her role as a counselor is most frequently helpful.

Among the nurse's therapeutic responsibilities as a counselor is the giving of reassurance. Many situations in the life of a patient require that someone give some reassurance. Sometimes the nurse may suggest that reassurance should more logically be provided by the psychiatrist, religious counselor, or social worker. The nurse needs to learn what services are available to the patient and how she can procure the assistance that he needs. However, more often than not it is up to the nurse to provide the needed reassurance. Such needs appear in every area of the patient's life. There is the patient who cannot sleep because he fears the treatment scheduled for the morning; the patient who is upset because her husband did not visit as he had promised and she is now sure that he does not love her; the

patient who believes that he is doomed forever because he has committed an unpardonable sin; and the patient who is afraid of everything. The list is endless and the needs for reassurance frequently appear at eleven o'clock at night or at three o'clock in the morning when no other professional help is readily available.

Obviously no set of rules or suggestions will serve as solutions in each of these many situations. Probably the most effective reassurance for fearful, upset patients is a staff of nurses and attendants who do not change frequently and who are consistently kind and accepting. Sitting beside a patient may in itself be reassuring. This may help the patient to feel that someone upon whom he can depend is there, ready to help in whatever way possible. Listening is one of the better ways of offering reassurance. Although logical, reasonable answers are frequently not helpful, they may be reassuring for some patients. Effective reassurance is dependent upon the situation, the nurse, her relationship with the patient, and his personality. Obviously a suspicious patient will require a different kind of help than will a depressed patient.

Another aspect of the nurse's counseling role is in helping patients find acceptable outlets for anxiety. The patient who is found lying in bed and sobbing into the pillow may be helped by a single suggestion that she walk up and down the hallway with the nurse. Another patient who is tense or excited may respond to the nurse's suggestions that she take a hot tub bath. Some other ways in which the nurse may help patients find outlets for anxieties include assisting the patient to participate in a simple task, to become involved in some group activity, or to talk about his feelings.

The nurse would be wise to seek the help and guidance of the psychiatrist when she realizes that she and his patient are involved in a significant interpersonal relationship. Developing a collaborative relationship with the psychiatrist who is dealing with the patient should increase the potential therapeutic effect of the total hospital experience.

THE NURSE AS A TEACHER

If hospitalization can provide the individual with opportunities to learn to live more happily and more successfully with other people, it will make a significant contribution to the patient's emotional growth. If the patient merely lives in the hospital to safeguard his family and the community and if he relies entirely upon the physician's treatment, it is questionable how worthwhile the institutional experience can be. It is in helping the patient to learn to cope in a more mature way with interpersonal relationships that the nurse has a role as a teacher.

Problems of behavior manifested by mentally ill patients are as varied as life itself and encompass every aspect of living. Some patients, like children, must learn many simple tasks involved in living. They need help in learning to dress appropriately for the occasion; to assume responsibility for tasks assigned; to care for physical needs so that they can be acceptable to others; to eat in socially prescribed ways; to accept a reasonably flexible schedule for eating, sleeping, and bathing; to avoid hurting other people's feelings; and to cope with many other aspects of group living.

The nurse may fill the role of teacher as she helps a patient learn a new game, dance step, or song in order for him to participate more actively in recreation. She may actually take the role of dance partner or may participate in a game to help a shy, frightened patient become integrated into a group. The nurse may participate in an activity requiring only two persons to help a hostile, suspicious patient learn that some people can be trusted. She may continue to participate with this patient over a period of time until she is able to help him move into some group activity without her supporting presence.

The psychiatric nurse in her role as a wise and understanding teacher helps patients learn to participate in more socially acceptable and satisfying living activities.

THE NURSE AS A
MOTHER SURROGATE

Traditionally in this culture the nurse has been a trusted person who performs personal services for sick people. Many of these services are similar to those a mother performs for children. Nurses who are permanently assigned to units in psychiatric facilities almost invariably become mother substitutes for some of the patients with whom they are closely associated. The role of mother substitute is part of the traditional role of the nurse and includes many mothering activities that may be required for some patients in a psychiatric situation. Although most mentally ill patients are able to bathe, dress, and feed themselves, there are a few who are too emotionally ill to carry out these simple tasks. For some psychiatric patients the nurse may need to assume the traditional protective, supportive, mothering role when she gives physical care.

The nurse, like a wise mother, realizes that it is important for patients to assume responsibility for their own physical care as soon as possible. Thus she gives physical care to emotionally sick patients in a sympathetic and understanding way but looks for and seizes every opportunity to encourage the patient to assume responsibility for his own care as soon as possible. The wise nurse withdraws from the task of feeding or bathing a patient just as rapidly as the patient is able to take over the responsibility for himself.

The psychiatric nurse not only carries out the mothering role in relation to the physical needs of patients, but she is also like a mother in relation to managing the house or hospital ward. It is she who develops many of the policies concerning the ward environment, which profoundly affect the lives of the patients. She is indirectly responsible for almost every aspect of the 24-hour day on the ward, from housekeeping to calling a physician if the patient needs emergency care. The nurse sets the tone of the hospital ward much as a mother sets the tone of the family.

One of the most therapeutic aspects of the nurse's traditional role as mother substitute is in assisting individual and groups of patients to set limits for their own behavior. This aspect of the nurse's role probably overlaps with the teacher role.

Patients who live together in hosiptal units may react toward each other as if they were members of the same family. These reactions are usually unconscious but are nonetheless real and may serve as a basis for much emotional and social unlearning and relearning. The nurse's role as mother substitute offers her an opportunity to provide patients with healthy experiences in the area of emotional relationships. She may be able to supply the warm, accepting mothering relationship that some patients require to move toward more mature behavior. She may serve as the object of many of the angry, hostile feelings that some patients cannot admit or express toward their own mothers. With the help of the psychiatrist who is directing the care of the individual patient, the psychiatric nurse may be able through her mothering role to supply an emotional experience that may be significant in the patient's total therapeutic regimen.

THE NURSE AS A THERAPIST

For several years some nurses who have had the benefit of an appropriate educational experience in psychiatric nursing have been developing the role of the nurse-patient relationship therapist. When the nurse functions in the role of nurse-patient relationship therapist, the principles developed through the practice of psychotherapy are being utilized.

Nurse-patient relationship therapy has developed differently in each situation, but basically it follows the same general guidelines.

The role of nurse-patient relationship therapist is carefully explained to all levels of the professional staff and to all patients in the clinical situation. Every attempt is made to be sure that the role is understood before any therapeutic activity is initiated. The nurse works collaboratively with the psychiatrists in the setting and confers regularly with those responsible for the treatment plans for the patients with whom she is working. The nurse's work becomes a part of the total treatment plan for the patient.

The nurse-patient relationship therapist strives, in a professional capacity, to help the individual with emotional problems that can benefit from her particular skills and knowledge. She works with patients who require help in improving their ability to cope with the daily problems of living. In contrast the psychiatrist more frequently works with patients who require help in making fundamental changes in the area of psychopathology or ego psychology.

Early in the initial phase the nurse-patient relationship therapist establishes with the patient the ground rules for the relationship. Thus the nature of the relationship and the responsibility of the nurse-therapist and the patient are discussed. The time, frequency, place for the sessions, and the approximate total number of meetings to be held are established.

The relationship passes through the same three phases experienced in the other relationship therapies discussed in this text. Thus there is an initial phase of getting acquainted and testing one another, a second phase in which the work of the nurse-patient relationship therapy is achieved, and a termination phase during which the emotional involvement in the relationship is decreased gradually. The length of each phase is dependent upon the individuals involved, the problems presented by the patient, and the patient's reaction to termination.

It is essential for the nurse's professional development, as well as for the patient's welfare, that she identify a skilled professional therapist to function on a regular basis as her preceptor or her supervisor while she is working in the role of a nurse-patient relationship therapist.

With this in mind, the therapist should record each nurse-patient therapy session in such a way that it can be used (1) to review the progress being made during the sessions, (2) to analyze the problems that have been presented, and (3) to evaluate patient progress against the established treatment goals.

THE TECHNICAL NURSING ROLE

The traditional role of the nurse includes those technical aspects involved in pouring and administering medications, carrying out medical and surgical treatments, and observing and recording patient behavior. Unfortunately, it is this aspect of nursing that many people identify as nursing care. The technical aspect of the nurse's role is of great value but is not always as therapeutic in the psychiatric situation as are some other roles that the nurse assumes or is cast in by patients and co-workers. Occasionally a mentally ill patient can accept a nurse as a helpful counselor or teacher only after her ability to carry out the technical aspects of the role has been demonstrated.

One of the nurse's most significant responsibilities is the accurate and perceptive observation and recording of the patient's behavior. In carrying out this function skillfully and meaningfully the nurse contributes to the understanding that all members of the psychiatric team bring to bear upon the patient's problem. Since nurses are the professional persons that live with patients for the entire 24-hour period, they have a unique opportunity to help other professional workers understand patients' needs through effective recording of samples of conversation, sleep patterns, interpersonal relationships, socialization activities, and descriptions of personal habits.

Two actual situations are reported here as examples of how the nurse functions in a variety of roles that are sometimes carried out almost simultaneously.

"Please take me back to the ward, Miss S., I feel sick." Tall, dark-haired 17-year-old Sam had walked across the dance floor and was pleading with the nurse in charge of the hospital unit where he lived to be allowed to leave the regular Wednesday evening dance. The dance was part of the recreational program for patients in a psychiatric hospital.

Both Sam and the nurse knew that patients were not usually allowed to leave the dance until it was over. She also knew that Sam had not made such a request before and intuitively she felt that something at the dance had been upsetting to him.

Miss S. quietly made the necessary arrangements with the therapist in charge of the dance and took Sam back to the homelike ward. Then she took his pulse, temperature, and respirations to be certain that he was not physically ill. When she found that these physical signs were within the normal range, she suggested that he help her make some sandwiches. Together they went into the ward kitchen where they prepared a snack for the other patients who would soon be returning from the dance. Sam seemed happy to help. He and the nurse chatted and joked together. He spoke at length about his mother's illness and his family's financial problems, but he did not mention feeling ill.

After finishing the sandwiches and cleaning the kitchen they went together into the ward living room and sat down on the couch. "Do you think that my face is changing?" he asked; "I just looked in the bathroom mirror and it seems to me that my nose is getting a lot longer."

The nurse looked carefully at his face and said, "It looks just the same to me. It seems to you that your nose is getting longer?"

Soon the other patients arrived from the dance. The ward was filled with the busy noise of twenty-five men discussing the dance, eating the evening snack, and getting ready for bed. Sam took part in all this activity but sought the nurse several times to ask questions: "Do you think you ought to call my doctor?" "Will I be able to sleep tonight?" "You think that I am going to be all right, don't you?"

Each time Sam came to ask a question the nurse took time to listen carefully to his questions and to answer truthfully and sincerely. She did call the doctor who was on duty that evening and told him about Sam's behavior. He agreed to come to see the patient. Because the doctor was not well acquainted with Sam, the nurse spent several minutes telling him briefly about Sam's family problems. She pointed out that the patient had been anxious and tense during the evening and had seemed to cling to her and to be asking for reassurance. The doctor talked with Sam. He felt that by allowing Sam to leave the dance, the nurse had been able to help him avoid an anxiety attack. The doctor told the nurse that her sympathetic listening and her efforts at reassuring Sam had been partially successful. The next day Sam's regular psychiatrist was able to help him look more objectively at the problem that had been so upsetting to him. With the doctor's help Sam was able to attend the dance the following week.

A few weeks later, the nurse was assigned to work with convalescent women patients. One Sunday evening she was welcoming all the patients as they returned from having spent a weekend at home. As the patients returned, they commented about the character of the weekend.

The nurse noticed that when Mrs. D. came back she was unusually quiet and that she looked as if she had been crying. The nurse spoke to her in a friendly tone and decided that she needed to spend some time with Mrs. D. later in the evening.

When the nurse had an opportunity to walk through the ward, she noticed Mrs. D. sitting alone and covering her face with her hands. The nurse sat down beside her and the patient began to pour out her story. "How much can one person stand? I can't take any more!" she sobbed. "What would you do if your husband told you to get out and that he didn't love you any more?"

The nurse thought to herself, "My! She *did* have a bad weekend. I wonder how I can help her with these feelings?" So she said, "Your husband says that he doesn't love you any more?" And with that invitation the patient continued to talk and tell about the problems that arose during the weekend at home.

The nurse knew from Mrs. D.'s social history that what she was saying was true, since the husband frankly admitted to the social worker that he was interested in another woman. Apparently he had stated his case directly to his wife during the weekend.

Many other patients were asking for help from the nurse, so she could not spend the entire evening with Mrs. D. However, as often as possible, she sat beside Mrs. D. or walked with her in the hall. She helped the patient unpack and put away her clothes. She got some aspirin when Mrs. D. complained of a splitting headache. The nurse called the psychiatrist and asked him to see Mrs. D. After the doctor had talked with the patient, the nurse gave her the sedative he had ordered.

Mrs. D. could not fall asleep even after receiving the sedative, so the nurse sat with her in the living room of the ward and listened without comment to a reiteration of the same problems.

These two brief situations are typical of patients' problems with which the psychiatric nurse is confronted daily. Some of the therapeutic opportunities available to the nurse are inherent in the nurse-patient situations just described.

IMPORTANT CONCEPTS

1. The nurse fills a variety of therapeutic roles while participating in the care of psychiatric patients.
2. The 24-hour daily living activities of the patient provide the unique oppor-

tunity that makes it possible for the psychiatric nurse to make a distinct therapeutic contribution.

3. Developing an accepting atmosphere in the ward is one of the major therapeutic contributions that the nurse can make to the patient's hospital experience.

4. The hospital situation can provide opportunities for patients to achieve greater success in social situations by helping them to develop feelings of security with other people.

5. There is no more important task for the nurse than listening to a patient in a positive, dynamic, sympathetic way without at the same time giving advice, stating opinions, or making suggestions.

6. The therapeutic role of the nurse concerns itself with the patient's reality problems that deal with here and now.

7. Probably the most effective reassurance for fearful, upset patients is a staff of nurses and attendants who do not change frequently and who are consistently kind and accepting.

8. The nurse may be able to supply the patient with a positive emotional experience that can substitute for one in which he has never before been able to share.

9. The nurse has a role as a teacher in helping the patient learn to deal in a more mature way with interpersonal relations and group living.

10. Patients who live together in hospital units may react toward each other somewhat as family members and gain some of the positive emotional experiences provided through family relationships.

11. The nurse's role as a mother substitute offers her an opportunity to provide patients with healthy experiences in the area of emotional relationships.

12. The technical aspects of the nurse's role are of great value but are not always as therapeutic in the psychiatric situation as some other roles the nurse assumes or is cast in by patients and co-workers.

13. The nurse-patient relationship therapist is one of the newest and most challenging roles being accepted by psychiatric nurses today.

SUGGESTED SOURCES OF ADDITIONAL INFORMATION

Black, Kathleen: Appraising the psychiatric patient's nursing needs, Amer. J. Nurs. 52:718-721, June, 1952.

Galioni, Elmer F., and others: Group techniques in rehabilitating "backward" patients, Amer. J. Nurs. 54:977-979, Aug., 1954.

Gregg, Dorothy E.: The psychiatric nurse's role, Amer. J. Nurs. 54:848-851, July, 1954.

Gregg, Dorothy E.: The therapeutic roles of the nurse, Perspect. Psychiat. Care 1:18-28, 1963.

Hays, Joyce Samhammer: The psychiatric nurse as a social therapist, Amer. J. Nurs. 62:64-67, June, 1962.

Holmes, Marguerite: The need to be recognized, Amer. J. Nurs. 61:86-87, Oct., 1961.

Kalkman, Marion E.: What the psychiatric nurse should be educated to be, Psychiat. Quart. (supp., part I) 26:93-102, 1952.

Morimoto, Francoise R.: The socializing role of psychiatric ward personnel, Amer. J. Nurs. 54:53-55, Jan., 1954.

Peplau, Hildegarde E.: Interpersonal relations

in nursing, New York, 1952, G. P. Putnam's Sons.

Prange, Arthur J., and Martin, Harry W.: Aids to understanding patients, Amer. J. Nurs. 62: 98-100, July, 1962.

Sabshin, Melvin: Nurse-doctor-patient relation-ships in psychiatry, Amer. J. Nurs. 57:188-192, Feb., 1957.

Schwartz, Morris S., and Shockley, Emmy Lanning: The nurse and the mental patient, New York, 1956, Russell Sage Foundation, pp. 201-284.

CHAPTER SIX

Making therapeutic use of self in one-to-one situations

The use the nurse makes of herself can be a therapeutic influence in the experience of the patient if she utilizes understanding and skill. It is the only tool that is uniquely hers and that she alone directs. The nurse may give dozens of daily medications and may assist with many somatic therapies, but these activities are medically directed. Aside from assisting the physician in carrying out therapeutic measures, there are two ways in which the nurse directly influences patient care. One sphere of influence lies in the use the nurse makes of herself as she deals with the patient in a face-to-face relationship. The other sphere of influence focuses upon the nurse-directed, 24-hour daily living activities of the patient. The key to success in both spheres is the use the nurse makes of her personality in interacting with mentally ill patients.

RELATING TO PATIENTS

All therapeutic relationships possess common elements, although they are developed differently by each person depending on the characteristics of the individuals involved. If a relationship is to become therapeutic, it is necessary to recognize the patient as a unique, important human being who experiences hopes, fears, joys, and sorrows as do all other people. It is necessary to understand that the patient has his own special set of problems and reactions to life. It is important for the nurse to develop a relationship with the patient so that she will understand, in a limited way at least, his emotional responses and the probable meaning of his behavior. Through her sensitivity the nurse can develop a recog-

nition of some of the patient's emotional needs and an appreciation for some of the ways in which she can be helpful to him.

The quality of the interaction between the nurse and the patient is closely related to the motivation that underlies her attitude toward nursing and her perception of her role as a nurse. It is important for the nurse to evaluate her relationships with patients. Because motivations are partially if not wholly unconscious, it is difficult to examine one's own motivations. Therefore the nurse will need guidance in evaluating her characteristic approaches to patients. It is suggested that this can be accomplished best through a series of friendly conferences with the psychiatric nursing instructor.

Some of the characteristic ways in which nurses relate to patients are discussed here in the hope of assisting the reader to examine the quality of her own professional behavior. Frequently the nurse relates to patients as a manager. The role of controller of the situation is an easy one for the nurse to adopt, since she has had some practice with this role in other settings. The nurse may believe that she is altering the authoritarian aspects of the role by acting toward patients as if she were the strong mother who knows best or by assuming the role of the physician's assistant who makes decisions about the patient's environment. Young nurses may adopt an authoritarian attitude because they pattern their behavior after that of older nurses who serve as role models.

It is important for the nurse to look objectively at her professional behavior with patients. If it has qualities of authoritarianism, she should ask herself why this is true. What secondary satisfactions are derived from this controlling attitude? Is this the best method of helping patients become more self-respecting and self-directing? Obviously the nurse who rigidly controls the patient's environment will not be able to create a hospital climate in which the patient can achieve maximum personal, emotional, and social growth. Development of emotional maturity is achieved only through practice in making decisions and in directing one's own behavior.

Inexperienced nurses sometimes relate to male patients in a seductive way. Actually this appears to be the only approach that some nurses are able to make to men. The nurse who chooses this method of relating to mentally ill male patients has confused her professional and social roles. She probably has given little thought to the meaning that her behavior has for the patient. Such an approach suggests that the nurse is not fully aware of the patient's psychological problems and does not realize that her seductive behavior may add to already disturbing feelings with which the patient is trying to cope. A nurse who utilizes seductive behavior in relating to mentally ill patients should seek the guidance of a mature counselor. She may need help in finding more appropriate channels through which she can express her own emotional needs.

Many nurses give little thought to the characteristic way in which they relate to patients. Some prefer to view their work role as a series of tasks to be performed. Such a nurse is probably seen by patients as a person who is busily engaged in performing tasks and avoiding patients.

She may relate to patients only when she is involved in performing a specific technical nursing task. Such a nurse should ask herself why she finds it necessary to remain aloof from patients. An evaluation of her professional behavior may reveal fears or an attitude toward mentally ill patients that can be altered.

Some nurses relate to patients solely through socialization. This approach might be called the role of the social technician. A nurse who utilizes this approach may spend much time initiating social activities and encouraging patients to participate. She may focus all conversation with patients on social activities. This approach makes it possible for her to avoid involving herself with patients except superficially and discourages patients from sharing emotionally upsetting problems with her. Patients need help in participating in social activities, but this is only one of their many needs. Focusing only on the social needs of patients limits the effectiveness of the nurse.

These are only a few of the ways in which nurses seek to relate to patients and are offered as suggestions to nurses who are exploring their own ways of interacting.

DEVELOPING A HELPING · RELATIONSHIP

The basis of all helping relationships is acceptance. This is a common word among nurses, although it is not universally understood or utilized by them. Other words that are equally important in psychiatric nursing are consistency and nonjudgmental. All these concepts are basic in developing a helping relationship

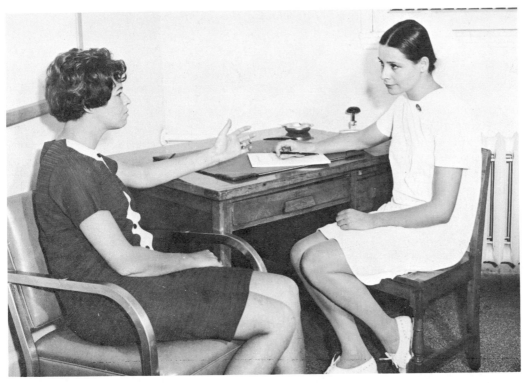

FIG. 6. *Acceptance is the basis of a helping relationship.*

with any patient. They are discussed here in the hope of helping the nurse to make effective use of them in caring for mentally ill patients.

Acceptance implies that the nurse treats the patient as an important person and not as a diagnostic entity or a set of psychiatric symptoms. Actually, the use of diagnostic terms may encourage the nurse to adopt an impersonal attitude toward the patient. The nurse implies that she is accepting the patient by calling him by name and by recognizing that he has the same basic personal rights she herself possesses. Acceptance implies that the nurse tries to understand the meaning the patient is conveying through his behavior. An accepting nurse recognizes that the patient handles his behavior as well as he is able at a given time. She allows the patient to express his feelings to her, realizing that in this way he is able to relieve emotional tensions. She does not censor the patient for statements and feelings that may not be conventionally acceptable, realizing that his behavior is an expression of his illness. She recognizes that his comments may not be directed toward her personally.

The word nonjudgmental is usually used in conjunction with the word attitude and is closely related to the concept of acceptance. Actually one cannot be achieved without the other. A nonjudgmental attitude is neither condemning nor approving. Through tone of voice and manner the nurse conveys to the patient a helpful attitude without morally judging his behavior. A nonjudgmental attitude toward the behavior of a mentally ill patient implies that the nurse recognizes that the behavior, like physical symptoms displayed by physically ill patients, is neither good or bad nor right or wrong but rather an expression of emotional need. She realizes also that the patient's behavior will change when his illness improves.

Acceptance of patients and their behavior is often difficult to achieve, and almost everyone occasionally falls short of the ideal. The behavior of some mentally ill patients is offensive at times. This is particularly true of the behavior of patients who are so confused that they soil themselves. It may be impossible for the nurse to avoid feeling repelled by the sight of a patient grossly soiled, but it is possible for her to avoid making him feel that he is an offensive person. Joking in front of a patient about his behavior or describing his shortcomings to others within his hearing is neither respecting nor accepting him.

Consistency is another important aspect to be considered in developing a helping relationship. The consistent nurse maintains the same basic attitude toward the patient day after day so that he learns what he can count on from her. Not only should the patient be able to expect the same positive attitudes and approaches from an individual nurse, but also the entire nursing staff should carry out ward routines, nursing procedures, and patient approaches with consistency from the standpoint of basic attitudes and overall policies. Consistency helps lessen the patient's anxiety by simplifying decision making and by avoiding uncertainties.

All mentally ill patients experience some loss of self-esteem and self-confidence. If a relationship is to be helpful to a patient, it must assist him in reestablishing his self-confidence and restoring his self-esteem. This is a slow process that requires consistent work over a period of time. Recognition of the patient as an important human being, genuine expressions of interest in him, spending time with him, conversing with him, and listening with understanding to his expressions of feeling are all ways of helping the patient to feel worthwhile, important and wanted. On the other hand, indifference, insincerity, and an impersonal attitude toward the patient reinforce his sense of unimportance and further convince him of what he may believe—that he is lacking in value as a person.

DIFFERENTIATING BETWEEN SOCIAL AND PROFESSIONAL RELATIONSHIPS

Sometimes it is difficult for nurses to differentiate between a social and a professional relationship when dealing with patients. The problem is even more complicated in a psychiatric setting because patients usually are not physically ill and are not bedridden. They frequently give the superficial impression of being socially and emotionally well. Nurses who have not developed an understanding of emotional illness may find it difficult to accept the fact that they are dealing with sick people. Thus their role confusion is understandable.

In a social relationship the needs of both of the involved individuals are considered. The needs of both must be met in a more or less satisfying way if the relationship is to continue. A social relationship usually develops spontaneously without a conscious plan. The goal of such a relationship is usually shared by the participants and is frequently limited to personal pleasure. The participants in a social relationship share mutual concern regarding reciprocal approval. It may develop more or less satisfactorily without conscious awareness of the emotional significance of the relationship.

In contrast, the professional relationship focuses upon the personal and emotional needs of the patient. The professional relationship is therapeutically oriented and is planned after consideration has been given to the needs of the patient and the therapeutic ability of the nurse. There is always a therapeutic goal toward which the nurse is working, but it is not always shared with the patient. When the nurse has accepted a professional role she must strive to be consciously aware of the developing relationship and its meaning. She should seek help in reflecting objectively upon the meaning of the interaction between herself and the patient so that she will be prepared to guide the patient in developing more mature behavior. In a professional relationship the nurse does not necessarily seek the patient's approval. She reevaluates the situation constantly so that she can distinguish between the patient's actual needs and his demands. When it is time for a professional relationship to be terminated, the nurse releases the patient emotionally and strives to help him move forward to more appropriate relationships.

Following are examples of the development of both a social and a professional relationship between a nurse and a patient.

A young student of nursing, Miss S., was assigned to a unit where she was to receive part of an initial experience in psychiatric nursing. The unit was populated by young men and women who were in their late teens or early twenties. The living quarters for the two groups were divided by a large living room. The patients gathered in the living room for group meetings, social activities, and conversations. Patients came and went freely in this unlocked unit. Some of the patients were employed during the day and returned to the hospital in the evening. Other patients were continuing their schoolwork in a nearby high school.

Miss S. participated enthusiastically in the social activities of the group. She frequently sought permission to participate in some of the activities planned for the evening hours. Permission was granted this request because it was the only possible way for her to become acquainted with several of the patients. When it was learned that Miss S. did not know how to dance, some of the young men volunteered to teach her. She learned quickly and was particularly successful in dancing with one young man, Jim. They were approximately the same age and had a few friends in common since they grew up in the same general area in the city. The student nurse began to focus a good deal of attention upon Jim. At patient parties she insisted that he dance with her most of the time. Because Jim was popular with the female patients, they became annoyed with the student nurse and complained about her to the physician in charge. When Miss S. was asked to stop attending ward parties, she arranged to meet Jim in the afternoon away from the hospital. She began writing Jim daily notes that were delivered by fellow students.

When the instructor became aware of this problem, she asked Miss S. to come to her office for a talk. Miss S. discussed the situation freely. She said that she enjoyed having the opportunity to associate with Jim and could see no reason why questions were being raised. She admitted that she planned to drop the relationship as soon as the psychiatric nursing experience was completed. Miss

S. said her friendship with Jim was an interesting interlude for both of them while it lasted. She was surprised to learn that Jim had requested a transfer from the unlocked unit to a unit where he would not be allowed so many privileges. She did not realize that Jim was desperately afraid of falling in love with a girl and that her relationship with him had reactivated many of his old fears and self-doubts.

In this situation Miss S. focused upon her own social needs and upon what she believed were Jim's social needs. Her stated goal for the relationship was immediate personal pleasure. Miss S. had given little thought to the meaning this relationship had for Jim or what effect her behavior would have upon her professional role with other patients. She did not seek guidance in evaluating the relationship. As a result of Miss S.'s failure to differentiate between a social and a professional relationship, her experience with Jim was not helpful to him or satisfying for her.

On this same unit another nurse was able to develop an effective professional relationship. Miss L., a young graduate nurse, came to work on the unit shortly after Miss S. left.

Miss L. became interested in Bill, a young man approximately the same age as Jim. He was painfully shy and avoided social contact with other people. He did not know how to dance and felt so inadequate that his only role in social situations was that of an observer. He did not take advantage of the privileges available to patients housed on this unlocked unit. He was intellectually very capable but had quit high school because of his shyness and fear of people.

Miss L. was sorry that Bill had not completed high school, and she decided that her goal would be to help him free himself of his fear of people to the extent that he would be able to return to school. She realized that this was a long-term goal and that it would be necessary for Bill to take many small steps forward before he could make such a move. She began her work immediately by sitting beside him for a few minutes each day. Getting acquainted with him was difficult because he was always deeply involved in reading. At first he was almost rude when she asked if she might sit down for a few minutes to talk. After many days Bill seemed to look forward to their daily chats. Finally she noticed that he closed the book when she approached.

After several weeks, Miss L. suggested that they take a walk together to the occupational therapy department to see what was going on there. He reluctantly accompanied her. On their tour of this department she talked about the many interesting available activities. She discovered that Bill had once done oil painting but feared criticism so much that he destroyed each painting before it was completed. Making use of this knowledge, Miss L. was able to obtain some oil painting equipment so that Bill could paint in a single room away from inquisitive people. Miss L. stopped to see his work daily and discovered that he had a great deal of talent. Other nurses came to praise his work. Finally, he was able to transfer his work to the occupational therapy department and eventually gave his consent to have several of his paintings hung in the lobby of the hosiptal.

One evening Miss L. gently encouraged Bill to accompany her to one of the social affairs given by the patients. During the first party he began to learn to dance. With encouragement and praise he learned to dance well and attended most of the social activities planned by the patients. He began dancing with other nurses and finally he felt sure enough of himself to ask young women patients to dance.

After Miss L. had known Bill for over a year she suggested that they go for a walk together outside the hospital. As usual he was reluctant to comply, but with encouragement he accompanied her. Several months after his first venture outside with Miss L., Bill began going out regularly with other patients to attend movies and football games and to visit art galleries. After working closely with Bill for two years, Miss L. suggested that they visit the high school near the hospital. As usual Bill needed much encouragement, but he finally made the visit with her. Eventually he was able to enroll as a student and completed his high school work.

Miss L. achieved the therapeutic goal she had established for the patient. When she first became interested in Bill, Miss L. discussed his problems with the physician, who approved her therapeutic goal and approach. She discussed each new development with the physician. Her work with Bill focused entirely upon his emotional needs. The relationship was carefully planned. From time to time Miss L. sought help from the physician in evaluating it and in understanding the relationship which was developing. She did not seek the patient's approval and actually did not receive it at first. As Miss L. worked with Bill she constantly sought to involve other people so that he was able to move forward in making more appropriate relationships in social situations and finally in high school.

TERMINATING A NURSE-PATIENT RELATIONSHIP

Much has been said and written about the importance of initiating a helping relationship with patients, and the elements of such a relationship have been analyzed in the hope of assisting nurses to accept a role in establishing a therapeutic climate for patients. Unfortunately, attention has not always been directed toward terminating such a relationship.

For many valid reasons nurses frequently leave a group of patients with whom they have worked in a psychiatric setting. This may be unfortunate if the nurse has been able to establish meaningful therapeutic relationships with them. Ideally, patients in a psychiatric setting should experience a relatively constant professional staff with whom they can establish meaningful relationships and work out emotional problems. When a nurse discovers that it is necessary for her to leave a group of patients it is important for her to share this information with them. Patients deserve to know the reason why they must lose a valued friend upon whom they have learned to depend. They will be able to accept the loss if they are told about it honestly and if they are given time to handle their feelings. The facts in the situation should be shared but not the nurse's feelings. Thus the nurse could say to a group of patients "I have just learned that I will be leaving this unit in two weeks. I am going to join the staff on Ward X. I am going to miss all of you. I am sure that we will see each other sometime at the hospital parties. Miss A. is replacing me on this unit and I hope that she will enjoy working here with you as much as I have." If the nurse is resigning for a personal reason she should share that information as honestly as possible. Whatever is told the patients should be factually true.

Patients, like all persons, will react to the loss of a valued nurse in a variety of ways depending on the characteristic way in which they respond, their unique emotional needs, and the relationship which they have developed with the departing staff member. Some patients may become depressed and unconsciously may feel that they have been responsible personally for the loss of the nurse. Other patients may not be able to accept the loss of this valued person and may repress the knowledge. The nurse may hear some of them comment that they were never told that she was leaving. Another group of patients may respond with anger and may demand that the nursing office change the transfer order.

When the nursing staff is prepared for a variety of reactions from patients, they can understand, accept, and cope with the behavior. This means that the nursing staff will need to spend time talking with the patients. They will need to make themselves more available than usual for listening to expressions of feelings about the situation. They will need to reassure patients that they are not being abandoned. Sometimes it is helpful if the patients are encouraged to channel their feelings into doing something constructive. One way of helping to redirect patients' feelings is to let them organize and carry out a party to honor the departing nurse.

The patients who have had an especially meaningful relationship with the departing nurse will need help from her in accepting the fact that she is leaving. She should help them look forward to accepting the new nurse who will come to replace her.

Sometimes patients are not given an opportunity to express feelings about such a situation or to handle these feelings. When this happens, as it does when a valued staff member simply disappears without any explanation, the feelings are not avoided but appear in many ways. A group of patients who have suffered such an unexplained loss may suddenly rebel against the entire nursing staff or the physician may find that many old symptoms that were being handled effectively by patients have been reactivated.

IMPORTANT CONCEPTS

1. The use the nurse makes of her personality is the key to her success in face-to-face relationships with patients and in directing their daily living activities.
2. In all therapeutic relationships it is necessary for the nurse to recognize the patient as a unique, important human being who, like all persons, experiences hopes, fears, joys, and sorrow and has his own special set of problems and reactions to life.
3. The quality of interaction between the nurse and the patient is closely related to the motivation that underlies her attitude toward nursing and her perception of her role as a nurse.
4. The nurse who rigidly controls the patient's environment will not be able to create a hospital climate in which the patient can achieve maximum personal, emotional, and social growth.
5. The basis of all helping relationships is acceptance that implies that the nurse treats the patient as an important person and not as a diagnostic

entity or a set of psychiatric symptoms.

6. The nurse who maintains a nonjudgmental attitude realizes that the unusual behavior of the mentally ill patient is neither good or bad nor right or wrong but an expression of emotional need.

7. Consistency in approach to patient care helps lessen patients' anxiety by simplifying decision making and by avoiding uncertainties.

8. If a relationship is to be helpful to a patient, it must assist him in reestablishing his self-confidence and restoring his self-esteem.

9. A professional relationship focuses upon the personal and emotional needs of the patient.

10. Ideally, patients in a psychiatric setting should experience a relatively constant professional staff with whom they can establish meaningful relationships and work out emotional problems.

11. Thoughtful attention should be given to terminating relationships with patients when it is necessary for the nurse to leave the unit where she has worked with them.

SUGGESTED SOURCES OF ADDITIONAL INFORMATION

Connolly, Mary Grace: What acceptance means to patients, Amer. J. Nurs. 60:1754-1757, Dec., 1960.

Bressler, Bernard, and Vause, Mary Ella: The psychotherapeutic nurse, Amer. J. Nurs. 62:87-90, May, 1962.

Hale, Shirley L., and Richardson, Julia H.: Terminating the nurse-patient relationship, Amer. J. Nurs. 63:116-119, Sept., 1963.

Hays, Joyce Samhammer: Focusing on feelings, Nurs. Outlook 10:332-333, May, 1962.

Kachelski, M. Audrey: The nurse-patient relationship, Amer. J. Nurs. 61:76-79, May, 1961.

Roberts, Dorothy I.: A psychiatrist helps them understand their patients, Amer. J. Nurs. 56:1302-1305, Oct., 1956.

Rogers, Carl R.: A counseling approach to human problems, Amer. J. Nurs. 56:994-997, Aug., 1956.

Schwartz, Morris S., and Shockley, Emmy Lanning: The nurse and the mental patient, New York, 1956, Russell Sage Foundation, pp. 218-230, 244-281.

Speroff, B. J.: Empathy is important in nursing, Nurs. Outlook, 4:326-328, June, 1956.

Therapeutic use of the self; a concept of teaching patient care, formulated by the Committee on Psychiatric Nursing of the Group for the Advancement of Psychiatry (Report No. 33), Topeka, Kansas, 1955.

CHAPTER SEVEN

The nurse makes therapeutic use of self in group situations

During World War II many members of the civilian population as well as large numbers of the Armed Forces required psychiatric help. It became obvious that the traditional treatment methods utilized at that time could not provide the help required by the large population of mentally ill individuals. To make maximum use of the psychiatrically trained personnel a plan was initiated through which patients were encouraged to talk out their problems in groups. Thus the concept of group therapy was born. As psychiatrists worked with this method and developed an effective technique that could be taught to others, it became obvious that group therapy had certain advantages for some patients that were not realized through the more traditional methods of individual therapy.

As more experience has been gained with group methods it has been recognized that group therapy has unlimited therapeutic possibilities in the treatment plan for a wide variety of individuals. It is now the treatment of choice for many patients and is frequently utilized in conjunction with individual therapy. A patient who seeks help at a Community Mental Health Center can expect to be encouraged to participate in some form of group psychotherapy.

NURSES AS GROUP THERAPISTS

As more is learned about the group approach to emotional problems, there seems to be a place for a variety of patient groups having a wide range of therapeutic goals and led by people with varied backgrounds and preparation. For several years psychiatric nurses have been actively involved in providing leadership for groups of patients in many different treatment situations. Some have chosen to function as the only therapist in the patient group. In such situations the nurse has usually had the benefit of leadership preparation before undertaking this role. However, a few nurses without previous experience or preparation have accepted the leadership role and have learned as the group worked together. In such situations it is wise for the nurse to seek supervisory guidance from a group psychotherapist in the treatment situation. Many nurses have functioned as a cotherapist with a member of another discipline. This is probably an ideal learning situation and provides an opportunity to reconstruct and evaluate the discussion after each session has been concluded. Sometimes two nurses may function as co-therapists with a group. This alliance also provides a learning opportunity when the therapy session is restructured and examined objectively.

CHARACTERISTICS OF A THERAPEUTIC GROUP

Everyone who has grown up in this society has been a member of many groups and realizes that they are almost always organized to achieve a specific goal. Thus the therapeutic group like other groups has a specific goal. It differs from a social group because its goal is to assist individuals to alter their behavior patterns and develop new and more effective ways of dealing with the stresses of daily living. To achieve this goal, individuals meet together regularly for a stated period of time to express

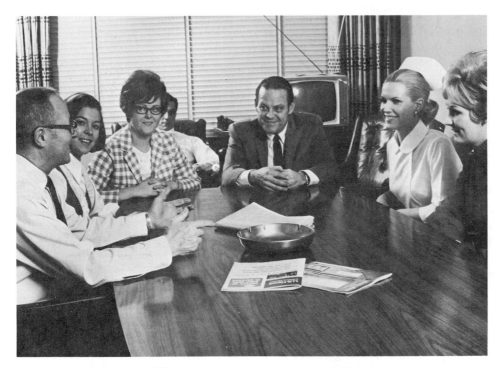

FIG. 7. *The nurse participates in group therapy.*

their ideas, feelings, and concerns; to examine their current ways of behaving; and to develop new patterns of living.

The group leader works to develop among the group members a sense of trust in her as an individual and as a group leader. She avoids being critical or judgmental of the behavior of individual members of the group and relies upon group action to control unacceptable behavior. The group leader strives to convey to the group members her acceptance of them as individuals and her respect for them as people. She avoids the appearance of controlling the situation or of being the authority in the situation.

CONSIDERATIONS IN ESTABLISHING
A THERAPEUTIC GROUP

Group psychotherapists differ in their approach to the question of selecting the ground rules when establishing a therapeutic group. Questions involving the size of the membership, the frequency of meetings and the characteristics of the participants must be decided. As might be expected, authorities answer these questions according to their personal treatment philosophies.

Some group psychotherapists insist upon a balanced group by which they mean that only individuals of the same age, sex, and diagnostic category should be included. Others do not believe that a balanced group is necessary or even conducive to the best possible group interaction. Another consideration is whether to include patients with limited intelligence quotients or verbal skills. Since group therapy depends upon effective communication skills this is an important consideration.

Certainly a decision must be made as to how large the group will be. Most authorities agree that a group should not be larger than ten but many group leaders prefer a group no larger than six. They also agree that the membership of a group should be stable.

A definite place in which to hold the group meeting must be identified. It should be quiet, comfortable, and private. The frequency and time of meeting must be decided as well as the date when group meetings will begin and end. When these decisions have been made and the group has come together for the first time, the ground rules should be shared with the members so that they will understand the nature of the contract they have with each other and with the group leader.

Many group leaders prefer to talk with potential group members before the actual group meetings begin. In this way each individual is acquainted with the nature of the sessions prior to the first meeting.

GROUP DEVELOPMENT

Every group, like every individual, progresses through several developmental phases. The first is the period of getting acquainted, during which time the members behave toward each other as strangers and are obviously distrustful of each other and the leader. This is a testing period during which the members are cautiously polite. Many groups move from the testing stage to a period of conflict and lack of unity, with hostility being directed toward individual members and the leader. Most groups move from the period of conflict into a period of sharing personal feelings and concerns about

emotional problems. This is the period in which the work of the group is achieved. During this period there is an opportunity for emotional reeducation and relearning. The members discover through the reactions of the other group members that there are many different reactions to their feelings and behavior. They come to realize how universal their problems are and that they are not as unique in their difficulties as they may have believed.

The last phase is precipitated by the approaching time for the group to conclude its meetings. Thus it is the phase of termination and may require six or eight meetings to work through the feelings of the individuals involved. During this period the members relive previous periods when they experienced the personal loss of someone very close to them. They may express feelings of being abandoned, rejected, or forsaken. The expression of these feelings provides an excellent opportunity to help the individual members of the group deal with these feelings and work through them.

ROLE OF THE LEADER

The leader is the key to a successful group therapy experience. The group leader needs to be aware of her own behavior and its effect upon others. The effectiveness of the getting acquainted period for the group is largely dependent upon the way in which the leader orients the members to the group process and to each other. The period of intragroup hostility and conflict can be successfully resolved if the group leader is able to be supportive to the members and successfully establishes a feeling of acceptance and respect. As the group moves into the working stage it is the leader who is able to involve the less verbal members by redirecting questions to them or by asking them how a situation seems to them. The leader sometimes provides essential factual information that is important in the resolution of an issue that has arisen. On occasion the leader may be useful in helping a patient learn exactly how others think about his behavior or his responses. The leader assists members in exploring situations they bring to the group from the outside and helps them to think through more appropriate ways of responding.

PSYCHODRAMA

Another type of therapeutic group experience that is sometimes provided for patients is called psychodrama. This technique was developed by J. L. Moreno, a psychiatrist, who began working with emotionally disturbed individuals in a theater in Vienna as early as 1941. Psychodrama is usually conducted by a leader who has been especially prepared to direct this type of activity. Although a variety of methods may be used, one of the more frequent techniques places the leader on a stage in front of an audience of patients and staff members. The leader identifies a situation in which interpersonal conflict is involved. He invites members of the audience to come to the stage for the purpose of acting out this human relations problem.

When members of the audience agree to accept parts in the drama, they are told the essential facts about the roles they are to play. The chosen situation frequently focuses upon a conversation with the significant members of a family. It is surprising how effectively patients and staff fill the roles to which they are assigned and how realistically feelings are expressed. The leader calls time when he believes the enactment has progressed far enough to provide the audience with a basis for a fruitful discussion.

Another method that has been used productively in psychodrama is for the leader to request a volunteer from among the audience to come forward and set up a situation that he wishes to portray. He is also asked to select individuals from the audience to play the parts required and to provide the role players with the necessary data about the roles they will enact. In some situations individuals from the audience are asked to come forward to play the roles of alter ego for the major characters in the psychodrama. This technique focuses specifically upon some personal concern of the individual who volunteered to develop a psychodramatic situation.

After the role playing is completed, the audience is given an opportunity to participate in a discussion of the situation they have witnessed and experienced vicariously. The participants from the audience may focus attention upon various aspects of the situation and frequently present similar life experiences.

Psychodrama provides patients with an opportunity to express feelings and concerns that relate to a personal human relations situation that is like, but not identical to, a personal problem of their own. Thus psychodrama has somewhat the same therapeutic effect as abreaction or the lessening of emotional trauma by re-enacting the situation. It also furnishes individuals with an opportunity for catharsis or an opportunity to freely express feelings. As in other group therapy situations, the individual is helped by the group to express feelings and consider them objectively.

The nurse is frequently involved in psychodrama as a role player or as a discussant. She will develop skill and understanding as she continues to participate in psychodrama. Eventually she may accept the role of the leader of the psychodrama sessions.

FAMILY THERAPY

A comparatively recent innovation in the area of group psychotherapy is family therapy. Three of the earliest proponents of this method were Nathan W. Ackerman at Columbia University, Gerald Caplan at Harvard University, and the late Don Jackson who worked at the University of California. Early in the 1950's these men wrote about the advantages of this method. Ackerman and Caplan continue to contribute to the literature about family therapy as they perfect their skills and develop new insights.

The basic assumption underlying family therapy is that the mentally disturbed family member is the sickest member of a sick family, having developed emotional pathology because of the negative relationships he has experienced with his family. Thus the proponents of family

therapy conceived the idea of bringing together the key members of the patient's family in a situation that might be referred to as a therapeutic confrontation. Like other group therapy situations the members of the group meet together regularly for a specific length of time and in a designated place.

The goals of family therapy are to assist in resolving pathological conflicts and anxiety, to strengthen the individual member against destructive forces both within himself and within the family environment, to strengthen the family against critical upsets, and to influence the orientation of the family identity and values toward health.*

Family therapy has become one of the most effective treatment modalities available for certain problem situations, especially in assisting disturbed adolescents to solve emotional problems. Some authorities believe that family therapy is the only effective approach to the problems of disturbed adolescents who are clearly rebelling against parental authority. It provides an opportunity for the parents and the adolescents, under the guidance of a sympathetic and knowledgable psychiatrist, psychiatric nurse, or social worker, to work together to solve the interpersonal conflicts that have developed within the family group.

Some family therapy sessions have been held in the home. As this trend develops it appears likely that the role of family therapist will become identified with the prepared psychiatric nurse, since she is comfortable in the role of family visitor,

*Ackerman, Nathan W.: Family therapy. In Arieti, Silvano, editor: American handbook of psychiatry, vol. 3, New York, 1966, Basic Books, Inc., Publishers, p. 210.

is knowledgable about family dynamics, and is skillful in group therapy.

STRUCTURED GROUP ACTIVITY

Psychiatric hospitals are frequently heavily populated with patients who appear to have lost interest in reality, to have lost a sense of personal value, and who seem to be unaware of the other patients with whom they come in daily contact. Group interaction is one of the most successful ways of stimulating these people and of rekindling their interest in their surroundings.

The nurse may be the only professional worker who is available or interested in developing some form of group experience that will encourage these patients to begin to communicate with each other and with the hospital staff. The goals of these group activities are chiefly social and recreational. If a few patients come together as a group and carry on an activity for a few sessions, the initial attempt has been successful.

The focus of the group activity depends almost entirely upon the individuals who are to be included as members. Their age, educational backgrounds, and physical health will greatly influence the choice of activities that can be suggested.

Some patients might be interested in a current events discussion group. Others who evidence no interest in reading the newspaper or listening to the television news reports would not be interested in such a group activity. Some patients might be interested in forming a poetry reading group, whereas others would abhor such an activity. Some women might enjoy sewing or knitting while they visit

together. Other women would frown on this suggestion.

In view of this wide variation in personal abilities and taste, the first rule to follow in initiating any recreational or motivational activity is to be well acquainted with the individuals who will form the group membership. The nurse will find that it is wise to encourage the members to participate in selecting the focus for the group meetings. The wise group leader will formulate some tentative plans for the first meeting but these need to be flexible and easily changed in case there are suggestions from the members.

The nurse leader will find that at first many patients will be reluctant to participate. Some individuals may require more than one friendly invitation to attend. Some patients who have lost interest in reality carry on an active phantasy life. Any group activity must compete with these phantasies for the patient's attention and enjoyment. Thus it is wise to offer patients something tangible such as refreshments during the initial group meetings. As the group becomes cohesive the members may assume responsibility for refreshments or their interest in the group activity may become great enough to overshadow the food as the major enjoyment of the meeting.

It is wise to vary the focus of the group activity from time to time in order to maintain the interest of the group members. As the members become acquainted with one another they themselves will suggest changes in the focus or the format of the meeting.

The following are some concrete sug-

73

gestions for planning an effective group experience:[*]

1. Develop a flexible plan that provides for change and spontaneity.
2. Encourage all group members to participate in the planning.
3. Keep the plan practical and within achievable limits.
4. Initiate activities that are within the abilities of the group members to handle.
5. Provide something specific such as refreshments that will give each group member some tangible satisfaction.
6. Avoid monotony by varying the focus of the group activity.
7. Maintain a consistency in the feeling tone of each meeting so that the expectations of the group members will be fulfilled.

IMPORTANT CONCEPTS

1. During World War II it became obvious that the traditional treatment methods utilized at that time could not provide the help required by the large population of mentally ill individuals among the armed forces as well as the civilian population.
2. The group method of treating people in need of psychiatric help was originally developed to make maximum use of the available psychiatrically trained personnel.
3. As psychiatrists worked with the group method of treatment it became obvious that group therapy had certain advantages over the traditional methods of individual therapy, and now it is recognized as having unlimited therapeutic possibilities.
4. There appears to be a place in the treatment plan for a variety of groups having a wide range of therapeutic goals and led by individuals with varied backgrounds and preparation.
5. For many years psychiatric nurses have been involved in providing group leadership for a variety of groups in many different teratment situations.
6. The therapeutic group has as its goal the alteration of the behavior patterns of the group members through the development of new and more effective ways of coping with stressful situations.
7. The group leader strives to develop among the members of the group a sense of trust in him and in each other.
8. Before the group meetings are initiated, decisions must be made about the size of the membership, the frequency of the meetings, the place and time of meetings, and the characteristics of the members.
9. Each group progresses through several developmental phases including the phase of getting acquainted, the phase of intragroup conflict, the period of mutual trust and sharing, and the period of termination.
10. Psychodrama provides an opportunity to express feelings and concerns about a human relations situation that is like, but not identical to, a personal problem and has

[*]Adapted from Brown, Martha, and Fowler, Grace R.: Psychodynamic nursing—a biosocial orientation, ed. 3, Philadelphia, 1966, W. B. Saunders Co., pp. 307-308.

an effect something like abreaction.
11. A basic assumption underlying family therapy is that the mentally disturbed family member is the sickest member of a sick family.
12. The goals of family therapy are to resolve pathologic conflicts and anxieties, to strengthen the individual member against destructive forces, to strengthen the family against critical upsets, and to influence the family orientation toward the values of health.
13. Family therapy is thought by some

to be the treatment of choice for disturbed adolescents.
14. Group interaction is one of the most successful ways of stimulating patients who have lost interest in their surroundings.
15. In view of the wide variation in personal abilities and tastes the first rule to follow in initiating any recreational or motivational activity is to be well acquainted with the individuals who will form the group membership.

SUGGESTED SOURCES OF ADDITIONAL INFORMATION

Ackerman, Nathan N.: Family therapy. In Arieti, Silvano, editor: American handbook of psychiatry, vol. 3, New York, 1966, Basic Books Inc., Publishers, pp. 201-212.

Armstrong, Shirley W., and Rouslin, Sheela: Group psychotherapy in nursing practice, New York, 1963, The Macmillan Co.

Baker, Joan M., and Estes, Nada J.: Anger in group therapy, Amer. J. Nurs. 65:96-100, July, 1965.

Brandes, Norman S.: Group psychotherapy in the treatment of emotional disturbance, Ment. Hyg. 53:105-109, Jan., 1969.

Brown, Donald I.: Nurses participate in group therapy, Amer. J. Nurs. 62:68-69, Jan., 1962.

Bueker, Kathleen: Group therapy in a new setting, Amer. J. Nurs. 57:1581-1588, Dec., 1957.

Bueker, Kathleen, and Warrick, Annette: Can nurses be group therapists? Amer. J. Nurs. 64:114-116, May, 1964.

Eddy, Frances L., O'Neill, Elaine, and Astrachan, Boris M.: Group work on a long-term treatment service, Perspect. Psychiat. Care 6:9-15, 1968.

Fagin, Claire M.: Psychotherapeutic nursing, Amer. J. Nurs. 67:298-304, Feb., 1967.

Gerrish, Madalene J.: The family therapist is a nurse, Amer. J. Nurs. 68:320-323, Feb., 1968.

Getty, Cathleen, and Shannon, Anna M.: Nurses as co-therapists in a family-therapy setting, Perspect. Psychiat. Care 5:36-48, 1967.

Glover, B. H.: A new nurse therapist, Amer. J. Nurs. 67:1003-1005, May, 1967.

Hargreaves, Anne G.: The group culture and nursing practice, Amer. J. Nurs. 67:1840-1846, Sept., 1967.

Kardener, Sheldon H.: The family: structure, patterns, and therapy, Ment. Hyg. 52:524-531, Oct., 1968.

Lego, Suzanne: Five functions of the group therapist—twenty sessions later, Amer. J. Nurs. 66:795-797, April, 1966.

Martinez, Ruth E.: The nurse as a group psychotherapist, Amer. J. Nurs. 58:1681-1682, Dec., 1958.

Pullinger, Walter F.: Remotivation, Amer. J. Nurs. 60:682-685, May, 1960.

Rohde, Ildaura Murillo: The nurse as a family therapist, Nurs. Outlook 16:49-52, May, 1968.

Schuurmans, Madelyn J.: Five functions of a group therapist, Amer. J. Nurs. 64:108-110, Dec., 1964.

Sink, Susan Mary: Remotivation: toward reality for the aged, Nurs. Outlook 14:26-28, Aug., 1966.

Stevens, Leonard F.: Nurse-patient discussion groups, Amer. J. Nurs. 63:67-69, Dec., 1963.

von Mering, Otto, and King, Stanley H.: Remotivating the mental patient, New York, 1957, Russell Sage Foundation.

Yalom, Irvin D., and Terrazas, Florence: Group therapy for psychotic elderly patients, Amer. J. Nurs. 68:1690-1694, Aug., 1968.

CHAPTER EIGHT

Utilizing the social milieu therapeutically

Since 1955 an impressive group of articles devoted to improving the care of mentally ill patients through the development of a therapeutic environment has appeared in the *American Journal of Nursing* and *Nursing Outlook*. Although the titles of the articles differ, all of them focus upon the therapeutic potential of the hospital experience. These articles reflect a national concern for increasing the therapeutic potential of hospitalization for mentally ill patients.

For many years the professional staffs of hospitals encouraged the belief that any actual therapeutic result in patient improvement was achieved by the efforts of the physician. As a result of this attitude nurses demonstrated a reluctance to accept responsibility for developing therapeutic relationships with patients or to accept credit for positive changes in patient behavior. Today, many physicians believe that a variety of people can provide therapeutic help for mentally ill patients. The time has come when the nursing staff must assume its share of the responsibility for providing the therapeutic experiences in living that are necessary for patients who need to achieve more mature patterns of behavior. It is interesting to note that this is not an entirely new or untried idea even in public psychiatric hospitals in the United States.

HISTORICAL BACKGROUND OF THE THERAPEUTIC ENVIRONMENT

The historical archives of American psychiatry include records of early, successful attempts to develop a homelike atmosphere for mentally ill patients with provision for social and recreational ac-

tivities. Doctors and their families joined other staff members in initiating and directing some of these activities. Early in the nineteenth century emphasis on a homelike environment, recreational activities, and a sympathetic approach to patients was referred to as moral treatment. In 1842, Boston State Hospital was reported to have placed emphasis upon moral treatment for mentally ill patients. At about the same time a similar approach was being carried out in Worcester, Massachusetts, at the public psychiatric hospital there. The superintendent of one psychiatric hospital in Massachusetts is reported to have taken Sunday dinner at the same table with patients. Intimate discussions of the patient's personal problems and difficulties were part of the therapy offered in those institutions at that time.

Some authorities believe that the era of moral treatment for the mentally ill ceased to exist as a direct result of the large numbers of immigrants who arrived in the United States after the Civil War. Many of these people could not cope with the problems of adjustment presented by the radically different environment they found in this country. Some could not accept the loss of the close family ties that existed in the European villages from which they came. Many immigrants reacted to these social and personal deprivations with such unusual behavior that institutionalization was necessary. When the patient population in mental institutions began to increase rapidly, the patients were no longer culturally homogeneous. Many of them did not speak English. Developing a homelike environment for people from such different backgrounds was difficult. The nation became preoccupied with the task of national growth and expansion. For reasons that are not entirely clear, the era of moral treatment for mentally ill persons passed. By 1940 our large public hospitals were filled to overflowing. Few patients recovered sufficiently to return to the community. Because of the ever increasing patient population the task of the hospital personnel was staggering. They were able to do little more than keep the patients bathed, dressed, and fed.

When the nation had time to evaluate national needs after World War II, attention became focused upon improving the care of mentally ill patients. Since 1945 many new approaches to care and treatment have been proposed. Among these was the old, partially forgotten idea that the hospital environment could provide therapeutic experiences for patients.

INFLUENCE OF PHYSICAL ENVIRONMENT UPON THE THERAPEUTIC CLIMATE

A therapeutic climate for mentally ill patients is dependent on the attitude of the staff toward mental illness and the needs of the patients and does not develop as the result of any fixed type of hospital architecture. It can be developed in any type of hospital if the staff focuses upon meeting the needs of patients. However, it is helpful if certain structural features are present. The needs of individual patients can be met more effectively if provisions for privacy, socialization, and planned activities are available. If such facilities are not already present in the unit where patients are to be housed,

some innovations must be introduced if a therapeutic environment is to be achieved. The goals of a therapeutic environment are to help the patient develop a sense of self-esteem and personal worth, to improve his ability to relate to others, to help him learn to trust others, and to return him to the community better prepared to resume his role in living and working.

If a patient's self-esteem is to be elevated, it is essential to provide an opportunity for privacy and a place where his personal belongings can be kept. In most situations a substitute has been found for the barracklike dormitories and public showers with which many large psychiatric hospitals were once equipped. The mass approach to the care of human beings destroys self-esteem and the sense of individual worth. The key to a therapeutic environment is provision for the unique needs of individual patients rather than dealing with patients as members of a crowd. The idea that nothing should be arranged for one patient unless it could be arranged for the group of patients has led many hospital staffs in the past away from treating people as individuals. This attitude sometimes increased the patient's difficulties rather than providing opportunities for him to solve problems.

If patients are to receive individualized care and if the environment is to be therapeutic, living quarters must be as attractive and inviting as modern college dormitories. In most instances no more than two or three patients should share the same room. If possible, single rooms should be provided for patients who have strong feelings about sharing a room with another person. Clothes closets and dressers or sastifactory substitutes for this equipment must be available. It is important for mentally ill patients to bring personal clothing and other equipment to the hospital to that they can be attractively and appropriately groomed. The use of hospital clothing may be necessary in isolated instances, but in the past this practice contributed to depersonalization of the patient population and reduced them to a group of human beings with a universal attitude of hopelessness. Because it is therapeutic for patients to assume responsibility for their personal cleanliness, laundry facilities should be available. This is particularly true on units where female patients are housed.

Dining room facilities are important in developing a therapeutic environment. Mealtime should be a leasurely experience and a time for sharing ideas and reinforcing friendly relationships. It is not merely a time for the intake of food. The nurses can profitably assume a therapeutic role by serving as hostesses at small tables that seat groups of four to six patients. The role of hostess is more effective if the nurse shares the meal with patients. This plan has been used successfully in some hospitals. As a hostess the nurse can encourage conversation and can help make mealtime a happy, relaxed, rewarding group experience. Such mealtime experiences cannot be initiated unless there is a dining room attached to the unit itself. Serving meals in large, noisy dining rooms where hundreds of patients are fed achieves the purpose of getting food to patients but negates the accomplishment of other therapeutic goals.

Bathrooms should provide privacy. Although locks on doors may not be advisable, it is possible to provide toilet doors that close and shower rooms that are equipped with screens. The old habit of showering ten or fifteen patients at one time contributed to reducing the patient to a member of a crowd and negated other attempts to help him feel like a respected human being. The therapeutic environment can develop most effectively when the physical surroundings lend themselves to helping patients feel that they are respected and their personal preferences are recognized, appreciated, and considered.

THE EMOTIONAL CLIMATE ESSENTIAL TO A THERAPEUTIC ENVIRONMENT

The physical environment of the hospital is vitally important in developing a situation in which the individual patient can feel comfortable and safe and in which he can develop more effective ways of coping with stress. Even more important in helping patients achieve the goal of improved emotional health is the interpersonal climate present in the unit where the patient is to live during his hospital stay. This climate is largely the responsibility of the nursing staff who are assigned to the unit.

Like all people who embark upon a new experience, patients need to be helped to become familiar with the hospital situation and to learn what the staff expects of them. One step toward helping newly admitted patients feel welcome and accepted is to provide a plan for introducing them to the physical surroundings, to the members of the nursing staff, and to the other patients. A plan of orientation for each patient will be helpful in encouraging a feeling of being accepted in the new environment.

Since a new environment is apt to be frightening to emotionally ill patients, a sensitive nursing staff will strive to develop a climate that encourages the patients to feel that the hospital is a safe place that will protect them from the dangers in the outside world. Some patients want and need reassurance that the hospital will protect them from their own impulses to injure themselves or others.

Providing safety for a patient includes safeguarding him against making significant decisions when he is not well enough to do so. Thus the nursing staff may find it necessary to help the patient avoid making legal decisions about a pending divorce or separation, about the sale of property or other financial matters, or about the choice of a school for his children.

The therapeutic emotional climate in a hospital is established by a nursing staff that is friendly, sensitive, and concerned about the welfare of the patients. Such a nursing staff is aware of the patient's individual rights and needs. They respect him as a worthwhile, important human being, even though his behavior may sometimes be unacceptable when judged by their personal standards.

A nursing staff striving to develop a therapeutic environment establishes as few rules and regulations as possible for patient behavior and restricts patient activity only when necessary.

Opportunities for freedom of choice are provided. As the patient demonstrates his ability to accept more responsibility for his behavior, opportunities for making choices are increased.

It is expected that as the patient's emotional health improves he will experiment with new mechanisms of adjustment and develop new ways of responding to others and of coping with stress. Some of these new methods of dealing with problems may not be appropriate. The patient will require encouragement to continue testing new patterns of behavior until he has achieved a more mature way of relating to other people.

The nursing staff fulfills a key role in providing the warmth, friendliness, acceptance, and optimism essential to the development of a therapeutic emotional climate.

The following characteristics of a therapeutic environment are adapted from Brown and Fowler*:

1. The patient is familiar with the situation and what is expected of him.
2. The patient feels comfortable in the situation and is free from a fear of danger.
3. Provision is made to meet the patient's immediate physical needs.
4. Provision is made for the patient to have clean surroundings and to be cared for with clean equipment.
5. The environment provides the patient with optimum safety from injury to his person from his own impulses or from the impulses of others, from anxieties related to his former environment, and from de-

---

*Brown, Martha M., and Fowler, Grace R.: Psychodynamic nursing—a biosocial orientation. ed. 3, Philadelphia, 1966, W. B. Saunders Co., pp. 295-297.

cisions beyond his current level of responsibility.

6. The personnel in the environment respect him as an individual, recognize his rights, needs, and opinions and accept his behavior as an expression of his needs.
7. The environment provides for a limited number of restrictions and for opportunities for freedom of choice.
8. The environment provides a testing ground for the establishment of new patterns of behavior.

SETTING LIMITS IN A THERAPEUTIC ENVIRONMENT

Words such as acceptance and permissiveness confuse some inexperienced professional workers and may encourage them to function in a psychiatric setting as if anything is allowed as far as patient behavior is concerned. Nothing could be further from the truth, and such an attitude is actually detrimental to patients who by their sick behavior may be asking for controls. Acceptance means that the hospital staff assumes an emotionally neutral attitude toward individual behavior and refrains from placing a judgmental label on it. It further means that the behavior is recognized as an expression of the patient's needs. Permissiveness refers to the prevailing attitude in psychiatric settings that allows a patient to behave as he needs to behave within limits of safety. It also allows a patient to experiment with new ways of behaving as he progresses toward more successful and satisfying behavior patterns. The staff cannot allow a patient to injure himself or others or to engage in behavior that will be le-

gally or morally detrimental to himself or others. When a patient's behavior cannot be permitted, the nurse should frankly tell the patient that the behavior cannot be allowed and should give him a logical reason for this decision.

Setting limits frequently becomes the responsibility of the nurse, although the psychiatric team usually makes the initial decision concerning the limit to be established. Certainly the nurse would be wise to seek an opportunity to discuss the setting of limits with other professional colleagues when such responsibility is entirely up to her. She will want to be certain that she is not imposing her own personal standards upon patients. If a form of patient government is operating, much of the limit setting can be established by this group.

An example of a limit frequently established in psychiatric settings is the requirement that all patients report for breakfast fully dressed and ready for the activities of the day. Usually this requirement is made because some mentally ill patients seem to prefer to stay up most of the night and remain in bed most of the day. This habit can help the patient avoid participating in most activities of the day and relieve him of the need to relate to people. If the patient is required to be up and dressed for breakfast he is then available to participate in group activities. This rule also requires the patient to establish some kind of living pattern that involves getting to bed at a reasonable hour in the evening. Some authorities argue that many well persons enjoy sleeping until noon and that they often skip breakfast. It seems reasonable to allow some patients to decide when they will retire and arise and what morning activities they will become involved in, including breakfast. It is apparent that before any rule that regulates patient activity is established all aspects of the result of such action should be considered, including the problem of enforcing the rule once it is enunciated. Consideration should be given to the way in which a rule assists or impedes the growth of mature attitudes on the part of patients.

The populations of modern psychiatric units are likely to include both men and women. This immediately calls for some limit setting concerning the relationship between men and women. Since sexual behavior is often a problem area for many mentally ill patients, they may feel much more comfortable if fairly specific limits are established for their going and coming on the unit where they are to live. The question essentially involves the limits that would be the most helpful to men and women who are fearful of each other but who should be helped to establish more mature behavior patterns in relation to the opposite sex.

The nurse can easily confuse limit setting with control of behavior. She may rationalize that many of the unnecessary controls that may have been imposed are limits placed on the situation for safety and security of patients. Sometimes unnecessary controls are placed on patient behavior because of one unfortunate incident. For instance, one psychiatric hospital refused to allow patients to go walking because several years earlier one male patient attacked a nurse with whom he was walking. The responsibility for setting limits should not be assumed by one individual until the proposed move has been discussed with other people and all possible alternatives have been explored.

THE NURSE'S ROLE IN A THERAPEUTIC ENVIRONMENT

It is not possible to develop a therapeutic environment without the strong, intelligent leadership of a nurse or, as reported in *The Therapeutic Community,* a strong leader acting in the role of the nurse.

When many of the traditional rules and regulations of the psychiatric hospital are discarded and the unit becomes a place that focuses upon meeting the needs of the individual and the group, the nurse is forced to accept a more active therapeutic role with patients. She finds it necessary to assign the clerical work, which formerly kept her confined to the nurse's station, to a ward secretary in order to free herself to give leadership to the personnel as they participate with patients in all the planned activities. Patients require mature help and guidance in initiating and carrying out social activities.

Patients will make use of the nurse as an understanding person with whom they can discuss the daily problems and emotional stresses that develop when they begin to experiment with new ways of behaving. The nurse needs to be more alert than ever to changes in patient behavior. In a therapeutic environment many of the traditional safeguards are removed, and therefore safety of patients depends more than ever upon an alert nursing staff. Thus it becomes the responsibility of the nurse to recognize changes in mood and behavior of patients and to intervene at appropriate times.

Skill in understanding group behavior and in directing groups is essential in the therapeutic environment. The nurse needs to work actively with patient government to solve many ward problems. Finally, active, functioning channels of communication are essential. The nurse's relationships as the leader of the nursing staff will be reflected in the total effectiveness of the psychiatric team and ultimately in the therapeutic climate of the psychiatric unit. To a large extent the effectiveness of the patient's total hospital experience will depend on the level of professional leadership provided by the head nurse.

HISTORICAL BACKGROUND OF THE THERAPEUTIC COMMUNITY

In 1953 a small book by Dr. Maxwell Jones entitled *Social Psychiatry* was published in England. It has been one of the motivating forces in the movement in the United States to utilize the hospital environment therapeutically in the treatment regimen of mentally ill patients. When Dr. Jones' book was published in this country, the title was changed to *The Therapeutic Community*. It is essentially a report of efforts at Belmont Hospital in England during and after World War II to rehabilitate neurotic patients through the use of group methods. That experience in group living at Belmont Hospital came to be known as the therapeutic community, and thus this name was applied to the report. Particular attention was paid to the development of the social structure of the hospital and to communication between patients and the hospital staff. Dr. Jones dedicated his book to "The Nursing Staff who have formed a framework around which our therapeutic communities have been built." Although the nurses to whom he referred were not registered nurses, they were intelligent, capable, mature women who utilized the interpersonal skill and understanding required in psychiatric nursing. The dedication is appropriate. Without a nursing staff with insight, understanding, personal warmth, and skill in directing groups, the concept of a therapeutic community could not have developed into a reality.

THEORETICAL CONSIDERATIONS UNDERLYING THE THERAPEUTIC COMMUNITY

The therapeutic community is a contemporary approach to the care of mentally ill patients through group activity. It is an attempt to introduce democracy into the hospital setting. The therapeutic community strives to involve patients in their own therapy, to restore self-confidence by providing an opportunity for decision making, and to focus the patient's attention and concern away from self and toward the needs of others. It has been organized somewhat differently in different settings. Sometimes the principles of the therapeutic community are utilized throughout the hospital, and in other situations it may be limited to one or two units where the patients are almost ready to be discharged.

One important aspect of a democratic situation is that the people who are to be influenced by a decision are involved in making the decision. Until recently, administrators and professional staffs of hospitals have taken the position that persons who require hospital care are incapable of making wise judgments and therefore must have all decisions made for them. Patients in most hospitals have been reduced to a dependent state when this philosophy was implemented. Recently there has been a growing realization that forcing an adult person into such a dependent role is not usually necessary and is not therapeutic. Of course, there are some completely dependent patients for whom all decisions must be made. This is obviously true of acutely ill or unconscious patients. However, in spite of the reason for hospitalization, a majority of adult patients are able to make valid decisions about many things involving their welfare. Forcing the dependent role upon some mentally ill patients may be particularly unfortunate. Some of these patients have spent a lifetime struggling against an unconscious desire to accept a dependent role. When hospitalization forces this role upon such an individual, he may never be able to relinquish it.

Today there is a growing belief that a therapeutic environment for mentally ill patients should provide an opportunity for the patients to participate in the formulation of hospital rules and regulations that affect their personal liberties. Following through with such a plan means that patients would be involved in formulating rules and regulations about policies that regulate smoking on the ward, bedtime, late night privileges, weekend passes, social activities, control of the radio, television, and piano, check-in time when returning to the hospital from a

weekend, reporting for meals, and the many other aspects of personal life that are influenced by rules in the usual psychiatric hospital. Also, it is thought to be therapeutic to involve patients in making decisions about patient behavior and relationships among the ward population. Thus patients in a therapeutic community might be given responsibility for rendering a judgment about the infringement of ward rules, settling arguments between patients, judging the appropriateness of granting weekend privileges for certain members of the group, and many other decisions regarding the regulation of life on the ward.

Careful preparation of both the hospital staff and the patients should be assured before a therapeutic community is initiated. The hospital staff may have a good deal of difficulty accepting the activities and responsibilities granted to patients. Before a therapeutic community is initiated, a thorough exploration of the implications of such an undertaking should be carried on through group discussions. All levels of hospital workers from physicians to attendants, kitchen helpers, and cleaning people should be involved in these group discussions because all will be affected by this new activity. All members of the staff need to have a thorough understanding of the goals and limitations of the undertaking. Patients in the units where the new philosophy is to be initiated should also have an opportunity to explore its implications through group discussions. These discussions should be directed by the physicians and nurses who will be directly involved in the future activities of the new organization. Both patients and hospital staff

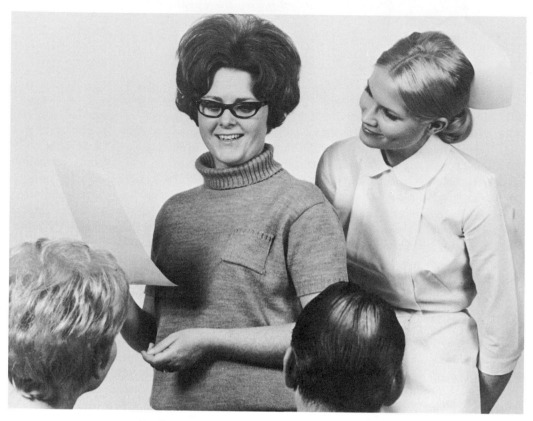

FIG. 8. *The nurse participates in patient government.*

need to understand what responsibilities they can and cannot assume.

Active administrative sanction, acceptance, and interest are essential if the therapeutic community is to be successful. Involving patients in decision making represents a drastic change in the entire administrative philosophy of many hospitals. The therapeutic community cannot be expected to function smoothly at all times, and problems will undoubtedly arise. Decisions made by patients will not always be correct or sound. Unless the entire hospital staff believes that involving patients in decision making is therapeutically valuable and worth the struggle, dissenting forces may destroy the undertaking.

Meetings of the therapeutic community should be held regularly and at specific times if they are to be effective. Meetings should not be allowed to deteriorate into a complaint bureau or to focus entirely upon what the hospital should do for patients. This can be avoided if the group has some real responsibility for solving problems relating to patients' needs.

Recently the members of a therapeutic community in a small unit of a large New York psychiatric hospital held a meeting to consider the problem of three suicide attempts that one young woman on the unit had made in one week. Their decision was to institute a buddy system so that she would be accompanied at all times by one of a group of patients, each of whom would be assigned to spend a specific amount of time with her daily. Several weeks after this decision was made the system was working well, and the patient had made no further suicide attempts. At this same meeting other problems considered were the problem of a patient who did not return on time from a weekend holiday, a fight between two patients, and the request of a new patient for a weekend pass.

It is far easier for the hospital staff to make all decisions for patients, but there is little that is therapeutic in this procedure. When patients have the opportunity to make decisions about their own and other people's behavior, they are presented with a realistic learning opportunity.

SIGNIFICANT ASPECTS OF A
THERAPEUTIC COMMUNITY[*]

1. The emphasis in a therapeutic community is placed upon social and group interaction, with both individual patients and staff being important members of the community.
2. The goal of the therapeutic community is to provide a favorable climate in which patients can gain an awareness of their feelings, thoughts, impulses, and behavior; try new interpersonal skills in a relatively safe environment; increase personal self-esteem; and realistically appraise the potentially helpful and destructive aspects of their behavior.
3. The work of the therapeutic community and the maintenance of an open

network of communication is achieved through a daily meeting attended by all staff members and all patients who work and live on the specific unit.
4. A successful therapeutic community requires that both staff and individual patients become fully aware of their roles, limitations, responsibilities, and authority.
5. Staff members in a therapeutic community make information openly available to patients with whom they share treatment responsibilities.
6. The treatment arena in the therapeutic community includes all relationships among the members of the community, with special attention being given to the network of communication between members.

IMPORTANT CONCEPTS

1. The nursing staffs in psychiatric institutions need to assume their share of the responsibility for providing therapeutic experiences in living for patients.
2. For reasons that are not entirely clear, the era of moral treatment for mentally ill patients, which was developed about 1840 and which emphasized a homelike atmosphere and sympathetic treatment, disappeared after the Civil War.
3. After the end of World War II the nation focused attention upon improving the care and treatment of mentally ill persons.
4. *The Therapeutic Community* by Dr.

---

[*]Data from Kraft, Allan M.: The therapeutic community. In Arieti, Silvano, editor: American handbook of psychiatry, vol. 3, New York, 1966, Basic Books, Inc., Publishers, pp. 544-547.

Maxwell Jones, published in England in 1953, has been a motivating force in the United States in focusing attention upon the contribution that a therapeutic hospital environment can make to care and treatment of mentally ill patients.

5. A therapeutic climate for mentally ill patients is dependent on the attitude of the staff toward mental illness and toward the needs of the patients and does not develop as the result of any fixed type of hospital architecture. However, it is helpful if certain structural features are present.

6. The goal of a therapeutic environment is to help the patient develop a sense of self-esteem and personal worth, to improve his ability to relate to others, to help him learn to trust others, and to return him to the community better prepared to resume his role in living and working.

7. The key to a therapeutic environment is to provide for the unique needs of individual patients rather than to deal with patients as members of a crowd.

8. The therapeutic community is a contemporary approach to the care of mentally ill patients through the sharing of treatment responsibility by patients and staff.

9. One important aspect of a democratic situation is that the people who are to be influenced by a decision are involved in making the decision.

10. In spite of the reason for hospitalization, the majority of adult patients are able to make valid decisions about many things concerning their welfare and should be provided with opportunities to do so.

11. Both patients and members of the hospital staff need to understand what responsibilities are involved in initiating a therapeutic environment.

12. Active administrative sanction, acceptance, and interest are essential to achieving a successful therapeutic community.

13. Limit setting frequently becomes the responsibility of the nurse, although decisions about what limits need to be established are usually made by group decision at meetings of the therapeutic community.

14. The work of the therapeutic community and the maintenance of an open network of communication is achieved in a daily community meeting attended by all staff and all patients who live and work on the specific unit.

15. The nurse can easily confuse limit setting with control of patient behavior.

16. It is not possible to develop a therapeutic environment without the strong, intelligent leadership of a nurse or some capable person who assumes the role of the nurse.

17. In a therapeutic environment the nurse will find it necessary to free herself from clerical work in order to give leadership to the ward personnel as they participate with patients in planned activities.

18. To a large extent the therapeutic effectiveness of the patient's hospital experience will depend on the level of professional leadership provided by the nurse.

SUGGESTED SOURCES OF ADDITIONAL INFORMATION

Bennett, Leland R.: A therapeutic community, Nurs. Outlook 9:423-425, July, 1961.

Bressler, Bernard, and Vause, Mary Ella: The psychotherapeutic nurse, Amer. J. Nurs. 62:87-90, May, 1962.

Briggs, Dennie Lynn: Social psychiatry in Great Britain, Amer. J. Nurs. 59:215-221, Feb., 1959.

Carleton, Estella I., and Johnson, Joan Canatsy: A therapeutic milieu for borderline patients, Amer. J. Nurs. 61:64-67, Jan., 1961.

Findley, Annie P.: They're learning to live again, Amer. J. Nurs. 61:84-86, June, 1961.

Greenblatt, M., York, R. H., and Brown, I. L.: From custodial to therapeutic patient care in mental hospitals, New York, 1955, Russell Sage Foundation.

Irvine, LaVerne F., and Deery, S. Joel: An investigation of problem areas relating to the therapeutic community concept, Ment. Hyg. 45:367-373, 1961.

Jones, Maxwell: The therapeutic community, New York, 1953, Basic Books, Inc., Publishers.

Lamb, Josephine T.: Freedom for patients in mental hospitals, Amer. J. Nurs. 58:358-360, March, 1958.

McCabe, Gracia S.: Cultural influences on patient behavior, Amer. J. Nurs. 60:1101-1104, Aug., 1960.

Ruhlman, Rose G., and Ishiyoma, Toaru: Remedy for the forgotten back ward, Amer. J. Nurs. 64:109-111, July, 1964.

Sabshin, Melvin: Nurse-doctor-patient relationships in psychiatry, Amer. J. Nurs. 57:188-192, Feb., 1957.

Sawatzky, Gordon, and Hardin, Harry T.: Making the most of the patient's ego assets, Nurs. Outlook 9:694-696, Nov., 1961.

Schaefer, Aileen: Participants—not patients, Amer. J. Nurs. 65:94-95, Feb., 1965.

Siegel, Nathaniel H.: What is a therapeutic community? Nurs. Outlook 12:49-51, May, 1964.

Simpson, George, and Kline, Nathan S.: A new type psychiatric ward, Amer. J. Psychiat. 119:511-514, Dec., 1962.

Stevens, Leonard F.: What makes a ward climate therapeutic? Amer. J. Nurs. 61:95-96, March, 1961.

von Mering, Otto: Beyond the legend of chronicity, Nurs. Outlook 6:290-293, May, 1958.

SECTION THREE
The nurse focuses on understanding her patients

CHAPTER NINE

Mental health and the cause and prevention of mental illness

On few topics is there so little exact information available as there is on mental health and the cause and prevention of mental illness. Completely satisfactory definitions of mental health and mental illness still remain undeveloped. To a large extent these concepts are culturally determined and are defined differently in different parts of the world. Behavior that might be characterized as abnormal or mentally sick behavior in one culture may be accepted and encouraged in another culture. For example, men who sit most of the day staring at the sun might be considered mentally ill in the United States, but in India they are considered to be holy and are provided for through the benevolence of the community.

Mental illness is a complex problem. It is thought to be a unique response involving an individual's personality as it interacts with his environment at a time when he is particularly vulnerable to stress. Early repetitive, negative interpersonal relationships within the family situation apparently influence the future emotional health of an individual in many unfortunate ways. Human beings who have experienced interpersonal stresses in early life are apparently more vulnerable during adolescence, the menopause, and old age than are individuals who have developed a basic sense of trust and security during the preverbal age period.

PERSONALITY ATTRIBUTES OF THE MENTALLY HEALTHY INDIVIDUAL

Although it is impossible to provide the reader with a definition of mental health that would be universally acceptable to all authorities in all cultures, it is possible to discuss the attributes usually identified as being present in the personality structures of those who appear to have successfully mastered their environments. The ability to cope with the recurrent stresses of living and achieve a relatively effective adjustment is referred to as mental maturity by many authorities, emotional maturity by others, and mental health by some.

Mental health is closely related to physical health because the body is a unified, integrated whole. The dichotomy of body and mind has persisted much too long among some groups because the cause and effect relationship between the two is not always demonstrable in specific medical terms.

Currently, different medical standards exist for evaluating mental health and physical health. Those applied to mental health are in terms of personality attributes, adjustment to stress, interpersonal capacities, and the ability to cope with reality. Evaluations in these terms are of necessity complex and imprecise. In contrast, much of the evaluation of physical health can be done in terms of precise measurement in the areas of weight, blood pressure, biochemical content of the blood, urine analysis, and so on.

Few people can be said to have achieved complete mental health or emotional maturity. Thus it is probably more helpful to evaluate the individual in terms of relative strengths or limitations in relation to the social norms and values existing in the community in which the individual lives. Because mentally ill people demonstrate some strengths as well as some limitations, it can be seen that the line of demarcation between mental health and mental illness is sometimes difficult to describe and is sharply defined in only a limited number of individuals. It also becomes clear that one can speak accurately of working with the healthy aspects of the personality.

Most authorities agree that one of the major attributes of the mentally healthy or emotionally mature individual is the capacity to love and to be loved in return. This capacity is usually thought to embrace the ability to establish a satisfying heterosexual love relationship and the ability to carry through this relationship to its usual eventual conclusion of marriage and the establishment of a safe home environment for the nurturing of children. It follows that the establishment of a home and the nurturing of children require the capacity to effectively cope with a work situation.

The ability to love and be loved also includes the many appropriate levels of love shared by the individual with parents, siblings, friends, and other individuals with whom he is involved. It is described by some authorities as adequacy in interpersonal relations.

The individual's level of self-acceptance and the way he perceives reality are usually mentioned as two other capacities significant in the development of mental maturity. These capacities involve how effectively the individual has learned to accept his own limitations and abilities. In other words, the capacity to live comfortably with ones' self is considered to be an important attribute. The way the individual perceives the world around him is equally important, since he copes with it in terms of his perceptions. Thus if the individual's view of the environment leads him to perceive it as a dangerous, hostile, threatening world, he will probably display attacking, suspicious, cautious behavior. On the other hand, if the individual accepts the world as a friendly, interesting, rewarding place in which to live, his method of coping with reality will be more acceptable, at least in this culture. Self-acceptance and the individual's perception of reality greatly influence another capacity, environmental mastery, which is almost always mentioned by authorities when writing about the mature, mentally-healthy individual. Environmental mastery suggests that the individual is highly motivated and has made an investment in living that has necessitated the high-level development of his inherent abilities.

In addition, the mentally healthy or emotionally mature individual will have developed the capacity for independent thinking and action. This capacity is described by some as efficiency in solving problems and by others as autonomy or self-determination.

A final capacity usually included in such a discussion is the ability of the individual to effect a balance or synthesis of all psychological functions and personal attributes, which provides a unifying, integrated outlook on life and a sense of direction to the individual in relation to his role in it.

Thus it can be seen that mental health or mental maturity is a highly individual attribute, that it cannot be defined in terms of the absence of disease, that it cannot be understood in terms of isolated symptoms, and that it is intimately related to the society in which the individual finds himself.

FACTORS THAT MAY CONTRIBUTE TO MENTAL ILLNESS

It is impossible to be definitive about the causes of a behavioral response that may be diagnosed as mental illness or to be specific about how this illness might have been prevented. The individual must be studied as a totality, as he is engaged with varying degrees of success in adjusting to his environment and as his environment affects him. No single set of facts can be considered separately when seeking the causes of mental illness. All of the facts must be studied together if the behavior of any individual is to be understood. The only reasonable approach to the study of the etiology of mental illness is a consideration of an individual's total life experience, with emphasis upon genetic, physiological, intrapersonal, interpersonal, and cultural factors, each of which may have contributed to the problem. The following discussion presents some of the cues concerning the possible role of each of these factors in producing mental illness.

Genetic factors

Current knowledge concerning human heredity has not developed to a state where definitive statements can be made about the influence of heredity upon the development of mental illness. About fifty years ago it was a generally accepted belief that mental illness was inherited and that the tendency to develop certain psychotic reactions was transmitted with regularity from one generation to another. These ideas seemed to be given validity when it was observed that manic-depressive and schizophrenic reactions did frequently appear in more than one generation of the same family. Today it is thought that the tendency to develop similar psychotic reactions among members of the same family may be a response to the environmental factors within the family rather than a result of heredity. It is reasonable to believe that children learn to behave in unusual ways when they are reared by parents who habitually respond in unusual ways to other people, to social situations, to work responsibilities, and to parenthood.

The question of the influence of heredity versus environment became a hotly discussed issue before Freudian theories became widely accepted in this country. People who were interested in the issue took sides, and two groups holding opposing views developed. For a time it appeared that the environmentalists had won the controversy. Today most well-read people take the rational view that both environmental and genetic factors significantly influence the way in which the individual reacts to life experiences.

More recently the work of a famous geneticist, Dr. Franz Kallmann, focused the attention of scientists once more upon the question of the role of genetic factors in the development of mental illness. His studies of identical twins with widely different environments were carried on for many years. He reported convincing evidence that may eventually lead to a greater understanding of the role of genetic factors in mental illness. Dr. Kallmann found in his study that when one twin developed schizophrenia, the other became ill with schizophrenia in 86% of the cases, even though these children were not reared in the same families and were not subjected to the same environmental influences. In the same study he found that when one twin developed manic-depressive psychosis, the other twin developed the same illness in 96% of the cases.

As scientific knowledge about human behavior evolves, scientists recognize the urgent need for more research and study of human genetics as it relates to the causation of mental illness. Disregarding the question of the genetic aspects of the cause of mental illness, the biological heredity of the individual is of great significance because body type, sex, intelligence, temperament, and energy endowment are largely determined by the combination of the genes that are contributed by each parent. These personal qualities that influence the new individual's life adjustment in specific ways are determined by his genetic endowment. In a sense, the individual also inherits the family milieu into which he is born and the cultural forces with which he will be required to deal. These factors surely influence an individual's total response to life and play a large part in his ability to maintain an emotional equilibrium throughout life.

Organic factors

A large number of patients suffer from symptoms of mental illness in conjunction with a physical illness, but because of the temporary character of most of these mental reactions they are not recognized as being psychiatric conditions. It is interesting to note that the same organic problem may produce a wide variety of mental reactions in different persons. This suggests that personality plays an important role in behavioral response even when brain tissue is involved.

Traumatic brain damage is one of the common organic problems to which the human organism reacts with abnormal mental symptoms. Such an injury may result in a variety of mental symptoms, depending on the location and severity of the injury and the age and personality of the individual. The aftereffects of brain injury are frequently serious because of a progressive intellectual and emotional degeneration that may occur and the possibility that this degeneration may be accompanied by convulsive seizures.

Brain tumor is an organic condition that may be accompanied by a variety of mental and physical symptoms. The symptoms are dependent upon the location of the tumor, its size, and to some extent upon the type of tumor. Surgery is frequently helpful but may result in the same sequelae that follow brain injury.

Before the advent of the antibiotics, late syphilis, technically known as syphilitic meningoencephalitis, accounted for approximately 10% of all admissions to psychiatric hospitals. Although syphilis may be congenitally acquired, it is usually acquired after the age of puberty. Many more men than women are affected by this disease. Today it is rare for a patient to develop syphilitic meningoencephalitis, although the incidence of syphilis is again on the increase. The mental symptoms said to characterize syphilitic meningoencephalitis are depression, expansiveness, or agitation. However, the symptoms vary a great deal depending on the personality of the patient involved.

Delirium resulting from toxins in the

blood or from a high blood level of certain drugs is a temporary condition that requires consideration and treatment of both the mental and physical symptoms. Barbiturate intoxication, delirium tremens, and delirium such as that which was once frequently seen in conditions such as pneumococcal pneumonia are examples of such problems. Individual reactions are marked in these conditions.

Cortisone and ACTH may produce psychotic reactions in selected individuals. The symptoms usually disappear when the drugs are withdrawn. Thyroid and pituitary diseases may result in overactivity, emotional lability, anxiety, and overt fear or confusion and depression. These symptoms usually disappear when the physical condition is corrected.

Encephalitis or inflammation of the brain may cause specific pathology and may lead to psychic and physical disorders, depending on the organism that caused the condition, the age and personality of the individual, and the treatment provided. The acute form of encephalitis is characterized by lethargy, delirium, confusion, and stupor. In its chronic form it is recognized clinically as paralysis agitans and is characterized by shaking palsy associated with increasing irritability, insomnia, and neurotic behavior.

Psychogenic factors

Psychogenic factors are involved with the individual's subjective and emotional feelings about himself. These include feelings of self-esteem, security, well-being, personal value, guilt, and inferiority. When an individual must cope with situations that increase negative feelings about himself, his anxiety level rises. Extremely high anxiety levels are unbearable and force the anxious person to seek defenses against these uncomfortable feelings. He may call upon a variety of unconscious mechanisms with which he is able to defend himself against feelings of guilt, inadequacy, and insecurity. Specifically, one of these defenses may be projection or an unconscious blaming of others. Thus an individual may relieve his guilt feelings about a sexual transgression by blaming his partner and claiming that it was not his fault but the fault of the woman whose behavior was seductive. A student may unconsciously defend himself against feelings of inadequacy by rationalizing and stating that although he failed a college entrance examination he can play football better than anyone on his team. These are simple examples of normal defense mechanisms utilized to help an individual maintain an emotional equilibrium and relieve anxiety when intrapersonal feelings are involved.

If intrapersonal feelings cause increased anxiety, it may become necessary for the individual to use more elaborate defense mechanisms. As time goes on the elaborate defenses may prove inadequate and he may begin to use bizarre ways of defending himself. When this kind of defense becomes necessary, the individual is said to be mentally ill. Some situations that produce intrapersonal conflicts that may require more adjustment than the individual is capable of achieving include serious financial problems, loss of a deeply loved friend or relative, a broken marriage, loss of a job, failure to receive an important promotion, or disappointment in the integrity of a trusted friend. The foregoing conditions are often referred to as precipitating factors because the individual seems to give up his usual defenses and substitutes psychotic behavior at the time the serious intrapersonal conflict develops.

Interpersonal factors

Interpersonal factors refer to the relationships that individuals develop with significant persons in their environment. Actually the development of positive feelings is dependent to a great extent upon the kind of interpersonal relations developed between the individual and the significant people in his environment during his very early life. Adult feelings of security, well-being, personal value, and self-esteem originate and are powerfully influenced by the relationship that was developed with the mothering person in the very earliest weeks and months of the individual's life. The feeding experiences are especially important in the development of an individual's attitude toward self and others. Likewise, experiences with other significant persons during the habit-training period of an individual's life influences his attitudes toward himself and others, especially in relation to developing unconscious guilt feelings about sexual expression. Similarly it is possible to relate most of the anxiety-producing situations in an individual's adult life to some faulty relationships that existed with significant adults, particularly the mother, during his early life.

The early family relationships, especially with mother and father, influence the individual's ability to cope with the problems of adult life. When faulty relationships in some aspect of the individual's early life have never been corrected, he may not be able to adjust successfully to all the future pressures of adult life. These faulty relationships that may influence the individual's future adjustment are referred to as predisposing factors. This suggests that they are dormant in the individual's unconscious life and may cause difficulty in the future, provided that a certain amount of intrapsychic stress occurs at a time when the individual is more vulnerable than usual.

A young man may be able to complete college, accept a responsible position, and carry on what appears to be a well-adjusted life until he becomes engaged to be married. The stress of assuming this additional financial and social responsibility added to the self-doubt that may develop concerning his ability to assume the masculine role in a marriage relationship may produce more anxiety than he is able to tolerate. At such a time his unconscious need for defense against anxiety may become so great that the individual may resort to unusual or bizarre ways of behaving.

Cultural factors

The culture into which one is born superimposes upon the individual many values and ideas with which he must cope for the remainder of his life. It presents the developing individual with many conflicts between bodily drives and acceptable ways of directing these drives. Young men are physically ready for marriage long before the culture sanctions marriage.

The culture in the United States imposes upon each person many ways of behaving simply because of the individual's sex. Sexual values are given to colors, furniture, occupations, hobbies, and almost everything else in life. A man may receive social disapproval if he wears pink trousers and a lace jacket because we have given a feminine value to pink and to lace. Likewise, a girl is likely to receive social disapproval if she chooses to work as a bricklayer because of our culture has given a masculine value to bricklaying.

In the past the roles of men and women have been clearly defined, but within the last two decades they have been changing rapidly so that there are people who now suffer from role confusion and who are not sure what their sexual role in life really is. This problem is related to early family life experiences because children learn role behavior by identifying with the parent of the same sex. Today children are not always sure what the distinct roles for mother and father are, since parents are apt to share the work of the home and the care of the children. Being unsure and confused about one's sexual role in life gives rise to feelings of insecurity and guilt and to a lowering of self-esteem.

Minority groups face problems superimposed upon them by the culture. Members of a group that is different because of race or religion may face many situations that cause them as individuals to feel unsure, inadequate, unwanted, and to fear for the loss of personal security.

High cultural values have been placed upon marriage, and a certain amount of disapproval is meted out to individuals who fail to marry after they have reached early adulthood. Single people eventually become members of a minority group and suffer some of the same discriminations with which minority groups must cope.

These examples are probably sufficient to suggest that cultural conflict can lead to adjustment problems that may result in such a high level of anxiety that the individual is forced to utilize abnormal defenses.

PREVENTION OF MENTAL ILLNESS

From the preceding discussion the reader has undoubtedly concluded that much of the emphasis upon the prevention of mental illness should fall within the area of family relationships. There are few if any facts upon which to base definitive comments concerning prevention of mental illness. Until there is a clear definition of mental illness it will be difficult to know exactly what preventive measures are required. However, there are some clues that suggest that children need to be provided with emotional warmth, support, and security in order to provide for the emotional and social growth of the child's personality. Much adult behavior is determined by responses that the child experiences from significant adults in the early months of life. It appears at this point in our understanding of human behavior that stable, secure, loving family life, especially during the earliest years, are essential to the development of attitudes about self and others that will make it possible for individuals to adjust to the pressures of adult life and live in a satisfying and productive way. It is the responsibility of the home and the school, both of which deal with children during their early and formative years, to help children develop the capacity to live mentally healthy adult lives and to provide corrective experiences for children who have had negative relationships with inadequate parents.

IMPORTANT CONCEPTS

1. Mental health or mental maturity is thought to be the ability to cope successfully with recurrent stresses of living and the achievement of a relatively effective adjustment to life.
2. Since few people can be said to have achieved complete mental or emotional maturity, it is more helpful to evaluate the individual's relative strengths or limitations in terms of social norms and values.
3. Mental health or mental maturity is evaluated in terms of personality capacities that involve interpersonal relations, self-acceptance, perceptions of reality, environmental mastery, self-determination, and resistance to stress.
4. Mental health and mental illness are culturally determined concepts and are defined somewhat differently in different parts of the world.
5. Mental illness is a complex problem that is thought to be a unique response involving an individual's personality as it interacts with his environment at a time when he is particularly vulnerable to stress.
6. The only reasonable approach to the study of the etiology of mental illness is the study of an individual's total life experience with consideration of genetic, physiological, intrapersonal, interpersonal, and cultural factors.
7. Current knowledge concerning human heredity has not developed to a level where definitive statements can be made about the influence of heredity upon the development of mental illness.
8. The tendency to develop similar psychotic reactions among members of the same family may be a response to the environmental factors within the family rather than a result of heredity.
9. Scientists recognize the urgent need for more research and study of human genetics as it relates to the cause of mental illness.
10. The biological heredity of the individual is of great significance because body type, sex, intelligence, temperament, and energy endowment are genetically determined.
11. In a sense, the individual also inherits his family milieu and the cultural forces to which he must adjust throughout life.
12. The same organic problem may produce a wide variety of mental reactions in different persons, which suggests that personality plays an important role even in individual responses to involvement of brain tissue.
13. Some of the situations that may produce psychogenic conflicts include serious financial problems, loss of a dearly loved friend or relative, a broken marriage, loss of a job, failure to receive an important promotion, or disappointment in the integrity of a trusted friend.
14. Interpersonal factors refer to the re-

lationships that individuals develop with significant persons in their environment and that exert a powerful influence on the mental health of an individual.

15. A stable, secure, loving family life as-

sists individuals to develop attitudes about self and others that make it possible to adjust to the pressures of adulthood and to live a satisfying and productive life.

SUGGESTED SOURCES OF ADDITIONAL INFORMATION

Barrett-Lennard, G. T.: The mature person, Ment. Hyg. **46**:98-102, 1962.

Engel, George L.: Psychological development in health and disease, Philadelphia, 1962, W. B. Saunders Co., pp. 161-165.

Galdston, Iago: The American family in crisis, Ment. Hyg. **42**:229-236, 1958.

Jahoda, Marie: Current concepts of positive mental health, Joint Commission on Mental Illness and Health, monograph series no. 1, New York, 1958, Basic Books, Inc., Publishers.

Kallmann, F. J.: Heredity in health and mental disorder, New York, 1953, W. W. Norton & Co., Inc.

Kolb, Lawrence C.: Noyes' modern clinical psy-

chiatry, ed. 7, Philadelphia, 1968, W. B. Saunders Co., pp. 116-135.

Korner, Ija N.: Mental health versus mental illness, Ment. Hgy. **42**:315-320, 1958.

Mechanic, David: Some factors in identifying and defining mental illness, Ment. Hyg. **46**:66-74, 1962.

Plunkett, Richard J., and Gordon, John E.: Epidemiology and mental illness, Joint Commission on Mental Illness and Health, monograph series no. 6, New York, 1960, Basic Books, Inc., Publishers.

Wedge, Bryant: Changing perception of mental health, Ment. Hyg. **48**:22-31, 1964.

CHAPTER TEN

Patients whose behavior is characterized by patterns of withdrawal

Patients who characteristically utilize patterns of withdrawal from reality in an attempt to achieve personal security are usually assigned the diagnosis of schizophrenia. This group of individuals seems to be incapable of investing enduring emotional attachment in any aspect of their environment.

Schizophrenia is one of the most serious illnesses with which any individual can be afflicted. Unfortunately, the majority of hospitalized mentally ill patients in the United States are afflicted with this baffling illness.

It is a psychosis that appears as a garbled reaction on the part of an individual who lacks the capacities and feelings required for handling the acute problems of reality. There is either a total lack of normal feeling tone or a perversion of the emotions. This problem results in a tendency to withdraw into a world of one's own subjective construction. Although individuals carry many of the characteristics of schizophrenia during their early years, the greatest number of its victims are found in the adolescent and earliest adult periods of life between the ages of 17 and 25.

Psychiatrists have classified schizophrenia into four major types, depending on the predominant patterns of behavior the patient utilizes in his attempt to achieve security. These subclassifications are the simple type, the hebephrenic type, the catatonic type, and the paranoid type.

The simple type of schizophrenia is characterized by indifference, inaccessibility, lack of interest in the opposite sex, and inability to accept responsibility. The hebephrenic type is characterized by severe personality disintegration, inappropriate behavior, and regression. Catatonic behavior is characterized by an acute stupor associated with a sudden loss of animation and a tendency to remain motionless in a stereotyped position. This behavior alternates with periods of excitement and explosive overactivity. The paranoid type is characterized by suspiciousness and ideas of persecution or of grandeur that are called paranoid delusions.

UNDERLYING CAUSATIVE FACTORS OF SCHIZOPHRENIA

Although there is no conclusive scientific proof of the cause of withdrawn behavior, many authorities believe that it is related to factors that are inherent in highly complex cultures such as that which exists in the United States. Most individuals who develop behavioral patterns that can be classified as schizophrenia have experienced highly unsatisfactory family relationships in their early formative years. They are almost always products of family situations in which it was impossible for them to develop warm, positive relationships with other significant members, particularly the mothering person. The individual has usually not learned to trust others and has not developed a self-image that makes it possible for him to feel secure in his relations with others. This failure to develop an integrated ego and the necessary strength to resolve conflicts between the id and the superego presumably derives from early, persistent tension-laden parental relationships. Schizophrenic patients may not accept themselves as having real value or an identity that is uniquely their own. Frequently such an individual has not been able to identify with the parent of the same sex and may be confused as to his sexual identity and role. Such handicapped persons often direct their love energies toward themselves since they are fearful of nonacceptance and rejection if they attempt to direct libidinal energies toward others. Because of their extreme sensitivity they develop patterns of *narcissism* and *introversion* that eventually lead to a life of activity and interest directed entirely toward satisfactions that focus upon self.

NURSING PRINCIPLES APPLICABLE TO ALL PATIENTS WHO UTILIZE PATTERNS OF WITHDRAWAL

The classification of schizophrenia into four types is only of academic interest and has no practical significance from the nursing standpoint. It is more important to recognize that the behavior of these patients is expressing a need and may fluctuate in an unpredictable manner. It is necessary for the nurse to attempt to understand the needs of patients who utilize withdrawal rather than to focus upon the diagnostic entities.

The problems of any schizophrenic patient are essentially an exaggeration of the problems of his prepsychotic personality. Because he has usually been a shy, aloof, and emotionally sensitive individual, he has been unsuccessful in varying degrees in coping with the emotional aspects of the day-by-day problems of routine living. Because of this defect such a patient has attempted a solution by withdrawing from everyday problems and adapting through the utilization of more satisfying

regressive or infantile behavior. To replace the world of reality, the patient often creates a phantasy world of his own that is devoid of certain emotional stresses. If such withdrawal into an unreal world continues, the patient finds more and more relief in dealing with an environment derived from his autistic thinking. This reduces his interactions with others to the dependent and simple adaptabilities of an infant, a process known as *regression*. All nursing activities should therefore be directed toward the prevention of regression and toward helping the patient to accept and to remain in contact with reality. It seems logical, therefore, that the nurse should strive to make reality as pleasant and as free of emotionally stressful situations as possible.

Back of the withdrawal tendencies in schizophrenic patients is a consistent affective indifference or emotional impoverishment. This lack of appropriate feeling makes it difficult for the nurse to express warmth and demonstrate spontaneous interest in the schizophrenic patient. It is helpful when the nurse understands that the schizophrenic patient feels lonely, isolated, and hungry for human contacts but is often incapable of inviting a friendly approach from another person. Only when the nurse approaches the patient with an accepting attitude and with friendliness can she be a source of therapeutic help.

Schizophrenic behavior is invariably difficult to understand because it is unconsciously motivated and may have little logical relation to the immediate environmental situation. Frequently the patient is said to be out of contact with reality. This means that he is motivated by his thoughts and is not sure what is the real world and what is a result of his phantasies. Thus he may fuse or confuse his fantasy world with the world of reality. Inappropriate and bizarre may be accurate descriptive terms for much of the patient's behavior, which is significant and meaningful only when considered from the standpoint of his emotional or instinctual needs. Although this behavior is often difficult to understand, it does have real meaning for the patient, and if the patient is closely studied, the meaning often becomes obvious. Many psychiatrists believe that the patient who is suffering from schizophrenia will eventually divulge his basic emotional conflict to the sensitive listener if given time. One of the most important aspects of nursing care is recording what the nurse observes the patient doing and saying.

DEVELOPMENT OF PATTERNS
OF WITHDRAWAL

Usually patterns of withdrawal have a slow onset, frequently developing over a long period of months or years, although the acute symptoms may appear in an abrupt fashion. Ordinarily friends and relatives observe a progressive indifference to normal interests, a blunting of the emotions, and a sullen, suspicious attitude. Odd and unpredictable behavior, silly postures, and excessive preoccupation with trivial things are common symptoms. Attempts to bring the patient back to a normal concern and interest in what is going on about him may produce inappropriate laughter, a stolid indifference, or a sudden and unexpected outburst of violence.

A disharmony between thought and feeling is a common problem. While talking of something that ordinarily would be associated with sorrow, the patient may laugh, or he may burst into tears when discussing some casual affair. Patients suffering from schizophrenia seem to have lost the ability to respond normally to joy, sorrow, or fear. They also suffer from the inability to communicate accurately to others.

Sooner or later the schizophrenic patient expresses ideas of persecution, and ordinary events begin to refer specifically to him. He begins to believe that his mind is being "read" by those about him and that passersby are talking about him. His beliefs are reinforced by the voices he hears denouncing him or controlling his behavior. In response to these voices he may become impulsive and unpredictable in his behavior. Reality and unreality are no longer differentiated, and there may suddenly develop wild panic, confusion, marked antagonism, and resistance to assurance. The patient may quickly retreat into a stoic silence and a frozen immobility and may sometimes stand for hours in a fixed attitude, mute, resistive, and with a stony expression on his face.

Just as suddenly the patient may become quiet and behave in what appears to be a normal way. At these times he demonstrates that no matter how mentally ill he may appear there is still a part of his personality which is not affected and with which a professional worker can begin to help him to interact with his environment in a positive way. Some of these healthy aspects of the individual's mind include the fact that his mental faculties are good, memory is intact, and general intelligence is unimpaired. Judgment, however, is poor, and generally the patient is not particularly aware of his abnormal behavior or its effect on others about him. This mental disorder has many other features. In general, schizophrenia means a serious disintegration of personality, because the symptoms develop from a fundamental defect in the basic personality structure. Social adaptation is extremely deficient, there is a turning away from reality, a complete domination of the individual by his unconscious needs, and a tendency to a return to certain childish or infantile modes of thinking and behaving.

MEETING THE NURSING NEEDS OF THE WITHDRAWN PATIENT
The newly admitted patient

For many reasons the nurse who has the responsibility for admitting mentally ill patients to a psychiatric facility should be skilled in the use of tact and reassurance. Initial admission to any hospital may be an upsetting and frightening experience. Mentally ill patients frequently fear other people and what other people may do to them. They cherish freedom and the ability to come and go at will. When they realize that they must remain at the hospital, many mentally ill patients develop a feeling of resentment. Sometimes patients are extremely upset by separation from family members. For these and many other reasons the nurse who admits a mentally ill patient to a psychiatric hospital needs to be kind, tactful, reassuring, persuasive, and patient.

The admission procedure, like all other experiences in the hospital, should be de-signed to strengthen the patient's self-esteem, to help him feel safe, and to build up his feeling of confidence in the hospital personnel. Unfortunately, not all admission procedures have had positive results, and some psychiatric facilities have developed admission procedures that do little or nothing to reassure fearful patients.

It is usually wise to postpone for an hour or two the activities involved in officially admitting the patient. This will give the nurse an opportunity to welcome him, to introduce him to other patients, to show him the physical arrangement of the ward, and to talk with him in an informal and friendly way so that he can begin to feel safe in his new environment. After the nurse has won the new patient's confidence and has answered his questions, he will probably be willing to accept the admission procedure without suspicion or fear.

Some hospital authorities may believe that assigning one nurse to spend a few hours with a newly admitted patient is too great an expenditure of time. Staying with a new patient does take time, but the positive results are worth the effort expended. If the patients are helped sympathetically and tactfully to get acquainted with the hospital setting, frequently they can accept the hospital routine without becoming anxious or fearful.

There are some patients who are so confused and upset on the first day of admission that it is not practical to attempt to introduce them to the ward setting or the other patients. With extremely upset patients it is very important to wait for an hour or so before trying to carry out the admission procedure. This lapse of

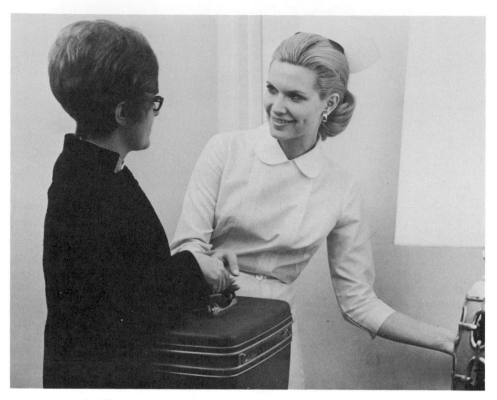

FIG. 9. *The nurse introduces the patient to the new environment.*

time gives the patient an opportunity to regain some emotional control and a chance for his fear to subside. It also gives the nurse time to reassure the patient and to begin to get acquainted with him. Any newly admitted patient who is waiting to have the admission procedure completed should be accompanied by a member of the hospital nursing staff.

Environmental requirements

The hospital is to be the patient's home for a period of time. If he is to benefit from this experience in living, it seems reasonable to believe that a congenial and pleasant atmosphere should be developed. It also seems important for the environment to be free from anxiety-producing experiences. Opportunities should be provided for the patient to participate in oc-

cupational and resocialization activities from the first day of hospital admission. It is therapeutically important for mentally ill patients to be allowed to wear their own clothing in the hospital, beginning with the first day of admission. Practices such as requiring that pajamas be worn during the first few weeks of hospitalization, even though the patient is physically well, makes it almost impossible to provide a variety of therapeutic experiences. The all too frequent plan of eliminating newly admitted patients from most or all hospital activities as a safety measure seems indefensible. The need to become self-destructive and to strike out against the environment will greatly diminish if patients are provided with challenging activities, if they are helped to feel secure and safe, and if the hospital personnel provide mean-

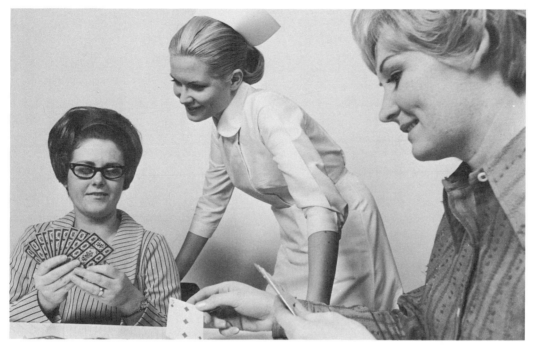

FIG. 10. *The nurse stimulates interest in recreational activities.*

ingful interpersonal relationships for them.

Maintaining a safe environment

Of course, it is necessary to exercise reasonable precautions to protect and safeguard both the mentally ill patients and the hospital personnel. Probably the most significant aspect of any combination of safety measures is an adequately prepared and interested staff provided in large enough numbers to ensure individual attention and a variety of therapeutic activities for all patients. Mentally ill patients, like all human beings, require individualized treatment if they are to recover and be able to resume a role in the community as a contributing member of society.

A serious mistake that has been made in the past in the care of mentally ill patients is the failure to realize that all persons need to be recognized as unique and important human beings. Because individualized care is so significant in the patient's total therapy, hospitals have defeated their own purposes by routinizing the care of the mentally ill.

Helping the patient develop social skills

Because of the patient's extreme sensitivity and fear of being unacceptable to others, the nurse should take the initiative in stimulating his interest in social activity and recreation. It is important that the nurse know something of the patient's background, and with this knowledge she can initiate conversation in which the patient can participate. When the patient develops a feeling of trust in the nurse, participation in some recreational activity can then be encouraged. This may be accomplished by extending an invitation such as "I need a partner for a game of table tennis; come and play with me."

It may be best for the nurse alone to play a game with the patient to help him feel secure. The nurse should provide opportunities for the patient to have some success experiences. Gradually other participants can be added as the patient develops more confidence. These participants should be other patients and staff members who relate well with the patient and will promote his sense of being accepted. Ward personnel should be a stable group, and the same individuals, including the nurse, should continue this program of socialization for several weeks or even months.

Providing corrective emotional experiences for patients

Although most schizophrenic patients show every outward manifestation of physical maturity, they are essentially struggling with many psychogenic conflicts that originated in childhood. Since the problems of the schizophrenic patient probably evolved at an early age from faulty emotional relationships between the individual and significant adults in his environment, corrective interpersonal experiences must be provided. Schizophrenic patients have often been bereft of a loving parent, or one parent was so rigid and unloving that identification with the parent of the same sex at the proper time was impossible. Such deprivation may have made it extremely difficult for the patient to trust or give love to a friend or a life partner.

A corrective family situation can be created, in a manner of speaking, when the doctor assumes the role of a kindly, understanding father, the nurse that of a wise, accepting mother, and other patients that of siblings. If such a synthetic family setting gives the patient sufficient love and acceptance over a long period of time, he can be helped to deal more realistically with his conflicts and can achieve some feeling of security.

Calling the patient Mr. Smith instead of John may be a way of suggesting that the patient is expected to assume an adult role. Using a title which connotes respect, whatever it may be, is usually an incentive to more acceptable behavior and may convey to the patient the idea that he is an important person.

Talking to the patient

The use of long and involved sentences should be avoided. Many schizophrenic patients are easily confused and have a limited attention span. Short phrases are more effective and specific words more helpful than generalizations. For instance, ice cream is more meaningful than dessert, and ham is more specific than meat.

The nurse may be tempted to exploit the negativism displayed by some patients. She may request the patient to walk backward when she assumes that the patient will do the exact opposite, which is the reaction actually desired. Utilization of negativism in such activities as feeding the patient and in giving medication may serve to increase the patient's confusion and encourage complete withdrawal.

Similarly, making use of delusions and hallucinations to direct the patient's behavior should be avoided. If, for instance, the patient hallucinates and believes that he hears the voice of his mother, the nurse may be tempted to say that his mother just told him to eat his breakfast. If the patient believes himself to be John the Baptist, it might seem at first that on that delusional assumption he can be persuaded to be more careful of his personal hygiene. The patient will cease to trust the nurse when such symptoms are utilized to accomplish the nurse's purpose.

If a patient asks for a confirmation of his hallucinations, it is better to answer truthfully. "No, Mr. Jones, I do not see the face of Christ on the wall." "No, Mr. Smith, your face is not that of a dog." It is wise to give honest replies that focus upon reality.

Meticulous honesty and fairness of the nurse are of primary importance. Should the patient make a request with which it is impossible to comply, a suitable answer is "I am sorry that I am not allowed to carry out such a procedure." Once a promise is made, the nurse is duty bound to carry it out. If possible, all requests and questions should be answered. If no answer is possible, the patient should be informed that his request will be referred to an appropriate person who can give an answer.

Caring for the suspicious patient

Like all other schizophrenic patients, the suspicious individual is essentially shy, sensitive, and unable to relate positively to others. Because he has never learned to trust, he resorts to the mental mechanisms of projection to cope with his environment and therefore places the blame for his inadequacies upon people and objects about him. Hostility is frequently a dominant attitude. Insight is poor, and usually the patient is convinced that he is being held illegally or without just cause. Consequently the patient may be threatening and dangerous.

Such a patient rarely desires to enter group activity. As a defense suspicious patients are usually aloof, sarcastic, and generally hostile toward everyone about them. This behavior is actually based upon intrapersonal fear and anxiety.

Suspicious patients usually take at least average care of their own personal hygiene. However, they may demand unusual privileges, such as complete bathroom privacy.

Such fearful, hostile patients must be approached with utmost tact and understanding. Solitary activities are more successful for them than are group activities. It is essential to realize that hostility and suspicion are aspects of the patient's illness.

Arguments with such individuals should be tactfully avoided, since any controversy is at once integrated into the patient's delusional system. To obtain the confidence of a paranoid person requires the most patient and persistent application of tact, tolerance of the patient's hostile attitude, and a quiet determination to establish a relationship with him.

Meeting the physical needs of withdrawn patients

When an individual withdraws from reality, one of the first changes in behavior may be a significant loss of interest in physical cleanliness and in personal neatness and attractiveness. The schizophrenic patient may be disheveled in appearance or may attire himself in bizarre fashion.

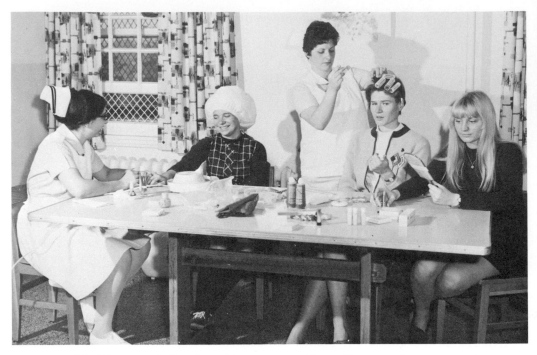

FIG. 11. *The nurse helps the patient improve her self-esteem by encouraging good grooming.*

One aspect of the nurse's responsibility lies in the supervision of personal hygiene and in encouraging the patient to bathe. It is important for the nurse to help the patient take responsibility for his own personal hygiene and grooming. When she herself assumes the responsibility for this procedure, she is in effect encouraging the patient to rely on his regressive behavior patterns rather than helping the patient to cope with the reality factors of living through his own efforts and initiative.

Female patients should be encouraged to look as attractive as possible. Nurses can initiate a positive relationship by helping them with all aspects of good grooming. The services of a hospital beautician are invaluable, and it may also be of great therapeutic benefit to have female patients arrange each other's hair. Male patients should be encouraged to shave, to keep their hair well-groomed, and to dress neatly.

Personal clothing rather than a standardized hospital garb promotes a sense of individuality and prevents a retreat into a colorless institutional environment that fosters regression. Praise and approval for efforts to look neat and to maintain correct grooming of hair and clothing is helpful to these patients.

Extremely withdrawn patients may be careless with regard to excreta. This means that the patient is so much out of touch with the demands of reality that he does not go to the toilet when he needs to void or defecate. This behavior is part of the regression to infantile reaction patterns shown by some schizophrenic patients. Initiating a toileting routine encourages the patient to cope with this problem.

Some catatonic patients withhold urine and bowel content, a condition that can result in a seriously distended bladder or in fecal impaction. Hence it is important to record daily bowel movements and to report to the physician when a patient has had no defecation for two or three days. Enemas should be avoided, since patients may misinterpret the enema procedure as a sexual assault. Most patients establish regular bowel habits in the hospital after receiving a balanced diet over a period of time. Women may suffer a concomitant loss of menstrual function when suffering from a severe schizophrenic illness. The menstrual cycle is usually reestablished after a few months of hospital routine.

Patients who retreat into a phantasy world often ignore physical illness and may offer no complaints even when the condition is a painful one. Acute mastoiditis, cystitis, lung abscess, and a broken bone in the hand or foot are examples of serious disorders that have been known to exist without complaint on the part of schizophrenic patients. The psychiatric nurse should be constantly alert to the physical condition of patients.

Catatonic patients sometimes alternate between periods of inactivity and periods of great overactivity. The overactivity may be initiated by upsetting thoughts or disturbing occurrences not necessarily related to the patient. Thus the behavior appears to be inappropriate and difficult to understand.

Standing and sitting in one position for hours may be observed frequently among withdrawn patients. Edema and cyanosis of the extremities are likely to develop. To avoid this the patient should be encouraged to take some exercise even if it is only to walk up and down the hospital corridors.

Adequate food intake for withdrawn patients is a major nursing responsibility. Tube feeding should be avoided except in extreme cases of food refusal, for the tube may have symbolic significance and may encourage complete dependence and more rapid regression.

Responses to hallucinations, delusions, and illusions are frequent reasons for the refusal of food by some mentally ill patients. The voices may tell the patients not to eat because someone is poisoning or contaminating the food in some horrible manner. This is a very difficult attitude to combat. Such a patient appears to be terrified at the thought of eating. Such suspicious patients may eat if they are allowed to have foods that are not easily contaminated. A list of such foods might include hard-cooked unshelled eggs, baked potatoes, unpeeled fruits, and bread from an unopened package. It is discouraging to hear some patients comment that poison could have been instilled in these foods if a hypodermic needle were used. Tasting the food in the presence of a suspicious patient who believes that the food is poisoned is another well-known suggestion. In this way the nurse may prove to the patient that she does not believe that the food is contaminated. Dietary problems that arise from illusions may be controlled by avoiding the offending food altogether. Some of the common illusionary problems involving foods include seeing tomato juice as blood, tapioca as living animal eyes, small whole potatoes as toes, and macaroni as worms. When refusal of food arises out of psychotic delusions, the problem is extremely difficult. One young patient refused food for several years because he believed that a little child could bring peace to the world by sacrificing himself. In spite of a variety of treatments this patient continued to refuse all food. He was kept alive by nourishment given through a gavage tube.

All but a few of the most acutely ill patients hospitalized in a psychiatric facility begin to eat soon after being admitted to the neutral, relatively anxiety-free environment of the hospital. It is helpful for these patients to be required to go to meals at regular, stated intervals even though they may not actually eat. Appetites frequently return when patients are encouraged to retire and rise at regular hours. Restoration of some semblance of an eating and sleeping schedule in the lives of mentally ill patients frequently does much to encourage food intake.

It is not a good plan to coax or threaten a patient in relation to his food intake. It is more therapeutic to invite the patient to come to the dining room or to serve the tray without comment. If the patient refuses to eat, it is wise to accept his refusal without comment. It is usually not therapeutically helpful to use any coercion, even persuasion, until the patient has gone two or three days without food. When the nurse first realizes that the patient is refusing food, it is a good plan to discuss the problem with the psychiatrist in charge of the patient's treatment. If the refusal of food becomes an actual health problem, the psychiatrist may feel that tube-feeding is indicated, although this procedure probably should be avoided if possible.

Patients, like children, sometimes respond positively to spoon-feeding. This is especially true if the patient is disoriented, confused, or tremulous.

It is probably never wise to force-feed a patient. Force-feeding rarely accomplishes anything positive, and it may be interpreted by the patient as an attack. When a patient persists in refusing food for days because of an irrational fear of eating or deep-seated self-destructive tendencies, it is futile to hope that anything can be accomplished by force-feeding. The following incident occurred after a patient had received a meal by force. When the entire meal had been ingested the patient induced an emesis and all was lost. The patient said "No one can make me eat." It would be well for nurses to remember that patients cannot be made to retain food even if they are forced to swallow it.

Mealtime as a pleasant experience

Because the first experiences human beings have in receiving love from the mothering person are associated with feeding, food is unconsciously associated with mothering and with receiving love and acceptance. It is important for the nurse who is developing a therapeutic environment for mentally ill patients to create and maintain a happy, friendly atmosphere during mealtime. There is probably never a time in the care of an emotionally ill person when it is therapeutic for anyone to become aggressive toward the patient concerning food. The mere physical acceptance of food is only part of the therapeutic significance of feeding a patient. Unless the feeding experience also provides a friendly, warm, accepting atmosphere, it has lost much of its potential value.

Mentally ill patients, like all people, deserve attractively prepared meals served

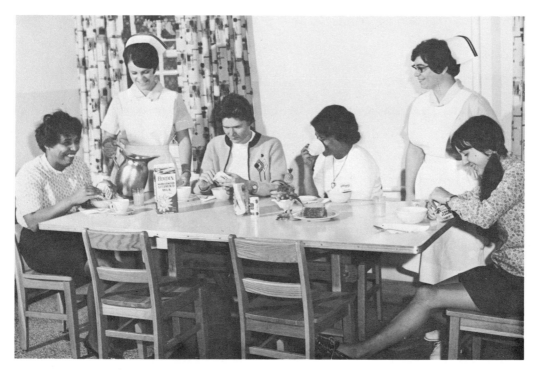

FIG. 12. *The nurse recognizes the importance of a friendly atmosphere at meal time.*

in pleasant, homelike surroundings that contribute to a therapeutic environment.

SPECIFIC TREATMENT APPROACHES TO THE WITHDRAWN PATIENT

Electroconvulsive therapy has been used in the treatment of schizophrenia with limited success. Its greatest usefulness appears to be with the catatonic patient. The main use of electroconvulsive therapy for schizophrenic patients may be in producing short remissions. Because it can be frequently repeated over a long period of time, electroconvulsive therapy can modify the most serious symptoms of early schizophrenia.

In all phases of schizophrenic excitement the ataractics or tranquilizers are of inestimable value. They are particularly useful in catatonic excitement and during periods of extreme agitation and dissociation. The result is a quieter, less apprehensive, and more cooperative patient who can be approached for more complete study and for psychotherapy.

Psychotherapy and emotional support are of great value in helping withdrawn patients learn to trust others and to develop a positive relationship with at least one other significant person.

Case report

The following case history presents the story of a young woman who resorted to catatonic withdrawal when she could no longer cope with the problems of daily living.

F. B. was 19 years of age when she was admitted to the hospital. The only child of missionary parents, she was born in a mission station in Africa. Her father was a quiet-spoken man, definitely esthetic and consistent in his practice of religious teachings. He had little patience with sensual matters and was very pious. The girl's mother was more practical and tolerant, but was dominated by her husband. They were so busy with the work of the mission that they had little time to spend with their daughter.

During the first five years of her life, F. B.'s only playmates were native children. Toward them, she had always taken an attitude of superiority. On entering a boarding school in the United States at the age of 5 years, she had difficulty with her classmates. She was inclined to be too critical with them and insisted on dictating to them about personal matters. In her twelfth year she had a long seige of pneumonia after which she lost weight and was chronically anemic and undernourished. She spent long hours in prayer, wrote endless letters to her parents, most of them consisting of long quotations from the Bible. She insisted on wearing old, worn clothing to the schoolroom and bitterly criticized classmates for not doing likewise.

Although her parents returned on furlough every five years, they could spend only a few days with her because they had many church meetings to attend while in the United States.

Her social behavior changed somewhat in her high school years, but she made few friends. She had a dog to which she was greatly attached, and, spent most of her free time in his company, taking long walks. She showed a preference for mathematics and Biblical history.

She entered the freshman year of college some eleven months before her admission to the hospital. Although her scholastic record was good, she was known as a strange girl who avoided company, smiled a great deal to herself, and had no interest in the opposite sex. Her parents, while on furlough from Africa, visited her during the Christmas holidays, and her mother expressed fear that she was not emotionally well. She manifested little interest in their visit, in spite of the fact that she had not seen her parents for over five years.

During the commencement festivities she disappeared from the campus for several days; later it was learned that she had spent the time at an evangelical camp meeting. She remained on the campus during the summer months to take some advanced courses in mathematics. During this interval she roomed with two other young women in the house of one of the faculty members. The latter were in the habit of discussing their love affairs in her presence, and she suddenly manifested an unusual interest in their conversations. Among other things, she inquired about various matters of sex and how to approach members of the opposite sex. A few nights later she informed one of the girls that she saw the face of her future husband in the light fixture. She scrutinized the fixture for several hours during which she sat in a trancelike state with a smile on her face. Early the next morning she spoke to a 13-year-old newsboy and informed him that she would marry him. When he made light of this proposal, she became upset, struck him in the face, and chased him down the street. Returning to her room, she tore out the light fixture, removed her clothing, and became unmanageable.

On being admitted to the psychiatric hospital she refused to answer questions. She smiled to herself and identified the house physician as "Herbert." She insisted on having the window opened because "they are playing the wedding march." Her speech was incoherent; she was definitely hallucinating and stated that she was hearing voices that questioned her moral standards.

For the first few days she talked a great deal about a phantasized courtship in which she was the central character. She carried on a dialogue, at one time representing the lover, at another time the maiden. After this she entered a long period of silence, during which she was mute, resistive, and refused food. Occasionally she said "if thy eye offend thee, cut it out." One evening she almost succeeded in enucleating her right eye with the thumb and forefinger of her right hand. She continued to talk incoherently, laughed a great deal, and made little attempt to keep her person clean. After several months she improved, but remained withdrawn, manneristic, and untidy. Five months after her illness began, her parents returned from Africa to visit her, but she manifested no interest in them. In fact, she showed no indication that she recognized them when they came into the hospital.

Discussion of case report

The case report is clearly the story of a young woman who failed to develop a stable, harmonious self-concept or to evolve an ego strong enough to resolve the conflicts between the id drives and the demands of the superego.

The history gives us little information about this patient as a child. We do know that her father dominated both the home and the mother and placed the welfare of the mission above all else. It is quite possible that her care even as an infant was relegated to employed native women who may not have remained in the household consistently. In the development of a sense of personal security the first five years of a child's life are crucial. The type of mothering person by whom the child is nurtured is of the greatest importance, especially in developing the ability to share and the ability to effectively cope with hostile, aggressive instinctual drives.

At the age of 5 years the child was sent away to a boarding school. Although this was probably the best plan the parents could develop, it was apparently not helpful to the patient. Authorities believe that the fifth year of a child's life is of great significance in the scheme of psychosexual development. During this period the child is beginning to identify with the parent of the same sex, has discovered that the sexual organ is a source of pleasurable sensations, and has recognized the structural difference between the sex organs of boys and girls. As has been mentioned in a previous chapter, castration fears or concern about the loss of the penis are sources of anxiety for children of this age. A boy may be concerned for fear he will be deprived of the penis as a punishment, and a girl may fear that she was deprived of a penis because of some earlier punishment or accident. When a child in this age period is removed from the parents, the child is apt to feel banished as a punishment for some transgression. Since sexual longings and phantasies have occupied some of the child's thoughts and since the child realizes that these are frowned on by the parents, it is natural for the child to feel that the banishment is related to "bad" thoughts.

The child being discussed in this situation undoubtedly felt banished by being sent to boarding school. Because of the father's strict and rigid attitudes toward any sensual matters, it is quite likely that the child was convinced that she was being punished. Even when parents are not a source of comfort and security for a child, the child mourns their loss when separated from them because they are the only significant reality known. Thus it is reasonable to believe that the child passed through a period of loneliness and bereavement at being deprived from the only mothering person she knew.

Initially, children protest this separation by crying or by other aggressive acting out behavior. After several days of hopelessness and withdrawal from activity, the child usually becomes detached and seems unwilling to resume a close relationship with any adult, even if the lost person returns. This detached attitude could be altered if the parent returned and remained with the child consistently. However, in the situation being discussed, the little girl undoubtedly developed a detached attitude toward other people and attempted to isolate herself personally to avoid anxiety resulting from fear of being cast aside and abandoned a second time. Her subsequent attachment to a dog suggested that she could not trust another person with her love and therefore gave it to an animal who made no demands and gave her unconditional devotion.

After the patient had a serious illness at the age of 12 years she began to spend long hours in prayer, wrote letters to her parents filled with quotes from the Bible, and wore her shoddiest clothing to school. This behavior suggests that she felt guilt-ridden for having been ill and was seeking to gain the favor and forgiveness of her parents, who in her phantasies may have been God's representatives on earth. Undoubtedly she felt unworthy of anything better when she chose to wear old and shoddy clothing to school and again was seeking to atone for phantasied sin.

Her unusual interest in the sexual affairs of other girls of her age and the inappropriate proposal of marriage was a reactivation of the very early problem of failure to develop an integrated ego. This patient developed a limited capacity to clearly evaluate the realities of the situation in which she found herself. In addition, the weak ego development made it difficult if not impossible to resolve the conflicts between the id drives (interest in marriage) and demands of the superego (the incorporated standards of her parents). Likewise she had never been able to effectively repress hostile aggressive drives and expressed these feelings freely in the hospital by tearing out the light fixture.

When the patient saw the face of her future husband in the light fixture, she was exhibiting a severe mental symptom called visual hallucinations. Hallucinations are one example of the personality disintegration that takes place in individuals suffering from an active psychosis. Hallucinations, like all symptoms, meet a basic need for the patient. In this situation the face supplied an answer for her that was an outgrowth of her unconscious longings and her inability to find answers to her own sexual needs through coping adequately with the social situation.

Hallucinations are an example of being out of touch with reality. This means that the patient is reacting to a stimulus from within the unconscious mind that is unrelated to the real situation. Her behavior might become even more confusing if she reacted part of the time to stimuli from the real world and part of the time to stimuli from within her own unconscious mind.

Planning nursing care for F. B.

When F. B. was admitted to the psychiatric hospital, she was acutely ill. She demonstrated severe pathological symptoms suggestive of acute schizophrenia. Communicating with her was especially difficult because she refused to answer questions or spoke in such an incoherent fashion that the professional staff was unable to understand the meaning of her statements. Her behavior vacillated between being excessively talkative and being mute and refusing food. On one occasion F. B. was self-destructive and attempted to enucleate one eye.

Nursing care for any patient must be focused upon the unique needs and abilities of the specific individual for whom the care is being planned. To achieve this the nurse needs to consider what the patient is attempting to communicate through the behavior that is being expressed. The nurse who was chosen to work with F. B. had to consider why it was necessary for her to behave as she was behaving before a helpful nursing care plan could be developed. When some understanding of F. B.'s behavior had been achieved, the nurse could decide how to respond therapeutically.

Since it was not possible to deal with all of her problems at once, the logical starting point was the establishment of a positive relationship with her. Hopefully this relationship would lead to the development of some communication with the patient.

Because the nurse knew that schizophrenic patients are highly sensitive individuals who isolate themselves interpersonally due to their fear of rejection, the approach to F. B. was unhurried, warm, friendly, and accepting. The nurse found it necessary to make repeated overtures to her before she was able to respond.

It was decided that the entire responsibility for the nursing care of the patient during the first weeks of her hospital experience would be assigned to a few carefully chosen nurses. This decision was made because the staff recognized that F. B. needed to develop a feeling of security and to learn to trust other people. Security can be enhanced by limiting the number of individuals with whom such ill patients come in contact and by keeping their daily routines much the same for several months. In the beginning, few demands were made upon F. B.

It was recognized that the attitude of the people with whom mentally ill patients come in contact during the early part of their illness has a significant effect upon their recovery. Patients such as F. B. require consistent acceptance, sincere interest, and constant encouragement from nurses and the other members of the professional staff.

Although communication with F. B. was difficult because she used language in a highly personal way, it was important for the nurse to spend time sitting with her and talking to her even though she rarely responded verbally. The nurse used simple, uncomplicated, direct statements when talking to the patient.

At the same time that the nurse was trying to help F. B. develop a sense of trust in others, feel secure and accepted, and feel safe enough to communicate verbally with other people, attention had to be given to the physical needs she exhibited when she was first admitted. According to the information provided she was withdrawn and untidy, refused food, and had self-destructive tendencies. This behavior was symptomatic of an individual who felt unworthy and guilty. It was obvious that F. B.'s self-esteem was badly shattered. Thus the nurse's efforts were focused upon trying to assist her to develop a more positive opinion of herself. This was partially achieved by the attention provided for her and the sincere, interested way in which it was given. Self-esteem was also enhanced through the mechanism of improving her grooming.

Early in F. B.'s hospital experience it was necessary for a nurse to assume a good deal of responsibility for bathing and dressing her, but in time she was encouraged to assume more and more of this activity herself. The nurses gently suggested that she would enjoy visiting the beauty parlor. At first they accompanied her on these trips and remained with her while she was there. As F. B. began to feel more secure in the situation, she was able to accept some responsibility for her own grooming.

The dietary intake for patients who refuse food is always of great concern. Because F. B. was regressed when she was first admitted, the nurses tried to help her in feeding herself by making suggestions such as "Pick up your fork" and "Put the food in your mouth." This plan was used because it was thought that she was unable to make the necessary decisions herself. However, it was eventually necessary to spoon-feed her. The nurses used an unhurried, relaxed manner and fed her from a tray in her own room.

During the spoon-feeding periods the nurses gave F. B. many opportunities to take the spoon in her own hand and assume some of the responsibility for feeding herself during a part of the meal.

After a few weeks she was encouraged to return to the dining room and take her meals with the other patients.

The problem of self-destruction was especially distressing. Criticism and reprimands for this behavior were withheld because the nurses realized that it would confirm her opinion that she was indeed a bad person. The close personal attention F. B. received when she was first admitted solved the problem of self-destruction during the early part of her hospitalization. However, F. B. was helped to reestablish her own inner controls, and the nurse served as an external authority until F. B. was able to accept responsibility for her own safety.

With such close association with the nurses, F. B. eventually became dependent upon them. Thus they realized that it was important to introduce a second patient into the situation as soon as possible. This was accomplished by including a second patient in some of the activities of daily living in which a nurse and F. B. were involved. A second patient began visiting the beauty parlor with her and the nurse.

Recreational activities were introduced into F. B.'s daily routine after a reasonable amount of time in the hospital had elapsed. The nurse and a second patient involved themselves with F. B. in finger painting and clay modeling. These activities were chosen because they have a special appeal for regressed patients.

In time the corrective emotional experiences provided for F. B. in the hospital made it possible for her to begin to relate to other people in a more mature way and to continue therapy while living at a girl's club.

IMPORTANT CONCEPTS

1. Schizophrenia is one of the most serious illnesses with which any individual can be afflicted, and it is the most prevalent of the mental illnesses.
2. The most distressing aspect of behavior exhibited by schizophrenic patients is their tendency to withdraw into a world of their own subjective construction.
3. Schizophrenia is classified into four major types, depending on the predominant behavioral patterns the patient utilizes in his attempt to achieve security.
4. There is no conclusive scientific proof of the cause of schizophrenia, but most authorities believe that it is related to the early and unsatisfactory family life the individual has experienced.
5. Schizophrenic patients are insecure in their relations with others, highly sensitive, lack a sense of personal value, and have a poor self-image.
6. Schizophrenic patients direct their libidinal energies toward themselves and are thus said to be narcissistic and introverted.
7. Patients suffering from schizophrenia seem to have lost the ability to respond normally to joy, sorrow, or fear.
8. Like all other schizophrenic patients, the suspicious individual is essentially shy, sensitive, and unable to relate positively to others.
9. Psychotherapy and emotional support are of great value in helping withdrawn patients learn to trust others and to develop a positive relationship with at least one other significant person.

SUGGESTED SOURCES OF ADDITIONAL INFORMATION

Andrews, Dixie: Process recording on a schizophrenic hebephrenic patient, Perspect. Psychiat. Care 1:11-39, 1963.

Arieti, Silvano: Schizophrenia. In Arieti, Silvano, editor: American handbook of psychiatry, vol. 1, New York, 1959, Basic Books, Inc., Publishers, pp. 455-509.

Carl, Mary Kathyrn: Establishing a relationship with a schizophrenic patient, Perspect. Psychiat. Care 1:20-22, 1963.

Field, William E.: When a patient hallucinates, Amer. J. Nurs. 63:80-82, Feb., 1963.

Goodman, Lillian: Regression—some implications for nurses in large public psychiatric hospitals, Nurs. Outlook 10:265-267, April, 1962.

Goodman, Lillian R., and LaBelle, Mary J.: The schizophrenic's mother, Nurs. Outlook 11:753-754, Oct., 1963.

Jackson, D. D., editor: The etiology of schizophrenia, New York, 1960, Basic Books, Inc., Publishers.

Kline, Nathan S.: Synopsis of Eugen Blueler's dementia praecox, New York, 1952, International Universities Press, Inc.

Kolb, Lawrence C.: Noyes' Modern clinical psychiatry, ed. 7, Philadelphia, 1968, W. B. Saunders Co., pp. 355-400.

McCown, Pauline P., and Wurm, Elizabeth: Orienting the disoriented, Amer. J. Nurs. 65:118-119, April, 1965.

Peplau, Hildegard E.: Loneliness, Amer. J. Nurs. 55:1476-1481, Dec., 1955.

Robinson, Alice M.: Communicating with schizophrenic patients, Amer. J. Nurs. 60:1120-1123, Aug., 1960.

Sechehaye, Marguerite: Autobiography of a schizophrenic girl, New York, 1951, Grune & Stratton, Inc.

Schwartz, Charlotte Green, Schwartz, Morris S., and Stanton, Alfred H.: A study of need-fulfillment on a mental hospital ward, Psychiatry 14:223-242, 1951.

Schwartz, Morris S., and Shockley, Emmy L.:
The nurse and the mental patient, New York,
1956, Russell Sage Foundation, pp. 90-138.

Schwartz, Morris S., and Will, Gwen Tudor:
Low morale and mutual withdrawal on a mental hospital ward, Psychiatry **16**:337-353, 1953.

Sister M. Rose Magdalen: Depersonalization,
Perspect. Psychiat. Care **1**:29-31, 1963.

Tudor, Gwen: Sociopsychiatric nursing approach
to intervention in a problem of mutual withdrawal on a mental hospital ward, Psychiatry
15:193-217, 1952.

Van Huben, Betty J.: Discussion of a process recording on a schizophrenic, hebephrenic patient, Perspect. Psychiat. Care **1**:40-44. 1963.

CHAPTER ELEVEN

Patients whose behavior is characterized by depression or elation

Some patients express anxiety through behavior characterized by overactivity, an elated mood, and excessive talkativeness. The elated mood may be so pronounced and sustained that the patient expresses the belief that every good thing is possible or will soon be consummated and every wish will be fulfilled. Ideas emerge in an easy, fluidlike manner; thinking seems to be effortless; memory is quickened; and the patient shows a quick but superficial wit. There is an apparent sense of self-security, and fears are pushed to the background. The patient is aggressive, cocksure in his opinions, and ready to talk with conviction on anything and everything. The ego is unrestrained, and ideas pour out so rapidly and with such ease that the tongue cannot give them full expression. Hence, the patient utters only segments of ideas and jumps from one to another in a rapid barrage. He has a quick recognition of persons and objects and a tendency to argue. The patient is apt to be domineering, will brook no restraint, and becomes irritable, denunciatory, and hypercritical of everything that interferes with his desire for free action. He is apt to become overactive, obtrusive, and may extend this excessive motor excitement into every direction. When limits must be set for his behavior, he sometimes becomes noisy, belligerent, and violent. His insight is always poor. The patient's interest is in the outside world rather than in himself. His ideation is concerned with his environment. In fact, the patient can almost be said to be at the mercy of his environment.

Surprising as it may seem, such an aggressive, overactive patient may also utilize quite different behavior to express anxiety. Within a few months he may be sad, may have difficulty in thinking and expressing thoughts, and may be very slow in his physical responses, or he may exhibit agitation.

Such a patient may have difficulty in formulating answers, may lose his ability to concentrate, and may be unable to choose a direct line of action. The patient may be tormented by a sense of insecurity or by ideas of remorse and self-abasement or may be overcome by a sense of guilt. He may complain of a total lack of affection and of a loss of interest in the things for which he formerly had much concern. He may feel that he is lost or being punished. The patient may have an overpowering sense of futility, a "feeling of emptiness," and a desire to retreat from everything, to seek oblivion, and to end his life. Danger of suicide is the outstanding feature of this condition, and this alone justifies the greatest caution and consideration from the standpoint of care and treatment.

Such symptoms as overactivity and elation or depression place the patient in the diagnostic category of manic-depressive psychosis. In 1896 Emil Kraepelin identified this condition and called it manic depressive psychosis, the name it bears today. If the majority of symptoms are in the area of elation and overactivity, the patient is said to be in the manic phase of this illness. If the symptoms are predominantly in the area of depression, the patient is said to be in the depressed phase of this psychosis. If the patient is in the middle years of life and for the first time is showing symptoms of deep depression, the diagnosis is likely to be involutional melancholia. Such midlife depressions are frequently accompanied with symptoms of agitation.

DIFFERENTIATION OF SCHIZOPHRENIC BEHAVIOR FROM BEHAVIOR IN MANIC AND DEPRESSIVE PSYCHOSES

It is sometimes difficult for students of nursing to differentiate between the overactivity demonstrated by some schizophrenic patients and the overactivity the manic patient exhibits. Both types of patients carrying these diagnoses may be physically overactive, and at times both may talk excessively. The schizophrenic patient who exhibits catatonic behavior may fluctuate from being almost stuporous to exhibiting explosive overactivity. Such overactivity is frequently described as a panic state. In such a situation the patient is probably responding to emotional thoughts and feelings that are not related to reality, but which are threatening, upsetting, and disturbing. This type of overactivity is especially difficut to understand because there is often disharmony between the mood and the ideas expressed. The patient may smile inappropriately or laugh while speaking of the disturbing thoughts that are uppermost in his mind. He may express terrifying visual or auditory hallucinations.

In contrast, the overactivity of a patient who is said to be behaving like a manic is characterized by glib argumentative speech that may be humorous but may change quickly to sarcasm and verbal abuse. Such a patient may appear to have boundless energy. He is usually irrepressible, demanding, and irritable. He frequently expresses ideas of grandeur and delusions of having great power and wealth. There is a dominant tone of euphoria even though the patient may demonstrate an underlying mood of sorrow. Authorities believe that the overactivity of the manic patient is actually a defense against depression. The professional person usually feels that manic overactivity is understandable because the patient maintains some contact with reality except in the most extreme examples of this illness.

Schizophrenic withdrawal and depression may be difficult for the beginning student of nursing to differentiate because patients suffering from either diagnosis are frequently physically inactive. However, the schizophrenic patient quickly demonstrates a disharmony of thought, feeling, and behavior. Although there may be a persistent mood it has little apparent relationship to the situation in which the patient finds himself or to his past experiences. In contrast, everything about the depressed patient conveys a depressed feeling to the observer. The way the patient sits, the facial expression, the voice quality, and the ideas expressed all suggest hopelessness and a sense of impending doom. Depressed patients remain well aware of reality, and their feelings seem understandable to individuals working with them.

Some authorities believe that the attempt to differentiate the behavior reactions of manic-depressive patients from those of schizophrenic patients is actually an artificial and unwarranted exercise. These authorities suggest that they may be aspects of one broad disease entity.

CAUSATIVE FACTORS

Manic-depressive psychosis has no specific causative factors that can be described with scientific certainty. Many scientists believe that there is an hereditary factor operating, since 60% to 80% of these patients come from families in which this illness has been prominent.

The psychiatrists who accept the theoretical explanations of behavior that have been developed by the psychoanalytic school believe that extreme mood deviations involving elation and depression are closely related to the early feeding experiences of the infant. During this period the mother who provides food and attention is both an object of love and a source of frustration for the infant. Ambivalent feelings of both love and hate for the mothering person may be initiated in this early period and may be carried on throughout life. In adult life ambivalent feelings are directed toward the environment and the significant persons in the environment. Individuals who develop the manic-depressive psychosis are thought to be reacting to the unconscious loss of a real or phantasied love object that was incorporated at an early phase of personality development. The individual first responds as if mourning for the lost love object and eventually begins to express hostility because he feels abandoned. The aggressive, overactive, elated individual directs his hostility toward the environment. The overactivity of the manic phase of this psychosis is thought to be a defense against the real problem of depression.

In the depressed phase of this psychosis the patient turns his hostility toward himself. He eventually concludes that he is at fault, that he is responsible for the loss of the love object, and that he is unworthy; thus he hates himself. He is said to be at the mercy of a punishing, sadistic super-ego. Such an individual has many narcissistic love needs. His adult relationships are likely to be immature and dependent.

MEETING THE NURSING NEEDS OF THE DEPRESSED PATIENT

The depressed patient expresses overwhelming feelings of guilt, ideas of self-depreciation, and self-accusatory delusions. The need that many inexperienced nurses feel to "cheer him up" is not helpful and often actually causes him to feel more guilty and unworthy than ever. When working with a depressed patient such statements as "Buck up." "Let's see you smile." or "There is a silver lining in every cloud." are not helpful. Gaiety and laughter have a tendency to make such a patient feel more guilty and thus more morose. The nurse can help this type of patient most by being friendly in a kind, understanding, businesslike way. Attempts at changing his mood through logical suggestions are fruitless and should be avoided. Sometimes just sitting beside the patient without trying to carry on a conversation is most helpful. At other times it is well to talk to the patient even though he may not answer. He will appreciate the personal interest being shown. Patience is the keynote in working with depressed individuals who are so greatly retarded in the spheres of thinking, feeling, and acting that every movement or word requires great effort and much time. The same question often needs to be asked more than once, and the nurse must wait patiently for the

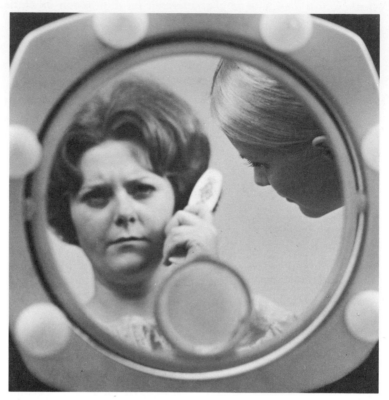

FIG. 13. *The nurse encourages patients to take pride in their physical appearance.*

answer. A large part of the therapeutic value of the hospital situation lies in the fact that decisions can be made for the patient. Thus the nurse should avoid asking such questions as "Do you want to take your bath now?" A more positive approach would be "Your bath is ready now. I will help you with it."

Physical care

Since depressed patients are retarded in thinking and action, most activity will need to be initiated for them. They are likely to develop certain distressing physical conditions because of inactivity. Some of the most common of these complications are fecal impactions, edema of the extremities, and pneumonia. Infections are common, and since such patients tend

to ignore the physical condition of their bodies, it is necessary for the nurse to be particularly alert during the daily bath.

Perhaps the most effective way of caring for a depressed patient is to place him on a simple daily schedule. Much encouragement and reassurance throughout each day will be required to help him follow the schedule.

These patients often need to be supplied with extra clothing. They exercise very little and frequently become chilled without appearing to realize it. The nurse should be vigilant in supplying sweaters, warm underwear, and warm stockings for the depressed patient.

Encouraging depressed patients to take pride in their personal appearance is part of their care. This is difficult because it is in opposition to their tendency to self-depreciation. Careful supervision of personal hygiene with attention to supplying clean clothing and helping the patients dress neatly is important in developing pride in personal appearance. Female patients need to be encouraged to accept appointments at the hospital beauty parlor, and male patients to go to the barbershop regularly. If a depressed patient is actively suicidal, it may be safer to ask the barber or beauty operator to come to the ward where the patient is hospitalized, rather than to send the patient to the operator.

Many depressed patients present a difficult feeding problem. It is helpful if the nurse can discover why the patient refuses food. It is not uncommon for these patients to refuse to eat because they believe they are unworthy of receiving food. Some depressed patients may say that they do not deserve food because they have not paid for it. Still others seek to destroy themselves through starvation. Many of these patients have simply lost a desire for food, along with all the other interests they formerly had in life. The inactivity of hospitalization also contributes to a lack of interest in food.

Finding a way to combat the depressed patient's failure to eat is dependent upon the reason for which the food is being refused. If failure to eat is caused by a feeling of unworthiness or the thought that the food has not been paid for, the patient may be reassured by being told that the food is prepared for all the patients because the hospital is interested in all patients regardless of whether they pay or not. It might be helpful to give the patient an opportunity to wash dishes or do some other simple tasks to give him a feeling of "paying" for the food. If the patient is attempting to starve himself, little can be done except to feed him mechanically.

Because depressed patients are susceptible to infection, it is important that their food and fluid intake be maintained. Every method of encouraging food intake should be employed. Some suggestions include providing physical exercise for the patient, serving him small attractively prepared meals, serving foods that the patient formerly enjoyed, allowing his family to bring in food, and to spoon-feed him if this seems to encourage him to eat. Although appetizers such as medicinal tonics, whiskey before meals, and small doses of regular insulin before meals probably should be tried, they usually have not been helpful in combating loss of appetite due to psychological causes.

Depressed patients often present a nursing problem because of their inability to sleep at night. Some of these patients become agitated during the night hours, and, because their tenseness and anxiety are increased, they may feel a need to pace the floor. The usual aids, such as warm sedative tub baths, cold wet sheet packs, and some hypnotic drugs, may be of benefit to individual patients. However, some patients do not seem to profit a great deal from any of these aids. If the physician believes in the use of electro-coma therapy, the nursing problems presented by the depressed patient will usually be decreased after this treatment is initiated. Many of the tranquilizing drugs are helpful in treating agitated patients.

THE SELF-DESTRUCTIVE SUICIDAL PATIENT

A mentally ill patient's need to injure or destroy himself is one of the most serious problems with which the personnel of a psychiatric hospital are confronted. The most effective methods for dealing with this problem vary, depending on the situation and the patient. However, there are some basic principles concerning care of the self-destructive patient with which every nurse should be fully acquainted.

Many psychiatric facilities take the position that they are primarily concerned with the patient's physical safety. This concern takes precedence over providing emotionally therapeutic experiences. Sometimes an attempt is made to ensure the patient's safety by removing from his environment all the equipment he might use to do injury to himself. This is extremely difficult because every piece of clothing, all eating utensils, cigarettes, furniture, bathroom equipment—literally everything an individual needs in the process of daily living—could be used if the individual wished to injure or destroy himself. One patient strangled herself by using a toothbrush to fashion a tourniquet from her long braided hair; another patient dived headlong into the toilet and suffered a serious head wound; the third patient destroyed herself by using the armhole of her knitted underwear as a noose; and a fourth patient injured herself seriously by setting fire to her dress with a cigarette. If the philosophy of making the environment safe is carried to its logical conclusion, the patient may be placed in an absolutely barren room with a pallet upon which to lie. To make self-destruction even more unlikely, hospitals have frequently followed the plan of placing the patient under constant observation so that he is observed by a hospital worker during every minute of the day and night. Variations of this procedure have been developed for patients who are thought to have less need to injure or destroy themselves. At best this procedure of environmental control and constant observation is only a preventive measure. Depriving patients of freedom to move about and placing them under constant observation may increase their self-destructive tendencies. This procedure may convince them that their worst fears are true and that they are worthless and unworthy or that they have committed an unforgivable crime and are being justly punished.

Some phychiatric facilities have attempted to handle a patient's self-destructive tendencies by developing a therapeutic environment to help build his self-esteem. Instead of removing all the potentially dangerous weapons from the environment, an attempt has been made to meet his emotional needs. This has been done by assigning a hospital worker, preferably a skilled nurse, to work constantly with the patient. The nurse helps him participate in occupational, social, and recreational activities. Subtly and appropriately she seeks ways to reassure the patient that he is a worthwhile, useful human being. The patient is constantly under close supervision, but the focus for the supervision has moved from watching him constantly as a preventive measure to helping him direct his drives and interests into constructive channels. The emphasis should probably be upon supplying safe opportunities for active participation in the daily hospital routine rather than upon removing all dangerous tools from the patient's environment.

It is essential that the nurse be thoroughly familiar with the self-destructive patient. She must be constantly aware of his every activity. In fact, nurses who work with psychiatric patients need to cultivate the ability to be constantly alert to all patients, their moods, their needs, and their minute-by-minute activities.

"A patient who talks about suicide never does it" is a common belief that every nurse should recognize as a serious fallacy. People usually talk about the thoughts that are uppermost in their minds. A patient alludes to suicide because he is thinking about it and immediately should be assigned to a hospital worker for special attention and help. All hospital personnel should be made aware of the patients on the unit who are thought to have self-destructive tendencies. Special attention should be given to any individuals who look or act depressed, who make statements about life not being worth living, who suggest that they may not be around much longer, or who have actually injured themselves during a previous illness. Some authorities believe that all patients give warnings of impending suicide. Hospital personnel need to be so well acquainted with the patients with whom they work that they will be able to interpret the cues that patients give.

If patients are able to feel that the hospital personnel are truely interested in them, if their needs for recognition and emotional support are being met, and if they are busily engaged in interesting occupational and recreational activities, the incidence of attempts at self-destruction will be greatly lessened.

Providing activity to relieve guilt feelings

Many authorities believe that depression is a problem involving hostility that the patient has turned against himself. Thus it is thought that the depressed patient has feelings of guilt and unworthiness that give rise to suicidal tendencies, refusal of food, inability to sleep, and loss of interest in personal appearance. The patient's guilt may be relieved when he receives what he feels to be adequate punishment for his "sins" and can thus "make atonement" for his guilt. This reaction may be the secret of the therapeutic value that electrocoma therapy has for such patients.

One of the methods by which a nurse may contribute to the care of the depressed patient is to provide him with tasks that will help relieve his sense of guilt. Depressed patients have been known to ask for such menial tasks as scrubbing the floor, scouring the toilets, washing dirty socks that belong to other patients, washing windows, or scrubbing the walls. Such tasks may provide a real therapeutic release for the guilt of the depressed individual and a means of atonement for sins. Although providing such experiences is contrary to the procedure followed in many hospitals, it has proved to be of great value to selected patients. Such treatment for depressed patients should not be carried out without the full approval of the physician.

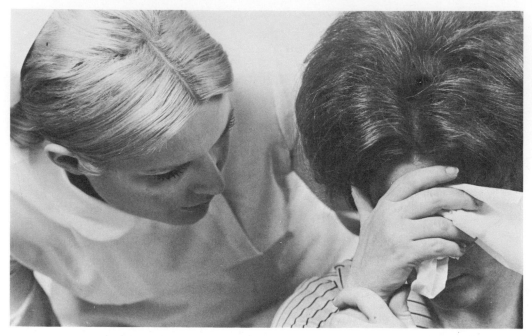

FIG. 14. *The nurse strives to understand the problems of the depressed patient.*

Recognizing cues to suicidal behavior

Electrocoma therapy and some of the more modern drugs have been successful, to some degree, in lifting the mood of many depressed patients. However, the problem of recognizing the potentially suicidal patient and safeguarding against the possibility of the patient's injuring himself is one of the most important responsibilities of the nurse.

Patients are usually thought to be potentially suicidal when they talk about death, speak about the uselessness of life, or conceal equipment that might be used for injuring themselves. All patients who appear to be depressed are also thought to be possible suicidal risks. It is important for the nurse to be well acquainted with her patients so that she can detect mood changes. Patients frequently provide cues to their feelings and to their intended behavior, but it is necessary for someone to be keenly aware of them as human beings to recognize the cues. If

the cue is recognized, the patient can be saved from his own hostile feelings by the provision of more vigilant care.

It is important to understand what the patient is communicating through his suicidal behavior. He may be saying that he is worthless and does not deserve to live or that life is meaningless and he does not want to live. He may be telling us that he feels angry and resentful toward other people or toward himself, or he may be saying that he feels so all alone that he cannot tolerate the situation any longer. In any case, his behavior is a cry for help.

When the nurse recognizes that a patient has self-destructive thoughts and may carry out these impulses, other members of the hospital staff should be alerted.

Intensive nursing care around the clock is required until the patient is no longer a danger to himself. A fine balance between allowing the patient enough freedom and at the same time being sure that he is safeguarded against his own hostile drives is a difficult but a necessary compromise.

Treatment of depression with drugs or electroconvulsive therapy

Many drugs have been used with depressed patients in the hope of elevating the mood of the individual, but few have proved to have any consistent or permanent value. Recently several of the newer drugs have been more or less successful in their action as antidepressants. Combinations of dextroamphetamine and a quick-acting barbiturate such as amobarbital have been most popular.

Although there are several so-called antidepressants, they all have undesirable and even dangerous side effects. When they are used, the nurse needs to be vigilant in watching for such untoward reactions as low blood pressure, dizziness, vertigo, extreme restlessness, blurred vision, dry mouth, sweating, edema, skin rash, constipation, and delayed micturition.

Far more successful and in many cases decidedly miraculous in its effects has been electroconvulsive therapy. A series of six to eight convulsions will frequently relieve the worst symptoms of depression and will induce the patient to assume a radically different and even optimistic attitude. Morbid ideas are no longer expressed, animation reappears, and sleep and appetite become normal.

Prolonged psychotherapy is required if the patient is to be helped to face his underlying emotional problems and work toward solving them in order to avoid a recurrence of the illness.

MIDLIFE DEPRESSION—INVOLUTIONAL MELANCHOLIA

The true involutional psychoses are based on deeper and more complicated factors than a mere diminution of sexual and endocrine activity, although one must concede that these play a minor or aggravating role. Probably more important are various temperamental and psychological elements in the personality of those who suffer with mental upset at the involutional period. A review of the life history of most of these patients reveals certain traits, habits, and dispositions that merely become exaggerated to the point where they must be regarded as abnormal. People who have lived narrow social lives, who have been overmeticulous, sensitive, and rigid in their daily habits are prone to develop a midlife depression. Depressions that appear for the first time in the middle years carry the designation of "involutional melancholia." For a time it was believed that the condition was merely another variety of manic-depressive psychosis. In a few cases the depressed phase that appears in the involutional period may be merely a duplication of previous attacks of manic-depressive psychosis. However, in most instances the agitation, the delusions of sin, and the extreme hypochondriasis appearing for the first time at the involutional period constitute a definite and separate clinical picture. Midlife depressions, like the depressive phase of manic-depressive psychosis, are precipitated by the loss of a love object, a change in status, such as a demotion or retirement, or the fear of loss of personal attractiveness. The dynamics are essentially the same as in other depressions.

The disease generally develops in an insidious fashion. The patient becomes progressively more tense and sleepless, has unprovoked spells of weeping, complains of a feeling of pressure in the head, and worries excessively about minor matters. Obsessive preoccupation with some trifling misdemeanor committed sometime in the past, a desire to confess unpardonable sins, and a marked agitation, with weeping and wringing of the hands, announce the acute phase of the mental upset. The patient may express the feeling that there is no hope, that she will be jailed and put to death. Suicidal impulsions are frequently demonstrated. The patient may refuse to eat because of somatic delusions such as a fear that she has no stomach or intestines or because of paranoid delusions such as fear that the food is poisoned. So-called nihilistic delusions, which deny the existence of things that no longer interest the patient, such as home, husband, and children, are outstanding. With all this agitation the patient usually realizes that he or she is ill; orientation is good, and memory is not badly impaired. Involutional psychosis occurs in both men and women but four times as often in women, who usually are in the late forties when the attack is recognized. Men are usually in the late fifties.

Prognosis

The outlook for the agitated and depressed types of involutional psychosis is fairly good, particularly if the prepsychotic personality is not badly warped. Approximately 80% of such patients improve, although recovery may not take place until after as many as eight years.

Electroconvulsive therapy is extremely beneficial in treating midlife depressions.

MEETING THE NURSING NEEDS OF THE ELATED, OVERACTIVE PATIENT
The nurse's approach

Individuals who are suffering from elation and overactivity require skillful and tactful nursing care. Most of these patients are acutely aware of reality and react strongly to environmental stimuli. Because these patients misidentify individuals with whom they come in contact, they may like or dislike a nurse because she reminds them of someone they once knew. Such patients are often bitingly sarcastic and pointedly profane and vulgar. Frequently they discover a physical or personality defect about which the nurse is sensitive and delight in repeatedly calling attention to this defect. Along with an elated affect they are extremely overactive in both the mental and physical spheres. Such patients are easily irritated and angered.

Whether the nurse can help elated, overactive patients depends to a large extent upon the attitude with which she approaches them. The tone of voice employed by the nurse in speaking to the patient is of primary importance. A firm, kind, low-pitched voice that carries a coaxing quality probably is most effective. The nurse who uses a loud demanding tone is defeated before she starts because this type of approach may cause the patient to become hostile and aggressive.

It is useless to attempt to hurry the elated patient because such an approach will result in anger and hostility. Thus the attitude of having all the time in the world to accomplish a procedure will be much more effective. Quiet persuasion is one of the chief aids in getting the elated patient to conform to the essential aspects of ward routine.

Consistent fairness and honesty in dealing with such patients are essential if one is to maintain rapport with them throughout a period of time. Although these individuals deserve and must have simple, honest explanations concerning their hospital environment, long discussions and explanations should be avoided, since such activities provoke irritability.

Because the elated, overactive patient's thoughts rapidly fly from one thing to another, he is described as being distractible. The skillful nurse makes use of the patient's inability to maintain sustained attention by directing his thoughts away from factors in the environment that encourage his destructive tendencies, provoke his irritability, or increase his excitement.

In dealing with the overactive, elated patient the nurse must recognize that the behavior she finds so difficult is a result of a mental illness and will be replaced by socially acceptable behavior when the patient is well again. The inexperienced nurse may be embarrassed by the loud talking, the vulgarity and profanity, the destructive activity, and the overt sexual behavior she observes. However, part of the skillful care of such a patient includes understanding why he needs to behave in such a way. With understanding will come acceptance of behavior.

The psychiatric nurse who is permissive and accepting of the behavior of the elated patient will not scold or shame him for his uninhibited actions or become angered by the patient's pointed, biting remarks because she will understand that they are a part of the patient's illness.

Simplifying
the environment

Since all elated, overactive patients are stimulated by environmental factors, one of the first responsibilities of the nurse is to simplify their surroundings and insofar as possible to provide a sedative environment for them. The nurse and the physician should decide together the best methods of accomplishing this simplification. Because other people irritate the elated patient and provoke him to engage in an excessive amount of talking, it is wise to place such an individual in a single room. The room should be as far away from the daily activity of the ward as possible and yet should be easily accessible to the head nurse who needs to be constantly aware of the patient and his behavior. Pictures and colorful drapes probably should be eliminated, since they may be too stimulating and certainly may be destroyed in a burst of excitement. Unnecessary furniture, such as a small table or a light chair, may be used by the patient as a weapon if he becomes extremely irritated. Care of the overactive patient must be individualized, depending on the degree of his elation and the amount of his excessive energy. It is usually wise to limit the number of persons who come in contact with him. Only a few persons, chosen because of their patience and understanding approach, should be assigned to his care.

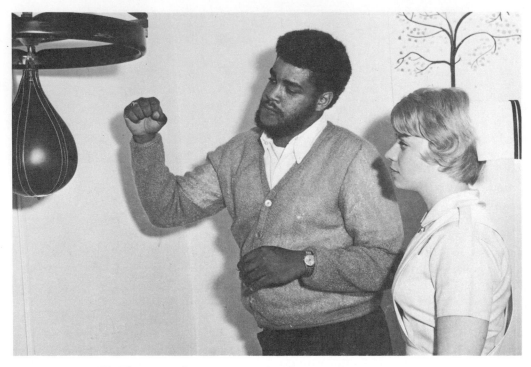

FIG. 15. *The nurse devises ways of redirecting excessive energy into acceptable channels.*

Controlling excessive energy

The overactive patient is suffering from a tremendous burst of energy for which he must find some outlet. Usually the patient has been admitted to the hospital because the outlets that he has chosen for his energy have been dangerous to him or to his family or offensive to other people. The nurse is confronted with the task of controlling or redirecting this excessive energy into more acceptable channels. She is guided by the written suggestions of the physician who takes into consideration the patient's physical condition, interests, and degree of psychiatric disability.

An excellent outlet for the excessive energy of individuals who are only mildly elated is writing. Most of these patients are eager to write their life story or to disclose the deficiencies of the hospital to the world and thus will readily put paper and pencil to use. Many mildly elated patients will be content to spend hours over their manuscripts.

Another outlet for excessive energy is provided by some of the housekeeping tasks of the ward. The nurse needs to be constantly aware of the possibility that the overactive patient may become physically exhausted. However, sweeping, dusting, and scrubbing are acceptable outlets for the excessive energy of certain patients, if careful supervision is provided. Tearing rags for rag rugs, folding paper napkins, folding linen, raking grass, and mowing the lawn are other activities that are useful outlets for energy. The activities chosen for these patients should require large sweeping movements, since they will become annoyed and lose interest in anything requiring fine, discriminative skills. Games such as table tennis, croquet, badminton, and medicine ball are often helpful as outlets for energy, provided there is no element of competition present. In competitive games the elated patient becomes overly stimulated and excited.

Formerly the sedative tub bath, the cold wet sheet pack, and various hypnotic drugs were administered to control excessive energy. Today overactive behavior is successfully controlled by chlorpromazine or one of the other tranquilizing agents.

At times, for the sake of the patient, it is essential to escort him to another part of the ward or hospital. Even after a simple explanation and much persuasion have been tried, some excited patients may resist this necessary maneuver and may even become combative if forced to cooperate. The issue should never be forced unless it is absolutely essential that he conform. When such an instance arises in which the patient must be helped to cooperate, the nurse should first obtain an ample number of people to assist in accomplishing the task. Then together, under the leadership of one professional person, a plan of approach to the patient should be formulated. After each worker is certain about his role, the group should approach the patient and put the plan of strategy into effect.

It is extremely unwise from a therapeutic point of view to threaten an excited patient or to suggest that he will be punished because of his nonconforming behavior. Such a maneuver usually results in increased hostility on the part of the patient. If the patient is directed in an understanding and sympathetic way and his behavior is accepted as part of his illness, it is usually possible to redirect

his energy without resorting to the use of restraints. With the advent of the tranquilizing drugs, mechanical restraint of overactive patients have been practically eliminated.

THE ANXIOUS, FEARFUL, DESTRUCTIVE PATIENT WHO IS IN A PANIC

A few mentally ill patients are admitted to the hospital because they exhibit behavior that is dangerous to themselves or others. Patients who suffer from intense feelings of fear, anger, hostility, or suspicion are said to be in a panic. Such feelings may cause patients to strike out against other people or the environment in general. Patients who strike out against others are dangerous and cause other patients to become frightened. Therefore it is essential to prevent this type of behavior, if possible, and to check it if it is precipitated.

Usually a patient who strikes out against his environment does so because he is terrified. He may be afraid of what he believes other patients and the personnel will do to him, or he may be undergoing terrifying hallucinatory experiences. If the latter is happening, the voices may be telling him what physical and mental tortures are awaiting him. It is obvious that a terrified patient can be helped only by someone who is in control of her own fear and can approach the patient calmly. Uncontrolled fear on the part of hospital personnel is extremely upsetting to patients.

When a patient becomes terrified, a calm, quiet member of the hospital staff should persuade the upset patient to enter a room that is away from the other patients. It may be that the disturbed patient will need to be carried away from the group if he is too upset to be persuaded. If the patient must be physically removed from the group, adequate personnel should be called together to make it possible to achieve this safely. The exact role that each of the hospital personnel is to carry out should be decided before any attempt is made to approach the patient. When the personnel are ready, they should approach the patient quietly and in a friendly way. An explanation should be provided concerning what the personnel believe would be best for him. He should be given every opportunity to comply with the request. If the patient is still unable to accept the persuasion of the group, it then becomes necessary for the personnel to pick him up and carry him, firmly but kindly, to a quiet room. If possible, some member of the staff who has a good relationship with the patient should remain in the quiet room. If the patient is considered dangerous or the personnel are afraid to remain alone with him, a second or even a third additional person should remain in the room until his fear or anger has subsided. When personnel are in short supply, it may be necessary to place the patient in a locked room alone. This is unfortunate, but if it is necessary some member of the staff should visit him at least every 15 minutes. He should be made as physically comfortable as possible and should be allowed to leave the quiet room as soon as he feels that he is able to do so or as soon as the staff feel that he can tolerate group living again.

More important than managing de-structive, threatening behavior is learning to avoid it. The first step in learning to avoid problem behavior is to discover the situations that are upsetting to patients and how to keep these from occurring. The nurse needs to learn to recognize the signs of an approaching emotional outburst and to employ measures that will help the patient to handle his negative feelings without acting out against the environment. Destructive behavior on the part of terrified, angry patients is rare in psychiatric facilities where an attempt is made to recognize and meet emotional needs and where the personnel recognize the importance of developing positive interpersonal relationships with patients.

Physical care

An overactive patient often loses a great deal of weight and may become severely dehydrated. This problem is exaggerated by the fact that he often does not take time to eat or drink and may sleep only 1 or 2 hours each night. He is often oblivious to physical injury or pain. Consequently the nurse needs to be vigilantly aware of such a patient's physical needs as well as his emotional ones.

Prevention of injury is one of the responsibilities of the nurse. Overactive patients are likely to injure themselves in a burst of elation and excitement and may disregard even such a serious trauma as a broken bone.

Keeping overactive patients warmly dressed during cold weather is sometimes a real challenge, since clothing may be an irritating factor to these people. Because clothing may impede the movement of arms and legs, excited patients may tear it off. Such patients often appear totally unaware of body temperature and must be safeguarded against becoming chilled.

Since constipation, fecal impaction, bladder distention, or other difficulties may be present but ignored by the patient, the nurse should observe the patient carefully.

Ensuring sufficient sleep for the excited patient is another challenge to the nurse. This is important, since exhaustion and even death have been known to result from long-continued failure of the patient to sleep. Many of these patients are so alert to all environmental stimuli that they sleep only 1 to 2 hours out of every 24. Some helpful measures to aid in producing sleep include either a sedative tub bath or a cold wet sheet pack just before the patient retires for the night. The choice of this type of treatment depends on the doctor's preference, the patient's physical condition, and the manner in which the patient accepts the treatment. Some hypnotic drugs are helpful, but occasionally they may increase the patient's excitement. The problem of wakefulness has practically disappeared with the introduction of the new tranquilizing drugs, particularly chlorpromazine.

Electroconvulsive therapy, which is employed by some physicians in treating excited patients, is often helpful in making it possible for these patients to sleep. In fact, this treatment may lessen the patient's elation and excitement to such an extent that all nursing procedures can be carried out effectively.

Excited and elated patients may not take time to sit down to eat. In such an instance it is wise to serve food that the patient can carry about in his hands. Sandwiches, fruit, and cupcakes are dietary items that he may "eat on the run." Sometimes the nurse is more successful if she follows the patient about with his tray and offers him food when she is able to obtain his attention for a moment. Elated, overactive patients require a high caloric intake and should have between-meal nourishment. Nurses are likely to disregard such a patient's need for fluids, since water fountains are usually available. However, the excited patient often does not take time to drink and should have water offered to him each hour.

If the patient is allowed to have his food on a tray and will take time to feed himself, the equipment on the tray should be very simple and unbreakable. As in every other aspect of the care of these overactive, elated patients, the nursing procedures must be individualized to meet the specific patient's needs. In some instances the elated individual may get along well in the dining room setting if he is under careful supervision. However, in most instances the elated patient is so stimulated by the dining room situation that it is more helpful if he is placed on tray service.

Although the patient should be encouraged to perform his own personal hygiene, he needs to be supervised closely. Some overactive, elated patients are too ill to assume any responsibility for their physical care and may need to have much of it given by the nurse. Other less excited patients can take a good deal of responsibility for their own cleanliness and grooming if a nurse stays with them and skillfully directs their activities. The nurse needs to remember that the patient may become playful and mischievous in the bathroom. Because of poor judgment these patients have been found washing their hair in the toilet bowl, throwing water about with gay abandon, or in various other ways reducing the bathroom to a shambles. It is for this reason that such patients should not be left alone in the bathroom.

The mouth of the overactive patient requires special attention, and lubrication should be applied to the lips regularly.

Most overactive patients require hospitalization, since both they and society need to be safeguarded against the results of their faulty judgment. These patients are likely to swing from elation into depression and must be guarded vigilantly against the possibility of suicide as the elation subsides.

Medical treatment

The tranquilizing agents, particularly the phenothiazines, have revolutionized the treatment of overactive, abnormally elated, and excited patients, and noisy wards in the modern psychiatric hospital are rapidly becoming a thing of the past.

The tranquilizing drugs have been so dramatic in controlling agitation, excitement, and increased psychomotor drive that the more drastic and cumbersome treatments, such as electrocoma, injections of convulsion-producing pentylenetetrazol (Metrazol), continuous baths, and prolonged narcosis treatments, have been virtually abandoned.

Psychotherapy is essential if the patient is to be helped to solve his underlying emotional problems and avoid a recurrence of the illness.

Case report of an overactive patient

The following is a fairly typical case history of a patient who was hospitalized because of overactive, elated behavior.

M. H., 48 years of age, was a real estate salesman by occupation. His mother had a mental illness at 46 years of age, which was probably a melancholia. He had been educated in private schools and earned a college degree in business administration. During his junior year in college, he failed to win a scholarship and became morose, sleepless, and nervous for a period of two months. A few years after finishing college he entered an auto sales contest and won first prize, a trip to Havana. While on this trip he became overactive and insisted on eating every meal at the captain's table, where he told obscene stories and embarrassed the women passengers. He participated in frequent brawls with the stewards and complained to the purser on the slightest provocation. On disembarking at New York, he refused to return to his home city. He demanded the most pretentious accommodations at the hotel, and, when these were unavailable, he entered into a noisy altercation with the manager that resulted in his being sent to a psychiatric hospital. He remained there for three months and then returned to his parents' home.

The present attack began about six weeks before admission. At that time he was engaged in selling real estate in a new subdivision. He became extremely active, arose early, and accosted prospective clients at bus terminals, waiting rooms, and hotel corridors. He talked in such a convincing manner that he made a good record in the first week of the sale. The patient continued to send in many deposits, bragged about his sales ability, argued noisily with his fellow salesmen, and finally was arrested because he failed to pay his fare on a city bus. He then entered a damage suit against the company for $100,-000. The attorney who was approached realized the absurdities of the patient's claims and filed the charges against the patient.

Immediately after admission he demanded to see the head physician and requested permission to use the telephone. He was fairly coherent but was circumstantial in his conversation. When asked a simple question, his reply was a long, rambling, and digressive account. After being continually reminded to answer the question pointedly, he did so, only to return to another long digression. He made unreasonable demands of the nurses and attendants and, if refused, became abusive, sarcastic, and irritable. At this time it was discovered that when a client had refused to make a down payment on a lot, the patient had drawn the sum out of his own bank account and had forged a signature on the sales contract. This explained his amazing sales success.

He spent much of his time in the hospital writing letters to the mayor, various attorneys, and influential citizens. He wrote on odd pieces of paper, with pencil and in a broad, sweeping hand, underlining almost every other word, and capitalizing others. Every day he met the physicians at the door of the ward and began to revile them. He particularly enjoyed arguing with the doctors, demanding evidence to prove that he was insane and consistently denying all charges of misbehavior. In a loud voice he promised to have the hospital superintendent removed, the doctors exposed as quacks, and the orderlies jailed for beating him. He was suggestively lewd in his conversation with all nurses except a student nurse to whom he proposed marriage. When it was pointed out to him that he was already married, he harshly announced that he would divorce his wife because "she leaves me in this crazy dump."

Throughout the ten weeks he remained in the hospital, he was the constant center of commotion, a chronic critic of everything and everybody about him, consistently refusing all medication, collecting and hoarding papers, combs, magazines, and all sorts of trash, and acquiring many bruises in frequent scuffles with other patients. Occasionally he was very agreeable and jolly, particularly if he was allowed to do all the talking. On these occasions he was fond of reciting cheap parodies of famous poems in a quick witty fashion. Some of these he had not quoted since his high school days.

Although he believed that he was wrongfully incarcerated and that he was being abused, he harbored no other delusional ideas and at no time was he confused or hallucinated. His intellect was keen and his memory, particularly for trivial things, remarkable, but he had no insight into his abnormal exaltation and irritability and his judgment was poor.

Discussion of case report

Elated, overactive behavior is thought to be an unconscious defense against depression in individuals fixated at the oral-sadistic level of psychosexual development. In very early life such individuals are thought to have sought acceptance from parents by becoming compliant, obedient, and hardworking.

The patient in this situation first experienced a depression at about the age of 21 when he failed to win a scholarship in college. To him this failure to achieve a prized goal represented a failure in life, and he became depressed in an unconscious effort to punish himself as his parents might have done when he failed to fulfill some expectation of theirs. For two months he had typical symptoms of a mild depression. He was morose, sleepless, and nervous.

A few years later he won a coveted prize in an auto sales contest. This award was a trip to Havana that eventually resulted in psychiatric hospitalization for three months because of overactivity. In this instance the patient probably developed anxiety over the future expectations of his company. He may have reasoned that they would undoubtedly expect more and bigger sales records from him now that he had been able to achieve the award of a trip to Havana. The anxiety about being able to fulfill the future expectations of his company changed into guilt feelings that in turn caused him to feel that somehow he should be punished. To guard against the depressed feelings that arise from a sense of failure and a need to be punished he developed overactivity and elation—the defense against depression.

Several years later he became involved again in a competitive selling activity. His unconscious need to succeed in order to fulfill introjected parental expectations started the chain reaction again. Thus anxiety about succeeding caused him to feel gulity about the possibility of failing, and this in turn caused him to expect punishment that led to the depressed feelings that accompany a loss. The loss was the failure in selling, which in his own mind had already occurred. Thus the unconscious defense against depressed feelings are again utilized. The patient became expansive, overactive, argumentative, sarcastic, irritable, made unreasonable demands, and became a constant center of commotion. In a sense of the word he did not give himself time to become depressed because he was too busy striking out against his environment in an orally sadistic way.

Typically he was not delusional, and he did not experience hallucinations. Thus he was constantly in touch with reality. His intellect was as keen as ever, and his memory was intact.

Some inexperienced people might conclude that the patient was not mentally ill. However, he was unreasonable and sometimes abusive when he did not get his own way. He also wrote letters to outside authorities because he believed he should not be hospitalized, and he constantly sought to expose the hospital personnel for their inefficient handling of the situation.

He had no insight into his condition, and his judgment was impaired.

This mild attack of overactivity lasted for ten weeks. At the end of this time he was able to return to his home.

This patient's mother suffered from a midlife depression. Too little is known about this situation to do more than suggest that the mother was herself fixated at the oral-sadistic level of psychosexual development, since she apparently directed hostility toward herself.

This type of personality structure undoubtedly made it difficult for her to give her son the sense of security he required as an infant to develop into a well-adjusted adult.

Suggestions concerning nursing care for Mr. M. H.

The members of the nursing staff assigned to care for Mr. M. H. were chosen carefully because his verbally hostile and physically aggressive behavior was difficult to accept. Not all nurses were able to control their feelings about his vulgar comments and understand objectively why it was impossible for him to control his behavior. In addition, he related more positively to some nurses than to others. Finally, some nurses enjoyed working with Mr. M. H., and others did not. All these factors were considered when choosing nurses to work with him.

The nursing staff decided that it would be best for him to be cared for in a unit of the hospital where a single room was available. In such a room it was possible to eliminate all but the essential furnishings. The single room was helpful in avoiding the overstimulation that might have resulted from his being assigned to a dormitory sleeping accommodation where he would have been involved with many other patients.

His recreational activities needed to be controlled because it was obvious that he became loud and disruptive when involved in competitive games. He became angry when he scored lower than other players in a game and accused them of cheating. These accusations usually brought on loud arguments and sometimes fights.

When it was necessary for the nursing staff to intervene in such an altercation, they took advantage of Mr. M. H.'s distractibility and subtly redirected his attention away from the argument to an activity that could be carried on in his room with only one other person, one who was able to tolerate his rapid conversation and accept his pointed criticism.

The members of the nursing staff were careful to avoid scolding or threatening Mr. M. H. when he initiated fights with other patients. They avoided comparing his behavior with that of other better controlled patients or even with his own behavior on a day when he was less noisy. The nursing staff realized that his problem behavior was part of his illness.

Mr. M. H. responded negatively to any member of the staff who attempted to speak to him somewhat sharply or who commanded him to do anything. They learned that he could not be hurried and that their approach was much more effective if they were quiet, friendly, and courteous to him and used a pleasant, businesslike tone of voice. On one occasion when a staff member did order him to comply with a hospital rule, he refused and never let the individual forget the incident.

They discovered that it was unwise to encourage Mr. M. H. when he was reciting or singing parodies or telling jokes. When some staff members did laugh at his jokes he became much louder and more ribald. It was necessary for them to intervene by accompanying him to his room before he became so excited that he could not be controlled.

In talking to Mr. M. H. the nursing staff avoided getting into long, complicated discussions or giving elaborate explanations. Instead, short sentences with specific, straightforward reponses to his questions seemed to satisfy him and avoided arguments.

The nurses were careful when giving Mr. M. H. praise. They found that he sometimes turned the words of praise around and used them in a different context to refute a point they had been trying to make with him sometime previously.

They were aware of his physical needs and realized that he frequently did not eat enough. This problem arose because his attention was distracted from the food or he left the dining room early before finishing the meal. Likewise, he sometimes had dry, cracked lips because he failed to maintain his fluid intake. Mr. M. H. was weighed every week, and when his weight had dropped below a desirable point for two consecutive weeks, his food was served in his room on a tray. A nurse remained with him during the meal and encouraged him to eat. Removing him from the dining room served to eliminate the many distracting features present in a large group. At the same time he was placed on a schedule so that fluids were offered to him every hour.

Crayons, paper, and pencils were made available to him in his room, and he was encouraged to write and sketch there in the hope that these more sedentary activities would lessen his hyperactivity. The nurses were careful to explain to him in an honest, straightforward manner why he was not encouraged to join the rest of the patients in the dining room. In like manner all other restrictions on his behavior were explained so that he could understand the reason for them and realize that he was not being rejected as a person.

Mr. M. H. gained some control of his behavior and became quieter and more amenable to suggestion without the use of electroconvulsive therapy or drugs. The professional staff did not believe that he was well enough to leave the hospital permanently. However, at the request of his family, he was allowed to go home at the end of ten weeks. The psychiatrist gave him a temporary leave and planned to see him twice a week during his visit at home. In this way Mr. M. H. could be returned to the hospital if his family felt that he needed more help than they were able to provide.

Case report of a depressed patient

The following case history is a fairly typical example of a patient who was hospitalized because of a depression.

Mrs. C. B., 29 years of age, had been married three years and had one child 14 months of age. Family history revealed nothing significant, except that her father was stolid and slow-going. He had a reputation for being a pessimist but was otherwise a stable, sober individual.

Five years before marriage the patient had had a period of nervousness and depression, which lasted about three months. This was precipitated by an unfortunate love affair. At that time she was attending a summer course in education at a local university where she met a young man. He had encouraged her to believe he was greatly interested, but at the school outing that terminated the summer session he ignored her and danced with another girl. The patient came home, said little or nothing to her parents, and the following morning was found in bed in a stupor. She had taken twelve 1-grain phenobarbital tablets. She was rushed to a hospital, given emergency treatment, and then transferred to a nursing home where she remained eight weeks.

The present attack began about six weeks before admission to the hospital. Again the onset was rather abrupt. Her husband returned home from work one evening and found her sobbing. After much urging on his part, she confessed that she was crying because she was a bad mother and a poor housekeeper. The husband naturally assured her that she was quite the contrary, but this only brought more sobbing and self-depreciation. She worried excessively about a small scar on her baby's temple that was caused by chicken pox. She accused herself of "marking" the child. The family suspected that she was merely tired from her spring housecleaning and hired a girl to come in and care for the baby. Her sister-in-law was called in to act as a companion. For three weeks she remained at home. She complained of inability to concentrate and prayed a great deal of the time. The well-meaning sister-in-law encouraged her by suggesting that she "snap out of it," and this merely served to agitate her. She was finally taken to her parents in the country. On two occasions she was found walking along the country road, and when questioned as to her destination, she merely stated that she wanted to "run away from everything." Her husband came to visit her one Sunday afternoon and took her for an auto ride back into the city. She requested him to stop at their home, since she wanted some extra clothes for the baby. She went to the kitchen and, before the husband could realize what she was about to do, cut both her wrists with a carving knife. She was brought directly to the psychiatric hospital after receiving emergency treatment for her wounds in the accident room.

On the day of admission she was able to give a clear account of her actions but responded in a dull, apathetic manner. She frequently interjected the remark that she should be dead, but that she was too big a coward to take her own life. She accused herself of being a rank failure and asserted that she should never have been born. She cried but did not shed many tears. She complained of a "numb" feeling in her head, of inability to sleep, and of loss of appetite. The physical examination was entirely negative.

For several weeks she remained apathetic,

withdrawn, and indifferent. She ate only when coaxed by the nurses. To every nurse she announced that there was no sense in bothering about her, since she would die on the morrow. She never inquired about the welfare of her child and was indifferent about her husband during visiting hours. Although she was not particularly untidy, she was rather slipshod in appearance and made no attempt to comb her hair or keep herself presentable. She took little or no interest in ward activities and in her fellow patients.

In the sixth week of her hospital stay, she was given the first electroconvulsive treatment. This was followed by four more, at the end of which she rapidly improved. After being in the hospital for three months she began clamoring for discharge, insisting that she must go home to take care of her family. She was cheerful and industrious, and in occupational therapy she was particularly adept in teaching English to a small group of foreign women.

Discussion of case report

The situation in the case report presents a young woman who is demonstrating a good deal of hostility, which she has directed toward herself. Thus it must be concluded that she has introjected a harsh, punitive superego. She is therefore suffering from a conflict between the instinctual impulses of the id and the rigid controls of the superego.

The history gives us very little information about the present attack of depression. However, it does tell us about the first attack, which came as a result of the failure of an interpersonal relationship of great importance to her and the loss of a beloved object—a cherished lover. At that time she attempted suicide by taking an overdose of sleeping pills. This may have been an unconscious attempt to kill the introjected lover.

Authorities tell us that individuals who resort to self-destruction are frequently fixated at the oral-sadistic level of psychosexual development. During the oral period of the child's development the loved object (the mother or the mother's breast) is unconsciously introjected.

Later in life a loved object may unconsciously represent the original object that was introjected. When an individual attempts suicide she is seeking relief from suffering, punishment for herself, or attempting to kill the introjected person.

This young patient's child is in the toilet training period. It is at this period in the child's development that he becomes more self-assertive and begins to defy the mother. It may be that this mother views the change in her child from a dependent, passive organism requiring constant tender guidance to a self-assertive individual as a loss. In a sense she has lost a dependent organism and gained a demanding child. She may be overwhelmed with the new responsibilities precipitated by the child's development. Thus she blames herself for being a bad mother, a poor housekeeper, and having caused a small scar on the baby's temple.

Her physical symptoms were those commonly found among depressed patients: inability to sleep, loss of appetite, dull and apathetic appearance, physical inactivity as evidenced by sitting in a dark corner with head bowed, complaining of a numb feeling in the head, and crying without tears. Her emotional responses were also those frequently found among depressed individuals: inability to concentrate, self-accusatory ideas, suicidal ideas, feelings of unworthiness, and loss of interest in child and husband.

Characteristically she was able to give a clear account of all the experiences relating to her illness.

As with many other depressed patients, a short course of electrocoma therapy changed her entire outlook on life. This may have been because she perceived electrocoma therapy as the punishment she unconsciously felt she needed.

Suggestions concerning nursing care for Mrs. C. B.

When Mrs. C. B. was admitted to the hospital her bandaged wrists and sad facial expression pointed to the fact that she was depressed and suicidal. Such patients require special physical arrangements and security precautions. In view of these facts, individual nursing care was provided for her. Nurses with proven ability to work sucessfully with depressed patients were chosen to be with her at all times until she recovered from the acute phases of the depression. They recognized the importance of establishing rapport with Mrs. C. B. and set about to achieve this. Their goals for her care were to protect her from her self-destructive tendencies and to care for her in such a way that she would be sustained until she was able to accept responsibility for herself.

These nurses adopted a kind, courteous, firm, hopeful attitude toward Mrs. C. B. In this way they tried to convey the impression that she was not a hopeless case as she insisted. They listened carefully to everything that Mrs. C. B. said and answered her questions carefully without disputing or agreeing with her expressions of worthlessness. They accepted her silences when she did not wish to talk. They avoided using meaningless statements such as, "cheer up" or "you know your family loves you!"

The nurses who worked closely with Mrs. C. B. were aware of her physical needs in the areas of food and fluid intake and rest. They found that she ate better if served food on a tray in her room rather than going to the dining room with the other patients. To help her sleep she was given a warm tub bath just before bedtime and a cup of hot chocolate to drink. Even these strategies did not always make it possible for her to rest at night. If Mrs. C. B. wanted to sit up and talk or walk up and down the corridors the nurse who was assigned to stay with her at night accompanied her in these activities.

When Mrs. C. B. accused herself of being a rank failure, the nurses tried to help her express her hostility verbally toward her environment and other people. In this way they hoped to improve her own self-esteem by redirecting her anger away from herself.

When Mrs. C. B. was given electroconvulsive therapy, the nurses explained the procedure to her. They stressed the fact that the treatment would help her feel better and that one of them would stay with her during the experience and bring her back to her room after it was over. They continued this reassurance before each treatment because they realized that patients have no memory for the experience and need repeated reassurance.

The nurses made decisions for Mrs. C. B. until she was able to make them for herself. They tried to develop a congenial, pleasant living atmosphere for her while she remained in the hospital. They encouraged her to become interested in some of the activities available in the occupational therapy department and accompanied her there whenever she felt well enough to go. They decided during a discussion with the physician to refrain from introducing the menial tasks that are said to be helpful in redirecting the guilt of some depressed patients. This decision was made because it seemed to them that mopping a floor would cause Mrs. C. B. to feel rejected and inferior.

PROGNOSIS IN MANIC-DEPRESSIVE PSYCHOSIS

For a single episode of elation or depression the outlook is usually good, but recurrences are to be expected. However, second and third attacks need not necessarily occur in every case. An attack of elation in early adult life generally means more attacks later. Depressions are more likely to occur in the later years of life.

It is never safe to predict the probable duration of any given attack, since there are great variations, and even the same individual may have both short and long periods of elation and depression. The average for all untreated attacks of elation is about six months; for untreated depressive episodes it is generally longer. When depressive periods show a strong element of fear, anxiety, and hypochondriasis, the condition may endure for many years. Likewise, elation may become chronic, particularly in older individuals if it is associated with organic changes in the brain, such as arteriosclerosis. Modern treatments have shortened the length of the attacks in both elation and depression.

An outstanding feature of manic-depressive psychosis is the fact that even after repeated attacks the intellectual capacities are rarely impared. In the free intervals the patient is usually able to carry on his regular occupation and live an entirely normal life.

IMPORTANT CONCEPTS

1. The manic-depressive psychosis is thought to have its origins in the frustrations that occur in the oral phase of personality development.
2. Patients suffering from this psychosis are ambivalent, dependent, and narcissistic and have difficulty in establishing mature patterns of adult interpersonal relationships.
3. Essentially, elated, overactive patients are venting their hostility upon their environment, whereas depressed patients have turned their hostility upon themselves.
4. Depressed patients suffer from a punishing superego.
5. Elated, overactive patients are acutely aware of reality and react strongly to environmental stimuli.
6. Simplification of the environment is a basic principle in the care of elated, overactive patients.
7. The tranquilizing drugs have revolutionized the treatment of the overactive, abnormally elated, and excited patient, and noisy wards in the modern psychiatric hospital are rapidly becoming a thing of the past.
8. The task of recognizing the potentially suicidal patient and safeguarding against the possibility of the patient's injuring himself is one of the most important responsibilities of the nurse.
9. The depressed patient suffers from overwhelming feelings of guilt, ideas of self-depreciation, and self-accusatory delusions.
10. The prognosis for single episodes of elation or depression is good, but recurrences are to be expected.
11. The dynamics of midlife depressions are essentially those of other depressive episodes.

SUGGESTED SOURCES OF ADDITIONAL INFORMATION

Arieti, Silvano: Manic depressive psychoses. In Arieti, Silvano, editor: American handbook of psychiatry, vol. 1, New York, 1959, Basic Books, Inc., Publishers, pp. 419-454, 540-545.

Bidder, George T.: Are drugs the answer in mental depression? Amer. J. Nurs. 61:60-63, Oct., 1961.

Bodie, Marilyn K.: When a patient threatens suicide, Perspect. Psychiat. Care 6:76-79, 1968.

Engel, George L.: Grief and grieving, Amer. J. Nurs. 64:93-98, Sept., 1964.

Farberow, Norman L.: Suicide prevention: a view from the bridge, Community Mental Health Journal 6:469-474, 1968.

Fernandez, Theresa: How to deal with overt aggression, Amer. J. Nurs. 59:658-660, May, 1959.

Hirsch, Joseph: Dynamics of suicide. Part 3, Ment. Hyg. 44:274-280, 1960.

Kolb, Lawrence C.: Noyes' modern clinical psychiatry, ed. 7, Philadelphia, 1968, W. B. Saunders Co., pp. 335-354.

Peplau, Hildegard: Themes in nursing situations, Amer. J. Nurs. 53:1221-1223, Oct., 1953.

Rykken, Marjorie B.: The nurse's role in preventing suicide, Nurs. Outlook 6:377-378, July, 1958.

Schwartz, Morris S., and Shockley, Emmy Lanning: The nurse and the mental patient, New York, 1956, Russell Sage Foundation, pp. 21-71, 167-181.

Shneidman, Edwin S.: Preventing suicide, Amer. J. Nurs. **65**:111-116. May, 1965.

Singer, Richard G., and Blumenthal, Irving J.: Suicide clues in psychotic patients, Ment. Hyg. **53**:346-350, 1969.

Tallent, Norman, Kennedy, George F., and Hur-ley, William T.: A program for suicidal patients, Amer. J. Nurs. **66**:2014-2016, Sept., 1966.

Umscheid, Sister Theophane: With suicidal patients: caring for or caring about, Amer. J. Nurs. **67**:1230-1232, June, 1967.

Wallace, Mary A.: The nurse in suicide prevention, Nurs. Outlook **15**:55-57, March, 1967.

CHAPTER TWELVE

Patients whose behavior is characterized by pathological suspicion

The tendency to be sensitive, to be hurt easily, and to assign base motives to the behavior of others exists in most people to varying degrees. This disposition to blame others for one's own dissatisfactions is more prominent in those who are highly sensitive and incapable of achieving at the high level they have established for themselves. There are thousands who go through life feeling that they are underrated, misunderstood, and abused and whose careers are blighted by bitterness, resentment, cynicism, and brooding over fancied wrongs and persecution. To obtain any sense of security, many such individuals establish the conviction that they are hounded by persecutors and that the responsibility for their failures belongs to others. Thus the suspicious person obtains relief from his feelings of inadequacy by blaming others for his shortcomings.

The patient whose behavior is characterized by suspicion and blaming others is reacting to a state of insecurity. Such a reaction is described as a paranoid condition. The individual's reason appears intact but is dominated by certain false convictions or beliefs. Such an emotional response springs from a basic personality that lacks the ability to cope with the social and work situations in which he is involved.

CAUSATIVE FACTORS

The personality that makes excessive use of the mechanism of projection is thought to have developed out of an early childhood, in which the individual experienced greater demands upon his ability to achieve than he was able to meet. In addition, the home and family environment is thought to have fostered chronic hatred, suspiciousness, and insecurity and the development of a rigid, narcissistic outlook on life. Thus the individual became highly sensitive, chronically insecure, haughty, sarcastic, hostile, and unrealistically proud.

DEVELOPMENT OF PROJECTIVE PATTERNS OF BEHAVIOR

The mental illness characterized by projective patterns of behavior develops very slowly, so that by the time the condition attains the proportions of a true psychosis the individual is generally well into the adult years. An early tendency in life toward excessive brooding and daydreaming may be followed by the development of delusional ideas. The individual suspects hidden meanings in things in the environment, and ideas of reference are formulated out of incidental remarks and trivial events. Slowly the patient amplifies his false ideas and distorts actual facts to fit his delusional scheme. His ability to successfully test reality becomes seriously impaired. From the persecutory stage the patient may develop ideas of grandeur. Endless persecution by others implies envy and jealousy of his own status, and it is necessary to his self-esteem for him to believe that he is an extraordinary person. He may develop the idea that he is a great prophet, a secret service operative, a mastermind, a great inventor, or a great religious leader.

The patient actually has an inadequate self-concept and therefore develops an unconscious feeling that he is personally inadequate. The delusions of persecution and grandeur are essential defenses to relieve his tension and his intolerable sense of personal and social inadequacy.

Some authorities believe that an unconscious homosexual conflict may be a frequent underlying cause. Similar types of projective maneuvers are commonly observed among so-called normal people who accuse others of having "dirty thoughts" when it is they who are dealing in obscene sexual phantasties. They suspect others of immoral behavior or accuse their marital partners of being unfaithful when it is they who have not always lived up to a high moral code.

Many patients find it necessary to enlarge upon their suspicious ideas constantly in order to lessen their feelings of guilt and to assure themselves that they are adequate. Patterns of projective behavior, like all other psychiatric symptoms, are of great significance to the patient and are developed as a result of an overwhelming unconscious need for them. Delusions of persecution or grandeur help the patient to feel as important as he needs to feel.

It is difficult for patients who utilize projective patterns of behavior to learn to adjust in a more positive way. In most instances projective behavior represents the patient's best effort in justifying his existence and placating his weak ego. Many individuals suffer with this distortion of personality, but possess enough self-control not to offend society. They may exist as harmless zealots, religious enthusiasts, or hermits. Occasionally institutional treatment, with its lack of competitive tension, may do much to alleviate the sensitivity of the paranoid person, and the major symptoms may become latent or disappear.

For those paranoid patients whose delusional state persists over a long period of time and in whom excitement and homicidal outbursts are frequent manifestations, long-term hospitalization may be required.

Psychiatric treatment of patients who use projective behavior patterns has been consistently unsuccessful. It is possible that large doses of chlorpromazine and other ataractics may reduce the emotional tension and the egocentric feelings of the patient.

MEETING THE NURSING NEEDS OF THE SUSPICIOUS PATIENT

It is not helpful to try to explain away the patient's false ideas or argue with the patient about them. Such an approach will cause the patient to become increasingly hostile and suspicious. If the nurse recognizes the significance of the delusion to the patient and the fact that life is intolerable to him without this ego-saving device, she will realize how futile it is to try to change the patient's ideas. It is a wise plan to listen respectfully to the patient without commenting upon the content of his conversation.

Most suspicious patients become hostile and aggressive toward their environment and almost universally believe that they are being held in the hospital illegally and unfairly. Such patients rarely ever develop any understanding of their illness or the fact that they need help. Often such a patient is diligently working to develop a plan for escaping from the institution. In fact, most suspicious patients deny that the institution is a hospital and refuse to accept their status as a patient. These in-

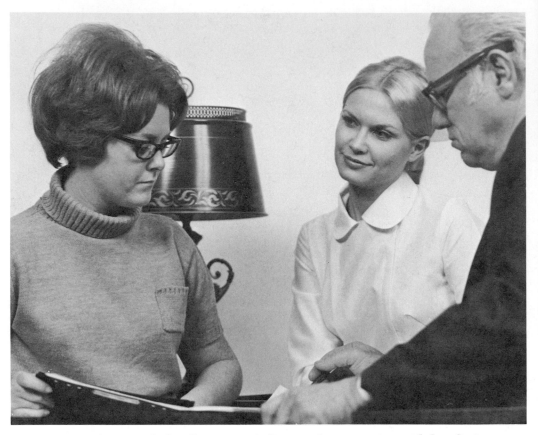

FIG. 16. *The nurse helps the patient feel secure by remaining with her during a testing session.*

dividuals frequently become verbally abusive and may actually be physically dangerous to people who represent authority. They may threaten the lives of those persons whom they blame for their incarceration.

The goal for the nursing care of patients whose behavior is characterized by pathological suspicion is to help them feel accepted and as secure as possible.

The nursing care plan should be individualized, depending on the needs of each patient. This individualized plan should take into consideration the patient's life history and his emotional needs. Occupational and recreational activities commensurate with his prepsychotic interests and abilities will be helpful.

Most suspicious patients present a cool, haughty, and aloof appearance. They usually remain apart from other patients and refuse to participate in group activity. Although it is usually a good plan to encourage patients to take part in group activities, it is often better to initiate solitary social activities for the suspicious patient.

It is helpful to provide the patient who has artistic or musical talent with materials with which to develop these interests. Many suspicious patients are intellectually capable and enjoy reading carefully chosen books and magazines. Such patients should be encouraged to enter into activities with the staff member or patient with whom a trusting relationship has been established.

It is usually more satisfactory to allow such an individual to occupy a single room instead of being assigned to a dormitory. Sleeping in a group situation may increase the patient's suspicion and hostility toward his environment.

The nurse needs to be alert to the extreme dislikes of the suspicious patient and should help him avoid others who seem to increase his irritability. The neutral environment of the hospital should be planned in such a way as to help the patient feel more secure, improve his self-esteem, and lessen his hostility toward his environment.

The sensitive nurse will avoid laughing or talking with another person when the suspicious patient can see her but cannot hear what is being said. Suspicious patients universally conclude that they are being discussed when they observe two people in a conversation. This situation is upsetting to them and usually evokes an outburst of tense, angry accusations.

The wise nurse is meticulously honest with suspicious patients. Sometimes it may not be wise to tell them all the facts when they ask about a situation that has occurred, but everything the nurse tells the patient must be true if she hopes to help the patient develop an attitude of trust in her and the staff.

Promises should be kept to the letter if they have been made to any patient, but the thoughtful nurse will be cautious in making promises, especially to suspicious patients.

When the patient is pouring out a long tirade against the hospital or complaining bitterly about the unfair treatment he is receiving, the nurse will be most helpful when she listens calmly without entering into a discussion or trying to convince him of his mistaken judgment. It is unwise to attempt to utilize logical reasoning with a suspicious patient because he will cling to his delusions even more tenaciously than ever when he is threatened by logic. Delusions are a protection and can be abondoned only when the patient feels secure and adequate in the situation.

Suspicious patients will respond more appropriately if a consistent approach of acceptance and friendliness is utilized by all staff members. Such patients need to feel respected and considered as worthwhile human beings. Their self-esteem can be enhanced by providing them with social and occupational activities in which they can succeed and for which they can receive merited praise.

Case report

The following is the history of the development of pathological suspicions in one individual.

A. T. was born of parents who were not of the same racial background. His father was an engineer and died as a result of an explosion when the patient was 10 years of age. He lived in a run-down part of the city with his mother. He made few friends among the other children who lived in that section of the city. Very early in his life he developed an interest in mechanics. He was a good student but rather aloof and decidedly sensitive to the jibes of his schoolmates. He spent his leisure hours studying chemistry and physics in the city library. At the age of 15 years he had a fight in the school yard with a boy who called his mother a foul name. After this affair he had very little to do with other young people, except those who were interested in a religious mission he attended regularly.

He was ascetic in his tastes, drank no liquor, did not smoke, and showed little interest in girls. On graduation from high school he worked for two years in a tile factory as a shipping clerk. At this time he was awarded a scholarship and matriculated in college. There his social condition was not improved, since the students avoided him and he displayed no interest in them. At the end of two years his scholarship lapsed, and having no resources of his own, he returned home and resumed his work with the same concern that previously employed him.

At the city mission during prayer meetings and on Sundays he gave long, testimonials and believed that he was a promising preacher. During the absence of the regular minister in the summer he expected to be asked to serve as a substitute. When another man was called, the patient expressed his resentment openly at the next meeting and resigned from the congregation. A few weeks later his mother passed away. He lived alone in a small upstairs apartment that he was able to maintain because his mother had left a small legacy. Here he secluded himself for many weeks and emerged only once a day to buy a few groceries and a bottle of milk. One day his landlady, who lived below, fearing that he was ill, climbed the stairs and knocked on the door. Receiving no answer, she obtained a key and upon opening the door was struck with a baseball bat. She managed to get to her rooms to call the police, who were compelled to use tear gas to subdue the patient.

When admitted to a psychiatric hospital, he refused to give his name. He wore a pointed beard and a loose gown resembling a monk's robe. He said, "Yes, I am an engineer—to be exact, I am God's own engineer. Do not concern yourself over my real name, it has enough stigma attached to it now. No, I am not married, but I have been tried by all the lures that women possess. No, I don't use rotten liquor or filthy tobacco—I am made for higher things. My enemies follow me everywhere I go and make obscene comments about me on the walls of public washrooms. I am offered only menial positions so as to keep me penniless most of the time. They put their heads together and scheme their dastardly plans.

"See this sore [pointing to a varicose ulcer]? This is where they inducted me with their electrical currents. That is why I slept in a 'nonconductor' bed. I made it myself and suspended it from insulators fixed in the ceiling. The landlady came up to destroy my devices because the bishop of her church had ordered her to do so. The modern church is determined to destroy me because I preach the older creeds. [Proudly] Why should I not be hailed as the second Christ?"

The patient's attitude and unusual ideas remained unchanged for many months. He showed little interest in or concern for other patients. He refused to shave or have his hair cut, had little interest in recreational or occupational activities, and spent most of his time staring out a window.

Discussion of case report

Unfortunately, too little is reported in A. T.'s case history to tell us much about his early childhood relationship with his mother, but there are suggestions about the results of that relationship from which certain conclusions can be drawn.

It will be clear to almost anyone reading this case history that the patient is gravely ill with a paranoid psychotic reaction and that he suffers from persistent and systematized delusions. These delusions can be classified as delusions of grandeur ("I am God's own engineer") and persecutory delusions ("Electrical currents have been run into my body").

This young man has developed these ideas to defend himself against the hostile world. However, his view of the hostile world is actually a reflection of his own hostile attitude (striking the landlady over the head with a baseball bat.)

As a child of a racially mixed marriage, he was faced with one of the most difficult social situations that a child can be called upon to face—he was socially unacceptable to children from both his father's racial group and his mother's racial group. Thus he was confronted with an essentially hostile world at school and became an isolate.

In this situation being an only child left him with no ally at home or at school. His father died when A. T. was 10 years old. Normally a child of 10 is beginning to emancipate himself from the family by seeking security and companionship from peer groups of the same sex. At this period in the child's psychosexual development he normally seeks a companion or chum with whom he can share some of his self-love. Thus the most important task in preparation for a normal love relationship is begun in this period and later focused upon someone of the opposite sex. Part of the tragedy of the patient's life lies in the fact that he did not develop a chum relationship with another boy of his age and did not belong to a peer group as do most 10-year-old boys. This defect in his development was caused in part by the cultural problem with which he was faced. However, it may also have been caused by the emotional relationship that developed between him and his mother. Some authorities believe that paranoid reactions have their developmental origins in the conflicts the child experiences with the mother in the first and second years of life. If the mother is overly possessive of the son, the child's psychosexual development may never advance beyond the homosexual level. Since his father died when A. T. was 10 years old and the boy had no companions, one may conclude that his relationship with his mother was unusually close. At any rate he sought refuge in the study of science and spent much time in a library, a place where everyone is usually welcome and equal.

At 15 years of age this patient fought with a boy who maligned his mother. This was a physical act of self-defense as well as defense of his mother. His anger was directed against a representative of one of the groups who had tormented him. After this event his social activities were confined to people attending a small city mission. Groups who attend missions are probably more accepting of individual differences than are other groups. Undoubtedly, the city mission was a social haven for the patient who felt that the world was a hostile, unfriendly place.

He began to develop ascetic tastes that may have been designed to assist him to be more acceptable to the mission group. He drank no liquor, did not smoke, and evidenced no interest in girls. These activities represent areas of personal life about which most religious groups have strict prohibitions. To live up to these rules was one way of achieving acceptance and approval by his church group.

After high school graduation this intellectually capable young man, who once had an interest in the sciences, went to work in a tile factory for two years. This move was undoubtedly made because of an economic need, but it must have been a dull, monotonous job and a great disappointment to one with academic aspirations.

After two years at the tile factory he obtained a scholarship and attended college. Here again he made no friends. When the scholarship ended, he returned to the tile factory, but soon the people at the city mission noticed that he was acting in an unusual way and thought himself ready to serve as the minister at the mission. When another man was chosen, he expressed hostility and resentment and resigned from the congregation. His mother's death was added to the blow of having to leave college, having to return to the tile factory, and not having been recognized by the city mission as the minister that he believed himself to be.

For this lonely, rejected young man the loss of his mother represented the loss of the only close human companionship he had ever known.

He attempted to carry on without his only companion and to live without working at the tile factory because his mother had left him a little money. Thus he secluded himself. This action eventually led to the incident of striking the landlady and being taken to a psychiatric hospital by the police.

When he entered the hospital, he was dressed as a monk and he refused to give his name. Since the world was so hostile and painful for him, he had assumed the role of a man of God and had withdrawn from it altogether. This patient, like all patients, had a reason for his behavior. He struck the landlady on the head with the baseball bat to protect himself against her because he believed that she had come on the order of the bishop of her church to destroy his protective devices (a nonconductor bed to avoid the electrical currents people were sending through his body). In addition, he believed that churches were persecuting him because his own mission had refused to accept him as a minister. The delusion of being God's engineer had a protective meaning for him. It provided an outlet for his mechanical interests, and since he was chosen by God to be an engineer, it was obvious to the patient that he must be excellent.

Thus, through his delusions, this patient had achieved those things that he could not achieve in real life. He was unconsciously utilizing projection (blaming others for his own shortcomings and deficiencies) to defend his ego and to establish his superiority.

In this patient we have an example of an individual who was ambitious but whose strivings were continuously frustrated. His continued failure to achieve highly valued goals and the need to enhance his own self-esteem caused him to resort to very unusual and paranoid defenses. With an already faulty personality development he was unable to cope with the many anxiety-producing factors in a life filled with problems over which he had little control.

Nursing care for Mr. A. T.

When Mr. A. T. entered the psychiatric hospital, the nurses allowed him to continue wearing the loose-fitting gown in which he arrived until he voluntarily exchanged it for a business suit. This concession was made in the hope of helping him feel accepted in the hospital setting.

The nurses allowed him to wear this unusual garb because they knew that suspicious patients respond negatively to any authoritarian approach and that flexibility should be maintained whenever possible.

The nurse who admitted Mr. A. T. avoided touching him because she realized that suspicious patients frequently misinterpret such actions and believe them to be sexual overtures. She went about the admission procedure in a calm, self-assured way in the hope that by her approach she could help him feel less insecure and frightened. She was careful to speak to him clearly and to enunciate precisely in order to minimize opportunities for misinterpreting her comments.

During his stay in the hospital the professional staff tried to be consistent in their approach to him and to be meticulously honest in answering his questions. They made a special effort to treat him with respect, since they realized that suspicious patients are easily offended. The staff avoided arguing with him about his delusions and made no comment when he stated that he was the lamb of God. They accepted the fact that he would not answer to his legal name and refrained from calling him by name.

The nursing staff meticulously labeled his personal belongings and were careful to see that they were never confused with those of other patients.

The nurses invited him to participate in group activities but accepted his decision without discussion when he declined. They kept a supply of recreational materials on hand, which could be used by him in his room without involving other patients.

When Mr. A. T. became hostile and falsely accused the nursing staff of misdeeds, they accepted his sarcasm without becoming angry and avoided adopting a punitive attitude toward him. They sought to provide for him as emotionally comfortable a situation as possible.

IMPORTANT CONCEPTS

1. The suspicious person obtains relief from his feelings of inadequacy by blaming others for his shortcomings.
2. The personality that makes excessive use of the mechanism of projection is thought to develop out of an early childhood that fostered chronic hatred and in which the individual experienced greater demands upon his ability to achieve than he was able to meet.
3. The pathologically suspicious individual has a rigid, narcissistic outlook on life and is overly sensitive and highly insecure.
4. The pathologically suspicious individual eventually loses his ability to successfully test reality.
5. Delusions of persecution and grandeur are essential for the suspicious patient to relieve his tension and his intolerable sense of personal and social inadequacy.
6. In most instances projective patterns of behavior represent the patient's best effort to justify his existence and placate his weak ego.
7. When an attempt is made to explain away the patient's false ideas or to argue with the patient about them, he becomes increasingly hostile and suspicious.
8. The goal for the nursing care of pa-

tients who utilize patterns of projective behavior is to help them feel as accepted and secure as possible in the hospital.

9. Suspicious patients will respond much better if a consistent approach of acceptance and friendliness is utilized by all staff members.

SUGGESTED SOURCES OF ADDITIONAL INFORMATION

Cameron, Norman: Paranoid conditions and paranoia. In Arieti, Silvano, editor: American handbook of psychiatry, vol. 1, New York, 1959, Basic Books, Inc., Publishers, pp. 508-539.

Chrzanowski, Gerard: Cultural and pathological manifestations of paranoia, Perspect. Psychiat. Care 1:34-42, 1963.

Kolb, Lawrence C.: Noyes' modern clinical psychiatry, ed. 7, Philadelphia, 1968, W. B. Saunders Co., pp. 401-412.

Schwartz, Morris S., and Shockley, Emmy Lanning: The nurse and the mental patient, New York, 1956, Russell Sage Foundation, pp. 113-138.

Stankiewicz, Barbara: Guides to nursing intervention in the projective patterns of suspicious patients, Perspect. Psychiat. Care 2:39-45, 1964.

Sullivan, Harry Stack: Conceptions of modern psychiatry, Washington, D. C., 1947, William Alanson White Psychiatric Foundation, pp. 56-60.

CHAPTER THIRTEEN

Patients whose behavior is characterized by neurotic symptoms

There is a large group of patients whose behavior is characterized by a constant effort to gain security and to control intolerable anxiety through the utilization of physical symptoms that have no organic basis. Another group of patients control anxiety by the utilization of repetitive, ritualistic maneuvers. All these individuals seek security in regression to a previous level of personality development where they were able to be comfortably dependent upon others. In contrast, the patient who suffers from a psychotic reaction achieves a retreat or flight from reality or, in the case of the overactive patient, a flight into reality.

The origin of these personality problems probably lies in the early childhood experiences of these individuals. In adult life the conflict has been repressed in the unconscious mind. The repressed conflict is between two or more divergent drives or desires. The symptoms of anxiety appear because of the inability of the ego to effect a compromise between these clashing desires. The result of these unresolved conflicts may be a flight into a state of physical illness that is functional and not organic. Ritualistic behavior may have a similar origin. Each inner drive or innate trend is represented by a group of ideas, which are held together by a strong emotional bond or common feeling and are known as a *complex*. Each complex demands expression in conscious activity, and in attempting such expression it may be working at cross purposes with another equally demanding complex. Thus one often senses in a psychoneurotic patient a struggle between the desire to express basic instinctual drives on one hand and to retain social and conventional approval on the other. In other words, a war exists in the emotional life of some individuals between the id drives and the superego.

The majority of people are able to live relatively normal, anxiety-free lives through the utilization of various unconscious strategies or compromises. It is here that many of the mechanisms of defense discussed in an earlier chapter come into play. As has been said, if the ego is unable to achieve a compromise between the id and the superego, the tension is relieved by some individuals by converting the emotional conflict into physical illness or ritualistic behavior.

MORE COMMON
NEUROTIC REACTIONS

Anxiety reactions are probably the most frequent neurotic manifestations observed in patients. The threat to the conscious level of personality arises from the energy of repressed emotions, such as deep-seated hostilities and resentments. Immediate external situations, such as loss of social prestige or love or a threat to personal and financial security, are regarded as important causative factors. Anxiety may be focused upon various visceral functions, frequently to the point of fearing imminent death or physical disaster, indicating that conscious control of primary or conscious anxiety is poor, diffuse, or incomplete. The physical symptoms expressed by individuals who are exhibiting anxiety reactions may be numerous but generally center about the vital organs of the body. Tightness of the stomach, fast-beating heart, a feeling that the heart may suddenly stop, no appetite, loose bowels, and heavy abdomen are frequent complaints offered by the patient. Palpitation, a feeling of shortness of breath, compression sensations in the head, tight sensations in the throat, numbness in the extremities, and a constant feeling of exhaustion are other typical experiences reported by patients suffering from anxiety reactions. These symptoms usually frighten the patient; he cannot concentrate on his work, feels depressed, and harbors fears of sudden death or insanity. Frequently many of these symptoms appear at one time and cause the patient to respond with a panic reaction or acute fear. He dreads being left alone, clings to his family, and avoids crowds and public places because he anticipates some dreadful form of collapse.

Conversion reaction is a purposeful, although unconscious, psychological mode of reaction by which the patient utilizes a physical symptom as a disguise in order to solve some acute problem or fulfill some desire, the open or conscious gratification of which is unacceptable to the individual. Conversion represents a primitive, instinctual mechanism to which a person resorts when he is incapable of adjusting through the usual methods of rational volitional activity.

The person who utilizes a conversion reaction unconsciously selects a set of symptoms, which are dictated by suggestion or by some previous acquaintance with persons who had the actual problem. Hence paralysis, blindness, stupor, epilepsy, and mental blankness are afflictions commonly presented by the person utilizing conversion. The symptoms presented by such a patient may therefore be either physical or mental.

Whether the symptoms are physical or mental, a characteristic feature of conversion is the patient's attitude of indifference toward his handicaps. There seems to be an air of contentment about the patient with conversion paralysis. He seems to be more relieved than distressed; an attitude that at once suggests that the patient prefers the physical problem to mental torment.

Phobic reactions are characterized by specific neurotic fears, which are symbolic of some anxiety-laden situation in the life of the individual. In the obsessive-compulsive reaction the defense against open anxiety is a preoccupation with a compelling ritual. In both these neuroses the mechanisms of displacement and symbolism are the major elements and, hence, are being considered as essentially one entity.

A *phobia* is a specific pathological fear reaction out of proportion to the stimulus. The painful feeling has been automatically and unconsciously displaced from its original internal source, to become attached to a specific external object or situation. The phobia is an obsessively persistent form of fear that is unrealistic and inappropriate.

An *obsession* is an undesirable but persistent thought or idea that is forced into conscious awareness. The thought is charged with great but unconscious emotional significance. Such a thought may include repetitive doubts, wishes, fears, impulses, admonitions, and commands.

A *compulsion* is an unwanted urge to perform an act or a ritual that is contrary to the patient's ordinary conscious wishes or standards.

It will be noted that all these intrusive ideas and compelling urges and fears appear in consciousness as though independently self-created.

The individual who suffers from an obsessive-compulsive neurosis is driven to think about or to do something that he recognizes as being inappropriate or foolish. There is an excessive preoccupation with a single idea or a compulsion to carry out and to repeat over and over again certain acts against his better judgment. Back of these compulsive or obsessive states is a personality that is usually conscience-driven, sensitive, shy, meticulous, and precise about bodily functions, dress, religious duty, and daily routine.

Obsessive-compulsive neurosis is a serious emotional illness because the imperative ideas so control the patient that he becomes a slave to his morbid preoccupation and can scarcely carry on his normal work and social activity. Dominating fears or phobias are the most outstanding feature of this illness. The patient may fear dirt, bacteria, cancer, or insanity. There may be an abnormal fear of open places, narrow corridors, small rooms, running water, staircases, high places, or various animals. In fact, the phobia may be focused on anything that in some manner suggests death, disease, or disaster.

The abnormal fear probably developed out of disagreeable and socially unacceptable ideas. Instead of an open anxiety or frank expression of id drives, the ideas and intense emotions attached to them are forced out of consciousness. Such repressed emotional energy attaches itself to an entirely different idea or activity and forces itself into consciousness as a tension that has little or no relationship to the original idea. The patient experiences a sense of relief after performing the compulsive act, since the symptom was developed for the purpose of relieving tension. The neurosis, therefore, is an example of displacement and symbolization. The original conflict because of unacceptable desires is replaced by tension over something that is more socially acceptable but that acts as a symbol for the patient.

Compulsive behavior and obsessive fears are substitution devices that relieve tension arising out of a sense of guilt or a feeling of personal insecurity. Unfortunately, the relief offered by the act is only temporary, and the ritual must be repeated at frequent intervals. Relatives lose patience and attempt to "break the patient of his habit." This only causes the victim to become restless, uncomfortable, and agitated because the act has become a fixed channel for the discharge of all tension arising out of his unconscious conflict.

MEETING THE NURSING NEEDS OF THE PATIENT WITH NEUROTIC BEHAVIOR

Many nurses who work skillfully and sympathetically with psychotic patients find that they are not nearly so effective when giving care to patients who express anxiety through physical symptoms or ritualistic behavior. A large part of the nurse's problem in dealing with anxious patients originates in her unconscious attitude toward persons suffering from neurotic problems and in her failure to understand the true nature of the illness. Because such an individual is aware of his surroundings, is not carrying on a conversation with unseen people, and complains of physical symptoms that have no organic basis, the nurse may feel unsympathetic toward the patient and may believe that he is "an attention getter" and that he could "snap out of it" if he really tried.

Such an attitude derives from a lack of knowledge and can destroy any possibility of the nurse being of therapeutic assistance to the patient. To achieve a more understanding attitude toward these individuals, it is important to develop some knowledge about the patient's emotional conflicts and the ways in which he uses the symptoms to cope with his problems.

It is significant to realize that all neurotic symptoms develop because of an overwhelming *unconscious* conflict and that the symptoms have tremendous unconscious meaning for the patient. The word unconscious has been stressed, since it is necessary for the nurse to realize that the patient does not clearly understand why the symptom has developed nor what he is gaining by using the symptom repeatedly. He does realize that the symptom helps relieve unbearable anxiety and tension.

It is also important for the nurse to realize that the physical discomfort and pain of which the patient complains is actually present even though there is no organic basis that can explain the existence of the symptoms. Experts are beginning to recognize that fear plays a significant role in causing pain. Since fear plays such a prominent role in the symptomatology of many anxiety-ridden patients, it is not difficult to realize that they actually feel the pain of which they complain. It is important for nurses to understand that emotionally conditioned pain is as distressing to bear as is pain that results from true physical disease.

Understanding the treatment goals

To make an intelligent and therapeutic plan of nursing care, the nurse needs to understand the nature of the patient's conflict and the meaning of his symptoms. Understanding the patient's needs can be achieved only through the use of the social and psychological information that is available about the patient. The plan for care and treatment of the patient should be developed collaboratively by the nurse and the psychiatrist who is treating the patient. The type of treatment the patient requires and the therapeutic goals the clinical team will establish need to be discussed collaboratively.

In some instances the physician may feel that the patient's recovery will be aided by allowing him freedom of choice as to his daily activities. In another instance the psychiatrist may feel that the patient would profit by following a schedule of daily activities in which most of the day is accounted for. Whatever the treatment goals may be, the patient requires a consistent approach from all members of the clinical staff.

General principles underlying nursing care

Although many of the specific aspects of nursing care for neurotic patients will need to be planned collaboratively, there are some general suggestions that apply to the nursing care of all fearful, indecisive, egocentric patients.

Such individuals need a warm, friendly, sympathetic nurse who accepts them as sick people in need of help and who helps them feel that they are worthwhile human beings. Scolding or sarcastic remarks di-

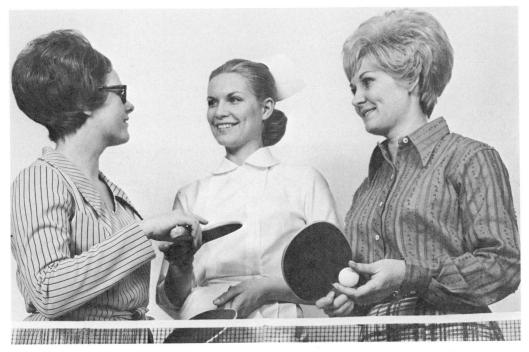

FIG. 17. *The nurse helps anxious patients to focus upon interests outside themselves.*

rected toward neurotic patients will serve only to reinforce their need to protect themselves by the utilization of their symptoms.

It is usually wise to listen completely and with an accepting attitude when the anxious patient describes his physical symptoms. Comments should be directed toward eliciting more information about the complaints. It is important for the nurse to remember that psychoneurotic patients can and do become physically ill and deserve medical attention if there is any reasonable doubt about the cause of the complaint.

Some nurses ignore the patient's neurotic symptoms, and in many instances this becomes synonymous with ignoring the patient. Since the anxious patient is using symptoms to make a bid for help or love, ignoring him makes it necessary for him to use his symptoms more frequently.

Avoid asking "How are you today?" For anxious patients this question is often an invitation for another outpouring of physical complaints. A much more helpful way to begin a conversation might be to comment upon some neutral topic that is of mutual interest to both the patient and the nurse.

In suggesting that an anxious patient participate in some social activity it is unwise to ask "Would you like to go swimming with the group?" Such a question will often bring the flat answer, "No," or a long recital about why the patient cannot possibly go. A better approach to this subject would be "The group is going swimming; I hope that you will go with us." If the object is to get the patient to participate in a game of table tennis, more positive results will be obtained if the tennis paddle is placed in the patient's hand by the nurse who might say, "We need one more person in order to play this

157

game. Come and play." This introduction is more apt to elicit results that if he is asked if he wishes to play.

It is helpful if the anxious patient is provided with an opportunity to succeed in the activities in which he participates. This is important because these patients need help in building self-esteem and self-confidence. Giving deserved praise and recognition for activities performed well is one way of reassuring and encouraging patients.

One of the most helpful approaches to the care of anxious patients is to assist them to develop interests outside themselves. Thus recreational and occupational therapy are particularly significant in their treatment. Many neurotic individuals have never been able to enter into games or group activities. It is therapeutically important to help these patients learn to play games and to participate in group activities. This gives them opportunities to release tensions as well as to develop new interests directed away from their physical symptoms. Recreational and occupational therapy will often be more successful if they are developed around old interests that the patient has had in the past.

The ability to carry on an interesting conversation about a wide variety of subjects is helpful if the nurse is going to work successfully with anxious patients. These individuals are often widely read and well educated.

Suggestions concerning nursing care of ritualistic patients

The patient who is suffering from morbid fears and compulsions is frequently found in a psychiatric setting and is usu-

ally a challenging nursing problem. Some nurses who have no understanding of the forces that play a part in developing such symptoms may assume the attitude that the many maneuvers of the patient are ridiculous. Nurses have been known to force a phobic patient to touch a doorknob even though it was well known that the patient was morbidly afraid of the dirt and germs he believed he would contact by touching the object. Other nurses have made it impossible for a patient to get into the bathroom to carry out the handwashing rituals that were so important to him in releasing tensions and fears.

When phobic and compulsive patients are not allowed to carry out the procedures they feel are necessary, they have no way of releasing tension. A high level of unreleased tension may culminate in a panic state. Unless the psychiatrist directs the nurses to adopt some other attitude, they should make it possible for the patient to carry out the anxiety-releasing rituals he has developed. These acute symptoms will usually become less prominent when the patient has become accustomed to a neutral, accepting environment.

The rituals carried on by these patients are essential for them if they are to develop any feeling of security in the situation. Because such rituals are time consuming, time must be allowed for the patient to perform his ritualistic maneuvers. If the patient is pressured to hurry through the ritualistic performance to save time, he may become terrified for fear the maneuver will not be completed perfectly. This will cause him to repeat the performance, and time will be lost instead of saved.

Many nurses, as well as the patient's

relatives, attempt to discuss the rituals reasonably with the patient in the hope of altering the behavior. This kind of pressure does nothing to help the patient and may actually cause him to feel more anxious and may increase his feeling of guilt.

Case report

The following case history is an example of how one individual began to utilize ritualistic behavior to defend himself against intolerable anxiety.

H. B., a man 47 years of age, came to the psychiatric outpatient clinic to ask for help with his problem after he had spent three months in a private sanitarium where no actual therapy was provided.

During his college days he had become emotionally upset and had worried excessively. His pastor was consulted, and after several conferences the patient was able to resume his schoolwork and graduated at the age of 21 as an accountant. He stated that he had always been very conscientious, worried a great deal about body cleanliness, and was known for his concern about keeping his room and clothing in perfect order. He was always prompt in appearing at his office and never left his desk before 5 o'clock. His fellow workers regarded him as very fussy, and his employer always remarked about the neatness of his desk and files—a comment that greatly pleased him. At home any irregularity in household routine upset him. His wife was fully aware of his rigid regard for rules and of his scrupulousness.

Four months before the present interview he had been assigned the responsibility of making out the income tax report for his firm, which dealt in stocks and bonds. This assignment was made on April 1, and he realized that he had but two weeks before the returns were to be filed. He worked under great pressure, and almost every day he remained in the office until late at night. With a day to spare, he entered the final figures on a roll of paper from an adding machine. Badly in need of sleep and rest, he seized this roll, thrust it into his overcoat pocket, and dashed for the midnight bus. He had intended to show the slip of paper to his wife as evidence that his job was completed. On reaching his home he could not find the roll. In a frenzy he searched his clothing, ran out on the street searching the sidewalk, but failed to find it. He was put to bed in an anxious, fearful state and remained under a physician's care for several weeks.

On returning to work, he found that he had developed an overwhelming compulsion. He could no longer pass a piece of crumpled paper on the floor or sidewalk without picking it up and inspecting it. During rush hour he was greatly humiliated and embarrassed by the necessity of bending over and picking up odd bits of paper. On several occasions while carrying out this compulsion he was knocked down by a hurrying passerby. A wastebasket full of discarded paper literally threw him into a panic. His only relief was obtained by waiting until after office hours when he could go over each item piece by piece. His physician recommended hospitalization in a psychiatric hospital. There he improved, but the obsessive idea remained, and for this reason he came to the outpatient department. He was well oriented, intelligent, had good insight, and otherwise appeared to be mentally normal.

Underlying this obsessive tension state was obviously a sensitive, overconscientious, fearful personality. The basic problem undoubtedly was concerned, in part at least, with his unresolved conflict about his need to be fastidious about body cleanliness and his role as a marital partner. Such problems probably originated in the attitudes that were taught during the habit-training period. The patient's wife spoke freely about the fact that their marital relations were unsatisfactory and disturbing. She had given up any hope of improving the situation by discussing it with the patient because he became extremely anxious when she introduced the topic.

The patient's mother was a fastidious housekeeper who was known in her community as a fanatic about maintaining correct standards of behavior and observing religious customs.

Discussion of case report

It is significant to note that Mr. H. B.'s mother was a fastidious hosekeeper and a fanatic about observing religious customs and maintaining correct standards of behavior. Undoubtedly, such a mother would insist that a child achieve perfection in toilet training at a very early age. In addition, she would rear him to behave in a rigidly correct manner and to repress instinctual thoughts and desires.

A young man who at the age of 21 is known as being overly concerned about orderliness, overly conscientious, and worried about bodily cleanliness is already well on the road to becoming a compulsive neurotic patient—one who controls unconscious anxiety by employing persistently repetitive acts. This behavior, like all human behavior, has purpose and meaning for the individual who employs it even though the forces producing it are unconscious. The patient *displaced* the anxiety arising from a feeling of guilt by engaging in ritualistic behavior.

In spite of Mr. H. B.'s early tendencies to be upset by household irregularities, he married. He and his wife managed to work out a relationship that could be tolerated. However, according to his wife the sexual relationship was unsatisfactory

and such an upsetting topic that he could not bear to discuss it.

It was not until he was 47 that Mr. H. B.'s symptoms became so severe that he required hospitalization. This was precipitated by the loss of a scrap of paper upon which was recorded a final total of a complicated accounting problem he had been assigned to complete. It is interesting to note that he was attempting to elicit his wife's approval for a successful task accomplished. Since he did not have her approval as a sexual partner, her approval about some other aspect of life was very necessary. The loss of the paper probably represented much more than simply the loss of a list of figures. Symbolically it must have represented the loss of the love and approval of his wife. This would account for his fear and anxiety. The tax report had been completed before he left the office. Thus there is little doubt that a duplicate of the figures could have been found. The problems precipitated by the loss of the figures could not possibly represent reality problems, but rather the loss must have been symbolic of the loss of something more important and irreplaceable.

In compulsive patients the repetitive act has a symbolic significance reminiscent of a magic ritual that is designed to eradicate the possible effect of unacceptable instinctual impulses. It also represents a type of self-punishment, since compulsive acts are recognized by the individual as being unreasonable and ridiculous. In spite of the patient's partial insight the tension and anxiety mount until the urge to repeat the act to control the tension becomes irresistible.

Like most severely neurotic patients,

Mr. H. B. was well oriented, intelligent and intellectually normal except for the compulsive behavior. This is an example of an individual whose personality is intact except in the one area that is involved with the compulsive behavior.

In spite of the normal aspects of the personality he was almost totally incapacitated by the need to examine every scrap of paper.

Essentially Mr. H. B. had a lifelong history of neurotic behavior. It became unmanageable at the age of 47. The treatment of such a severe, long-standing neurosis requires an intensive, psychoanalytic approach to the problems. The outcome is guarded.

TREATMENT OF PATIENTS WHO EXHIBIT NEUROTIC BEHAVIOR

Hospitalization in a psychiatric setting is usually helpful for patients who exhibit severe neurotic behavior because the environment is neutral, they are removed from the significant members of the family who may be the source of much emotional tension, and they are able to feel more secure where the routine is simple, makes few demands, and can be fairly accurately anticipated. Hospitalization in a general hospital setting may be unfortunate for some patients who have already focused most of their attention upon physical symptoms that have no organic basis. Such patients may become more tense, anxious, and fearful in a setting where the emphasis is placed upon physical problems.

Some of the new psychopharmacological agents have been helpful in reducing tension and providing the patient with a degree of emotional comfort. However, the only permanent relief for patients suffering from intolerable anxiety and fear lies in discovering the basic cause of the problem and helping the patient understand the actual source of his symptoms.

There are several methods of helping patients achieve insight and self-understanding. Most of these methods require knowledge and skill such as the psychiatrist possesses. However, well-prepared nurses are beginning to work in this area and have been successful in helping individual patients through a one-to-one relationship or as discussion leaders with groups of patients.

A discussion of these therapeutic methods will help the nurse to understand the treatment that patients receive in psychiatric settings and to better identify her role in working with a patient when he is participating in one of these therapeutic activities.

Psychotherapy

Psychotherapy is any procedure that promotes the development of courage, inner security, and self-confidence. The most effective methods in psychotherapy are suggestion, analysis, and reeducation. It consists of an effort to help the patient to understand himself, the particular nature of his illness, and how his physical problems are caused by the conflicts in his emotional life. Psychotherapy is not a fixed technique; it is more an art than a science, and its methods must be adapted and modified to fit the individual situation. In plain language, it is a form of mental exploration. It is universally acknowledged that one cannot standardize psychotherapy, that it must be individual, and that it will vary from patient to patient.

The patient must have confidence in the physician and some respect for his knowledge and experience. A word of assurance alone may be the deciding factor in relieving many anxious patients of their fears. Such a relationship is dependent upon positive *rapport* between the physician and the patient.

The patient is encouraged to talk about his life experiences. He is encouraged to talk freely about anything that comes to his mind, as long as he relates his own ideas and concerns. This random talk allows the patient to follow freely the associations that come into his mind and are accurately described as *mental ventilation*. The physician will note that there are certain occasions and events that the patient dismisses quickly or avoids mentioning except in a slurring way. These sensitive areas are then explored more fully. The patient is encouraged to talk about them more freely until they no longer cause excess emotion, a process known as *desensitization*.

The patient is guided to an understanding of how his repressed feelings produced his condition. This is done in a simple, clear style, thereby helping the patient to gain insight into the exact nature of his illness. Thus begins the process of *reeducation*.

The patient is encouraged to face his distressing problems; he is urged to think of them instead of running away from them, to become familiar with them rather than to "forget" them, and to approach their solution in a candid, open manner.

Prerequisite for any form of psycho-

therapy is to identify the chain of events and situations that caused or contributed to the mental or emotional illness. No period in the patient's history should be overlooked. Information should be gathered concerning inheritance and experiences of early life, as well as current or recent happenings, and conditions in the social environment—domestic, occupational, or other.

The purpose of psychotherapy is to educate the patient about himself and to emancipate him from his conflicts and from an abnormal dependence upon others. From the beginning of the treatment, or shortly thereafter, the patient is encouraged to take an active part in his own therapy. If all goes well the patient should take more and more constructive steps in the management of his own case. He can then answer some of his own questions and can make his own decisions. The physician measures his therapeutic success by the degree to which he makes himself less and less necessary.

Psychotherapy falls into two general types, supportive psychotherapy and "uncovering" psychotherapy. Supportive therapy helps the individual to cope with his problems and includes such techniques as diagnosis, advice, education, guidance, counseling, assurance, and medication. Uncovering therapy involves exploring and bringing to consciousness the source of repressed and forgotten conflicts and experiences that operate at unconscious levels to cause nervous tension. Uncovering therapy gives meaning to abnormal or irrational feelings and maladjustments in normal life situations.

The most important element in the doctor-patient relationship is the unconscious attitude of the patient toward his doctor. The latter is cast into the roles of a father or mother. The patient's attitude may be rivalrous or even erotic. This shifting toward the doctor of desires, feelings, and relations originally experienced by the patient with regard to his own parents, siblings, and other persons is known as *transference*. Hence, every nuance of feeling, ranging from trustful dependence to open hostility, may be directed toward the psychiatrist. When the patient's attitude toward the psychotherapist appears to be favorable, the transference is regarded as being positive. Resistant or antagonistic attitudes of the patient toward the doctor imply a negative transference. The unconscious attitudes of the doctor himself toward his patient is called *countertransference*.

The therapeutic process is dependent upon the interpersonal experience between the patient and his physician. The therapy can be a success only if the physician succeeds in getting the patient interested in promoting his own well-being on his own behalf rather than to please a third person. The relationship between the two must remain at a professional level and never at a social one.

Psychoanalysis

Phychoanalysis is something more than assisting the patient to recall some childhood experience, such as being locked in a dark room, or the recalling of some long-concealed hate of a sibling. Such exhuming of old memories by suggestion, narcosis, or hypnosis may relieve the symptoms of a deep-seated emotional problem, but it rarely dissolves the basic difficulty.

The analyst by a long and often tedious program looks for clues to the fundamental disturbance—in free association, in the content of dreams, from the nature of the patient's transference, and from those matters the patient appears to avoid because of resistance to their open recognition. The analyst leads the patient back to forgotten events and emotional crises, to his childhood fears, frustrations, and other residuals that operate at unconscious levels and cause the individual to be a nervous and unhappy person. As one exponent phrased it, "the patient acquires a more conscious knowledge of his inner conflicts and gains freedom from the tyranny of the unconscious."

Group psychotherapy

Group psychotherapy is a psychological means of treating emotionally disturbed individuals in a group setting. Group psychotherapy uses some of the concepts and techniques of individual therapy, particularly of psychoanalysis, and of social psychology. It can be didactic, inspirational, or analytical.

Transference relationships are formed and intensified in the group between members and the therapist and between member and member.

The physical requirements for conducting a group are simple and easily met. A large quiet room with some comfortable chairs arranged roughly in a circle is all that is required.

In group therapy new relationships are formed, multiple transferences are established, personality structures are revealed, and a feeling of belonging and changing is achieved through the immediate experience. The technique encourages members to express their feelings, to reveal themselves, to be frank and direct, and to give support and comfort.

Psychodrama

Psychodrama is a form of mental exploration and treatment largely developed by Dr. J. L. Moreno. In the role of an actor, the patient is given a specially selected part that affords him an opportunity to give free expression to his inner conflicts in relation with other performers who symbolize or represent persons who are the real objects of his loves or hates. For example, a son who normally represses his hostility toward a father may freely express it as an actor and may even reveal the cause. On the other hand, if he is induced to take the father role, he may, after doing so, tolerate his own father's point of view in a more objective and understanding manner.

IMPORTANT CONCEPTS

1. Physical symptoms with no organic basis are unconscious maneuvers utilized by the patient to gain security and to control intolerable anxiety.
2. The symptoms of anxiety rise to conscious awareness because of an inability of the ego to effect a compromise between two clashing desires.
3. Anxiety reactions are probably the most frequent neurotic manifestations observed in patients.
4. Conversion is a purposeful, unconscious reaction through which a patient utilizes a physical symptom as a disguise to solve some acute problem or fulfill some unacceptable desire.
5. In the obsessive-compulsive reaction the preoccupation with a compelling ritual is the individual's way of defending himself against anxiety. The performance of the ritual provides a release of tension.
6. All neurotic symptoms develop because of unconscious conflict and have a great significance for the individual.
7. Because fear plays a significant role in pain, physical discomfort and pain may actually be present even though there is no demonstrable basis to explain the existence of the complaints.
8. Patients who utilize neurotic behavior patterns need a warm, friendly, sympathetic nurse who accepts them as worthwhile human beings who are ill and who are in need of help.
9. One of the most important aspects of the care of all anxious patients is to help them develop interests outside themselves.
10. The nurse should make it possible for the ritualistic patient to carry out the anxiety-releasing maneuvers that are so essential to his security operations.

SUGGESTED SOURCES OF ADDITIONAL INFORMATION

Abse, D. Wilfred: Hysteria. In Arieti, Silvano, editor: American handbook of psychiatry, vol. 1, New York, 1959, Basic Books, Inc., Publishers, pp. 272-292.

Chrzanowski, Gerard: Neurasthenia and hypochondriasis. In Arieti, Silvano, editor: American handbook of psychiatry, vol. 1, New York, 1959, Basic Books, Inc., Publishers, pp. 258-271.

Engel, George L.: Grief and grieving, Amer. J. Nurs. 64:93-98, Sept., 1964.

English, O. S., and Pearson, G. H. J.: Emotional problems of living, ed. 3, Philadelphia, 1963, W. W. Norton & Co., Inc.

Friedman, Paul: The phobias. In Arieti, Silvano, editor: American handbook of psychiatry, vol. 1, New York, 1959, Basic Books, Inc., Publishers, pp. 293-306.

Kolb, Lawrence C.: Noyes' modern clinical psychiatry, ed. 7, Philadelphia, 1968, W. B. Saunders Co., pp. 458-500.

May, Rollo: The meaning of anxiety, New York, 1950, The Ronald Press Co.

Schwartz, Morris S., and Shockley, Emmy Lanning: The nurse and the mental patient, New York, 1956, Russell Sage Foundation, pp. 182-198.

Sullivan, Harry Stack: Conceptions of modern psychiatry, Washington, D. C., 1947, William Alanson White Psychiatric Foundation, pp. 54-59.

CHAPTER FOURTEEN

Behavior disorders resulting from toxic and organic brain disorders

The human brain is sensitive to a wide range of poisons. Their effect is to cause the patient to respond with varying degrees of behavior disturbances. As a highly specialized organ, it requires an unfailing amount of oxygen and has an elaborate blood supply that cannot be seriously disturbed without creating physical, emotional, and psychological problems. Like other organs of the body, the brain suffers whenever some systemic disease elaborates poisons or impairs circulation. Whenever the brain function is affected by some general physical disease, the mental condition is known as a *symptomatic* psychosis.

DELIRIUM

While symptomatic psychoses are not particularly frequent, the causes are many. The most common mental reaction is a delirious state. The delirium may be mild or severe. It implies some degree of clouding of consciousness and a tendency to tremor and to fumbling movements of the hands and fingers. In the severe forms there are vivid hallucinations of sight. The delirious patient may see terrifying images of animals, human faces, dancing objects, or merely flashes of light. There may also be hallucinations of touch, as if insects were crawling over the body. If the patient recovers from a delirium, he generally fails to recall any events that occurred during the period of confusion.

The nurse should remember that delirium may be of fleeting occurence. It may last but a few minutes, to be followed by a lucid period, and frequently may be manifested by merely a frightened look or a muttering of a few unintelligible words.

Psychoses with acute infectious diseases

Very young children, chronic alcoholics, and elderly people develop dilirium very quickly if an infection is severe and the fever is very high. Delirium is more likely to occur at night. If a patient with a high fever becomes restless, tires easily, and seems to have difficulty in grasping simple statements, one should be on guard and should suspect an impending delirious state. The delirious patient wanders in speech content, seems dreamy, dazed, and apprehensive, may fumble with the bedclothes, and generally looks about in a bewildered manner. He may not clearly recognize persons, or he may look at his visitors with apparently unseeing eyes. If the delirium deepens into deep stupor or coma, the condition is undeniably grave.

Occasionally the delirium resulting from an acute infection may include agitation and sudden irritability. The patient may even climb out of bed and walk about in a confused manner.

Treatment. It is obvious that the treatment of symptomatic delirium is essentially the treatment of the infection or circulatory defect that is the disturbing factor. Bed rest and seclusion from any external stimulation are essential. To this end such sedatives as chloral hydrate or paraldehyde are recommended. Delirium in the presence of very high fever may be controlled by giving sodium salicylate or aspirin in 10-grain doses three times a day, which will usually bring the temperature down. Because delirium may be an expression of vitamin deficiency, the administration of 10 to 50 mg. of vitamin B_1 daily may be effective in eliminating the psychiatric symptoms.

Delirium tremens

Delirium tremens is an acute reaction to a heavy and consistent intake of alcohol for a period of several weeks without an adequate intake of food. In an individual who has been a chronic alcoholic for several years, delirium tremens may be precipitated by a head injury or a surgical procedure without the patient having taken alcohol at the time of its appearance. Delirium tremens consists of confusion, excitement, and delirium. It is usually of relatively short duration and does not cause a profound and permanent change in the personality.

The delirium is preceded by loss of appetite, restlessness, and insomnia. Slight noises cause the patient to jerk with fear, and moving objects lead to great excitement and agitation. Gradually, consciousness becomes clouded, friends are no longer recognized, and designs in the wallpaper appear as insects or crawling animals. The patient becomes terrified. Imaginary threads are picked off the bedclothing and creeping insects are felt and seen on the skin. There is a ceaseless fumbling and picking movement of the fingers and hands. The face has an anxious or terrified expression, and the eyes are bloodshot. The skin is moist with perspiration; the tongue and the lips are tremorous. The pulse is rapid and weak, and there is always some elevation of temperature.

The death rate in delirium tremens is high: 10% to 15% of these patients die. Heart failure and bronchopneumonia are the most frequent causes of death. Autopsy reveals an edematous brain.

Case report

The following history furnishes an example of how such a problem can develop.

M. M., male, age 29 years, was admitted to the hospital from a boardinghouse where he was found suffering from delirium tremens. He was unmarried, worked intermittently as a dock laborer, and shared his room with a fellow worker with whom he often drank at a nearby saloon. He had been drinking excessively for three weeks. The day before admission he was excitable and quarrelsome and accused his roommate of throwing sand down his neck. During the night he mumbled to himself, rolled about, and fell out of bed. He claimed a dozen dogs were looking in at the window. Toward morning he was stuporous, shaky, and incoherent.

On admission he was put to bed. He wore a terrified expression on his face. Constant supervision was necessary. He picked incessantly at the bedclothes. He was able to mumble his name, but little more. During short lucid moments he said he had been drinking too much and asked for another "shot." He insisted that he saw leering faces on the walls and that there was a leopard under the bed. He was dehydrated, feverish, his eyes were bloodshot, and his gaze shifted constantly from one corner of the room to another.

Twelve days after admission his sensorium cleared. He was able to give a clear account of his past but remembered nothing of the first ten days of his hospital experience. In fact, he was greatly puzzled to find himself in a hospital bed and inquired into the identity of the institution.

Nursing care of delirious patients

Irrespective of the cause, the delirious patient is critically ill and requires constant and understanding care. The patient should be secluded in a quiet room, and visitors should be limited to one or two members of the family or very close friends. Restraint should be avoided. Instead, the patient should receive constant supervision to avoid injury to himself or others.

Applying an ice bag to the head may serve to reduce the excitement and mental confusion. A cool sponge bath in bed very frequently will induce sleep. The skin is usually dry and hot and should be closely watched for abrasions and pressure spots. Cold cream applied to the lips prevents fissuring. The mouth and tongue should be cleansed several times a day.

Feeding should begin with high-calorie fluids, and, as rapidly as the patient can tolerate it, semisolid and solid foods should be added. Water in ample quantities should be given at frequent intervals, particularly if the fever is constant and dehydration is present.

Insofar as possible, all procedures and treatments should be carried out at one time. It is important to keep in mind that the patient should be subjected to a minimum amount of stimulation and that rest is a most essential part of the care of a patient who is toxic, restless, and delirious.

Recovery from any systemic condition that causes delirium is necessarily slow. Relapses into a confusional state are not at all uncommon. Except for some simple forms of occupational therapy, exercise and mental concentration are contraindicated for several weeks after the acute illness.

GENERAL PARESIS OR MENINGOENCEPHALITIC SYPHILIS

General paresis is due to a progressive syphilitic infiltration of the brain tissue that results in a degeneration of nerve elements and produces typical neurological and mental disturbances. Since the use of penicillin in the treatment of early syphilis, paresis has become relatively uncommon.

General paresis develops within two to twenty years after the first stage of the syphilitic infection. It is much more frequent in the male. Before adequate treatment was developed, about 10% of all admissions to mental hospitals carried the diagnosis of general paresis.

The early signs of this disease are so insidious in appearance that they may be unrecognized even by intimate friends until an acute episode of some sort occurs. This may be a convulsion, or the full-blown symptoms may appear only after an injury to the head. Gradual changes in personality are the principal features of the very early phase. The patient becomes forgetful in keeping appointments, is careless of his dress, and shows a general deterioration of his ability to perform in socially approved ways. Judgment becomes poor, and there is a tendency to evade important issues and to show a smug indifference or apathy to critical problems. General loss of mental acuity is covered by shallow rationalizations, by outbursts of irritability, and by moods of depression or elation.

In the complete mental picture of a patient suffering from general paresis, a feeling of grandeur is frequently the most outstanding symptom. Delusions of wealth or power and euphoric ideas about the future are freely expressed. The basic personality of the patient influences the reaction to meningoencephalitic syphilis, and some patients may be depressed rather than elated. Memory defects are prominent, and irritability is easily evoked when attempts are made to control the expansive ideas. The mood is unstable, and the patient laughs and cries easily.

The physical signs are equally typical. The pupils are irregular. There is marked tremor of the lips and tongue. The speech function is seriously affected—words are slurred, syllables or even words are omitted, and certain phrases are incomprehensible. Writing is likewise affected. Tendon reflexes are usually overactive. Incontinence of urine and absence of the tendon reflexes generally indicate that the syphilitic process has involved the spinal cord. This form of the disease is called tabo-paresis.

Laboratory tests are most valuable in confirming the diagnosis. In the majority of cases the blood shows a positive Wassermann reaction. The critical test lies in an examination of the spinal fluid, which is almost universally Wassermann-positive. The so-called collodial test performed either with gold chloride or gum mastic reveals the paretic curve, which is recorded generally as 5555542100.

Unless the patient with general paresis is radically treated with large doses of penicillin, the outcome is a progressive degeneration of mind and body. Death usually occurs within six to eight years after the mental symptoms appear. These patients have little resistance to infection.

CONVULSIVE DISORDERS (THE EPILEPSIES)

The term "epilepsy" is to be avoided because it connotes a personality stigma that in most cases is unwarranted. The most common feature of all convulsive seizures is a lapse of consciousness of varying duration that is accompanied by changes in motor, sensory, and visceral functions. In brief, convulsions are disturbances in the electrophysiology of the brain, and the symptoms depend on the areas of the brain producing abnormal electrical discharges. A vast amount of new knowledge has been gained through study of the brain with the electroencephalogram (EEG).

The *grand mal seizure,* perhaps the most common type, and certainly the most disturbing, is a generalized discharge from all parts of the brain causing a sudden and complete cessation of consciousness associated with alternating extension (tonus) and flexion (clonus) of all four limbs, respiratory arrest with cyanosis, biting of the tongue, foaming at the mouth, and occasionally incontinence. After each seizure there is usually a short period of mental clouding and agitation. When such seizures appear in rapid succession the condition is known as *status epilepticus.* In grand mal the EEG tracings show very high and very fast spikes during a seizure, and during free intervals a breakdown of normal rhythm can be induced by hyperventilation.

Since convulsions are a symptom, the grand mal seizure may be caused by brain injury, tumors, toxins, or infections, but by far the greatest number of these generalized attacks have an unknown cause. They may first appear in early infancy but more often in puberty and endure throughout adult life.

The *petit mal seizure* and its variants consist of momentary lapses of consciousness marked by a staring or blank expression with some deviation of gaze in an upward direction. These spells sometimes appear in early childhood as often as one hundred times a day but may be so fleeting as to escape the attention of parents and teachers for several years. They may disappear in early adult life. The EEG usually shows a striking three per second spike and dome configuration.

Perhaps the most interesting seizures from the psychiatric standpoint are the so-called *psychomotor attacks* because they contain a wide variety of psychic phenomena. In EEG studies the abnormality is a random spike that appears to be in one or both temporal lobes. The most common lesion is a small area of degeneration believed to be caused by birth injury. The warning sign is often a peculiar sensation ascending from the gastric area associated with an intense feeling of fear. Again it may be a familiar and unpleasant odor or taste. There is rarely a complete loss of consciousness; instead the patient seems to be reacting to some situations in his past in what seems to be a bizarre manner and performs inappropriate acts such as undressing in public. These are known as automatisms. Occasionally during an attack the patient reacts with smacking of the lips, tongue licking, chewing, gulping, and excessive salivation. The function of memory is also involved, and in one type the patient undergoes strangely familiar experiences or dream states called "déjà vu." When consciousness is restored, the patient does not recall the content of his dreams except to state that they were familiar.

Jacksonian seizures are caused by specific focal lesions in the cerebral cortex. They are partial seizures involving only one side of the body, beginning in one hand, arm, or leg.

Treatment of convulsive disorders is possible through the use of a large number of anticonvulsant drugs. However, each patient responds differently, and treatment must be highly individualized. Some of the side actions of these drugs may be a health hazard, such as depression of bone marrow function, ataxia, and mental stupor.

Most effective, particularly in grand mal and psychomotor attacks, are Dilantin, 100 mg. three or four times daily, Mysoline, 250 mg. three times a day, Mesantoin, 100 mg. two or three times daily, and phenobarbital, 100 mg. (preferably at bedtime to control nocturnal attacks). Tridione or Paradione (300 mg. capsule three times daily) is usually prescribed for petit mal seizures, but evidence that these drugs are highly specific is lacking.

Psychopathology in patients with convulsive disorders

The nurse needs to understand the ego struggles of the patient who is subject to unpredictable convulsions. The numerous restrictions imposed by the illness, such as being deprived of driving a car, swimming, or working with machinery, the ever present possibility of an attack in the schoolroom, factory, or a public place, and the onerous necessity of regular and unrelenting medications that often dull the senses, may lead to an irritable neurotic state with bouts of depression, rebellion, and hysteria that at times overshadow the disease itself.

TRAUMATIC BRAIN DISEASE

Traumatic brain disease implies that the patient has received a definite brain injury, which has resulted in either brain contusion, laceration, or compression or damage to the cerebral blood vessels. The impact to the head has been sufficiently severe to produce varying degrees of surgical and traumatic *shock*. The brain responds to injury as does any large visceral organ, such as the stomach, intestines, or liver. Hence the patient is not only rendered unconscious but also becomes very pale and cyanotic and has shallow, irregular respiration and a feeble, rapid pulse. The pupils are usually widely dilated, different in size, and respond poorly to light. Vomiting of a projectile type may occur within a short time after the injury.

Bleeding from a large vessel, particularly an artery, causes a rapid rise in intracranial pressure. The spinal fluid may be grossly bloody.

Individuals with severe brain laceration or slow bleeding within the cranial cavity may often appear to be normally conscious and alert. However, there may not be a clear consciousness but a condition called *automatism*. In this state the patient appears to be answering questions correctly and coherently, but on closer inquiry it will be discovered that he is not aware of having been injured, his insight is poor,

and he gives a falsified or garbled account of the accident. He may also be abnormally elated or facetious. After recovery is complete, he will recall none of this immediately posttraumatic experience.

When the patient does recover from the immediate effects of the trauma, he not only fails to recall the events that followed the time of the injury but also fails to remember events and experiences that occurred several hours or days before the time of the accident. This is called *retrograde amnesia*. Some authorities regard this symptom as a better criterion of brain damage than the duration of the period of unconsciousness.

Posttraumatic deterioration or encephalopathy

Even after apparently complete recovery from severe brain injury, gradual degeneration of brain cells and overgrowth of glial tissue may develop over a period of several years, and the patient may deteriorate mentally.

Encephalographic changes that confirm the clinical signs of chronic dementia can be detected. The brain rhythm is irregular, with slow waves and bursts of rapid, high-voltage discharges typical of epilepsy.

Convulsions may appear in the person with a traumatized brain as late as five years after the injury. Marked personality changes display themselves through a greatly altered personality, emotional instability, and outbursts of rage that are contrasted against a general mood of indifference. Memory defects can be demonstrated, as well as inability to focus attention upon any productive work.

In addition to true epileptic seizures,

the person suffering from posttraumatic brain deterioration may also be subject to recurring attacks of automatism. The patient may have "wandering states" or may have explosive outbursts of violent and homicidal behavior that are not recalled when normal conduct is resumed.

Treatment and nursing care

The treatment and nursing care of the patient with psychosis or "personality change" following severe brain damage is largely a matter of sensible, understanding management. It is better that such patients occupy quiet quarters away from relatives and other patients to prevent outbursts of petulance and paranoid reactions. Emotional demonstrations of any sort should be avoided as much as possible. Some simple form of occupation that makes little demand for sustained physical or mental effort does much to keep the patient contented and free of wide mood swings.

PSYCHOSIS WITH EPIDEMIC ENCEPHALITIS

Psychoses with epidemic encephalitis are probably caused by a virus infection of the brain. In the acute phase the patient is delirious and feverish and often complains of diplopia. These symptoms are usually followed by a long period of lethargy that may last for several days and in rare instances for several months. In adults the symptoms that usually become progressively more severe include gradual spasticity of the limbs, constant tremor of the hands, a masklike expression, and drooling of saliva from the

mouth. This condition is called Parkinson's syndrome. The mental disturbances are usually secondary to the patient's muscular rigidity and general physical helplessness. Irritability, moroseness, frequent bodily complaints, and insomnia are the most common features. True mental deterioration rarely occurs except in very advanced cases.

Treatment of parkinsonism with hyoscine does much to relieve the stiffness, fatigue, and drooling. Hyoscine hydrobromide can be given by mouth, 1/150 grain two or three times a day. Stramonium, in 5-grain doses three times a day, has the same beneficial effect.

Sedatives are helpful for irritability and insomnia. The nursing care of the patient with the chronic form of encephalitis requires patience, understanding, and thoughtful guidance. Mild exercise should be alternated with long periods of bed rest. The patient should be encouraged to feed himself, even though the procedure requires an extra amount of time. The food should be solid because the patient has difficulty in swallowing soups or semisoft material. Because of constant tremor, the patient suffering from Parkinson's disease should not be hurried, and much patience is essential on the part of the nurse when she assists him. Occupational therapy is recommended when the tremor is mild and the medical treatment provides muscular relaxation.

PSYCHOSES WITH HUNTINGTON'S CHOREA

Huntington's chorea is a hereditary disease involving the brain. It was first described by an American physician in 1872.

The symptoms usually develop in middle life, with twitching of the face and purposeless movements of the trunk and limbs. In severe cases these movements become so pronounced and constant that the sufferer can no longer feed or dress himself. There is frequently evidence of slow intellectual deterioration and personality changes expressed by irritability and outbursts of temper. Occasionally the patient expresses ideas of reference and delusions of persecution. Attempts at suicide are common because patients soon become aware of the hopelessness of their condition.

There is no specific treatment for this disease.

BEHAVIOR DISORDERS ASSOCIATED WITH CHRONIC ALCOHOLISM
Korsakoff's psychosis

In some respects Korsakoff's psychosis, an interesting form of alcoholism first described by Korsakoff in 1887, is an acute alcoholic reaction. It is regarded as evidence of brain damage because it results in a certain degree of personality change and blunting of intellectual capacity. In this condition the patient may appear to be delirious, but more accurately the picture is one of memory defect concealed by falsification. The patient has a memory gap for recent events and fills in these gaps with confabulations. In addition, there is peripheral neuritis with tingling of the extremities, or in severe cases there may be wristdrop and footdrop.

Characteristically, there are pronounced changes in the brain cells, as well as degenerative disease of the peripheral nerves. All these disturbances are due to a deficiency of vitamin B, particularly niacin. Treatment with thiamine, niacin, brewer's yeast, and a vitamin-rich diet of milk, fruit, and meat generally restore the patient to nearly normal physical and mental health.

Alcoholic dementia or deterioration

Alcoholic dementia or deterioration is the end result of prolonged and excessive drinking and is essentially a chronic dementia. The onset is gradual, and a personality change, which becomes more evident to the family than it does on the street or in the shop, occurs slowly. The patient lacks perseverance, becomes maudlin, and is careless as to appearance. He will not tolerate any criticism of his drinking and becomes touchy and irritable. He indulges in shallow rationalizations to explain his drinking. There is a certain guile and superficial poise in contacts with outsiders and a fawning respect for authority, but at home the chronic alcoholic is a petty tyrant. His capacity for work suffers greatly, and he not only neglects his family but also becomes dependent upon them for support. Chronic alcoholic degeneration represents one of the most common and bitter social tragedies that blight family life. Its malignant influence may extend to many innocent individuals, particularly the children, upon whom it may leave a deep psychological impression.

BEHAVIOR DISORDERS ASSOCIATED WITH CEREBRAL ARTERIOSCLEROSIS

While senile dementia and arteriosclerotic psychosis are considered as being two separate ailments, the two conditions quite frequently exist side by side. Arteriosclerotic brain disease generally appears much earlier than does true senile deterioration, the symptoms beginning sometimes as early as the fiftieth year. Actually, disease of the arteries may be found in relatively young individuals. A patient suffering from this condition may expire with failure of coronary circulation, failure of kidney function, or a massive hemorrhage in the brain long before he attains old age.

Mental symptoms of simple arteriosclerosis

Simple arteriosclerosis is the arteriosclerosis of the more elderly patient. The blood pressure is not very high; in fact, it may be normal. The disease involves the larger arteries of the body and the brain. Large patches or plaques of fatty and calcified material appear in the inside layers of the blood vessels, gradually closing down or narrowing the channel or lumen. In the brain this may lead to anemia and sluggish circulation.

The mental symptoms are not unlike those of true senile dementia, but they may appear rather suddenly. The patient may experience attacks of unconsciousness, confusion, loss of speech, and temporary paralysis of one side of the body. These symptoms may gradually disappear only to recur at irregular intervals. In the meantime, general mental efficiency becomes lessened, speech shows some defects in articulation, and irritability increases. Finally, an attack of unconsciousness occurs, fever develops, and, if the patient does not expire, recovery is in-

complete and a permanent hemiplegia may cause the patient to be permanently disabled.

The lesion in the brain is not generally a true hemorrhage in this type of cerebral arteriosclerosis. More often it is a large area of softening where the brain tissue has degenerated because of total blocking of the artery that supplies the particular part. The process of acute softening is therefore caused by a thrombosis.

IMPORTANT CONCEPTS

1. Like other organs of the body, the brain suffers whenever some systemic disease elaborates poisons or impairs circulation.
2. The treatment of symptomatic delirium is essentially the treatment of the infection or circulatory defect that is the disturbing factor.
3. Irrespective of the cause, the delirious patient is critically ill and requires constant and sympathetic bedside supervision.
4. General paresis is caused by a progressive syphilitic infiltration of the brain tissue that results in degeneration of nerve elements and produces typical neurological and mental disturbances.
5. The brain responds to injury as does any large visceral organ, such as the stomach, intestines, or liver.
6. Even after apparent complete recovery from severe brain injury, gradual degeneration of brain cells and overgrowth of glial tissue may develop over a period of several years and the patient may deteriorate mentally.
7. Korsakoff's psychosis is an acute alcoholic reaction, but, because it often re-

sults in a certain degree of personality change and blunting of intellectual capacity, it is regarded as evidence of brain damage.

8. Although senile dementia and arteriosclerotic psychosis are considered as being two separate ailments, the two conditions frequently exist side by side.

SUGGESTED SOURCES OF ADDITIONAL INFORMATION

Amendt, Janet A., and White, Reginald: Continued care services for mental patients, Nurs. Outlook 13:56-60, July, 1965.

Block, Marvin A.: Alcoholism is many illnesses, Nurs. Outlook 13:35-37, Nov., 1965.

Brown, Mary Louise: Helping the alcoholic patient, Amer. J. Nurs. 58:381-382, March, 1958.

Burton, Genevieve: An alcoholic in the family, Nurs. Outlook 12:30-33, May, 1964.

Cohen, Sidney, and Klein, Hazel K.: The delirious patient, Amer. J. Nurs. 58:685-687, May, 1958.

Elliot, Alta: Parkinson's disease; nursing care, Amer. J. Nurs. 55:817-818, July, 1955.

Expert Committee on Alcohol and Alcoholism: Alcohol and alcoholism; report of an expert committee, Geneva, 1955, World Health Organization, Technical Report Series No. 94.

Family-centered approach to the control of alcoholism; a conference for public health nurses, Boston, 1959, Massachusetts Department of Public Health.

Fitzig, Charmaine: Nursing in an alcohol program, Amer. J. Nurs. 66:2218-2221, Oct., 1966.

Holehouse, Edna: The alcoholic in industry, Amer. J. Nurs. 59:206-207, Feb., 1959.

King, A. R.: Basic information on alcohol, Mt. Vernon, Iowa, 1958, Cornell College Press.

Kolb, Lawrence C.: Noyes' modern clinical psychiatry, ed. 7, Philadelphia, 1968, W. B. Saunders Co., pp. 193-210.

Magee, Kenneth R.: Parkinson's disease; neurological management, Amer. J. Nurs. 55:814-817, July, 1955.

May, Philip R. A., and Wilkinson, Mary A.: Neurological nursing in a psychiatric hospital, Nurs. Outlook 12:56-58, Aug., 1964.

McCarthy, Raymond G.: Alcoholism, Amer. J. Nurs. 59:203-205, Feb., 1959.

Moser, Doris: An understanding approach to the aphasic patient, Amer. J. Nurs. 61:52-55, April, 1961.

Parry, Allen A.: Alcoholism, Amer. J. Nurs. 65:111-115, March, 1965.

Pirnie, Florence A., and Baldwin, Maitland: Observing cerebral seizures, Amer. J. Nurs. 59:366-369, March, 1959.

Platke, Frederick: Modern trends in the management and control of syphilis, Amer. J. Nurs. 55:1482-1484, Dec., 1955.

Schwartz, Morris S., and Shockley, Emmy Lanning: The nurse and the mental patient, New York, 1956, Russell Sage Foundation, pp. 149-156.

CHAPTER FIFTEEN

Patients whose behavior is classified as a personality disorder

Patients whose behavior places them in the category of having a personality disorder present a wide range of personality maladaptations. Their behavior reveals the existence of inner conflicts and difficulties expressed through a lifelong pattern of repetitive disturbances in the areas of social and sexual adaptation. Their expression of conflict differs from that of the other psychiatrically ill individuals in that they do not exhibit the gross disturbances of thought, feeling, or behavior observed among psychotic patients or the fixed psychological defenses observed among neurotic patients. Instead, they demonstrate pathological trends and inner conflicts through their maladaptive relationships with others. Characteristically they demonstrate the minimum evidence of anxiety.

The standard nomenclature of the American Psychiatric Association classifies the personality disorders as *personality pattern disturbances,* which include the inadequate personality, the cyclothymic personality, the schizoid personality, and the paranoid personality; *personality trait disturbances,* which include the compulsive personality, the passive-aggressive personality, and the emotionally unstable personality; *sociopathic personality disturbances,* which include antisocial reaction, dyssocial reaction, sexual deviation, and addiction to alcohol and drugs; and *special symptom reactions,* which include learning disturbance, speech disturbance, enuresis, somnambulism, and others. This chapter will focus its attention upon the group of individuals who are classified as exhibiting sociopathic personality disturbances.

Formerly, most patients now classified as antisocial personalities under the larger heading of sociopathic personality disturbance were labeled with the term constitutional psychopathic state or the more familiar label of psychopathic personality. This diagnostic terminology suggested that the patient's problem was a part of his basic constitutional makeup and thus discouraged an attempt to identify the underlying psychodynamics of his behavior. This viewpoint discouraged a search for an effective treatment for the condition and encouraged a feeling of hopelessness in relation to the patient's prognosis. Finally, the term psychopathic personality became a wastebasket designation into which antisocial behavior that did not fit logically into other diagnostic categories was placed. In spite of a change in nomenclature and an official dropping of the old terminology, the classification of psychopathic personality continues to be used.

THE ANTISOCIAL PERSONALITY
Description

Patients who are said to possess antisocial personalities seem incapable of conforming to social or legal standards. They constitute a threat to society because of their ruthless attitude toward others and their lack of a sense of responsibility. They usually test within the normal range on an intelligence test, and many are intellectually superior. In spite of this ability, they seem incapable of making a satisfactory social adjustment. These people are usually self-centered and selfish; they lack the ability to develop lasting and meaningful relationships with other people; they possess poor judgment and insight; they do not profit by experience or punishment; and they are unreliable and devoid of a sense of responsibility.

Development

The reason for the inability of individuals with antisocial personalities to develop satisfactory social relationships is unknown. The defect seems to lie in the emotional and volitional aspects of the personality rather than in the intellectual areas.

In studying the longitudinal histories of many of these patients it is usually obvious that they were emotionally impulsive and maladjusted children. They have apparently failed to develop a socialized superego. The personality appears to be dominated by the primitive demands of the id. The ego has failed to establish a constructive identity or to evolve socially useful adaptations and controls. In some way these individuals have failed to make a positive identity with parents or parental substitutes who should have provided the love, security, recognition, and respect that a child requires if he is to develop into an emotionally healthy individual. Failure to make a positive identification and to accept socially useful controls may have been the result of a faulty parent-child relationship. At any rate the psychopathological forces that were initiated in the individual's early life experiences have continued throughout adulthood. Thus most of these patients seem to possess an inherent ego defect that causes them to basically distrust others and to respond to primitive id impulses regardless of society's disapproval.

Treatment

If patients with antisocial personalities are to be treated with any hope of success they will require institutionalization. Because their early childhood relationships with parental figures have not resulted in the development of essential ego controls or a socialized superego, an opportunity to correct this defective development should be provided. The institution should provide a friendly, accepting, human environment, where there are firm, reasonable, consistent limits and controls placed upon behavior. A permissive atmosphere is usually not helpful for these individuals. They need to be helped to develop a socialized superego, and such growth may be fostered by an organized, structured, controlled environment.

The treatment goals for these patients should include helping them to accept and utilize more socially approved attitudes and standards in their relationships with other people. To achieve this they must be helped to trust other people. Hopefully this can be achieved through the development of a therapeutic relationship with one of the members of the professional team. Since the psychiatrist is usually the ultimate authority in the hospital, it would probably be helpful if the therapeutic relationship could be developed with a psychiatrist who could provide the necessary discipline.

The treatment goals can be promoted through a system of rewards and prohibitions, with socially acceptable behavior being rewarded with privileges and less acceptable behavior being responded to by the withholding of privileges.

If the antisocial behavior has developed out of social and cultural influences, the patient should be helped to cultivate a more acceptable social situation. Certainly he should not be allowed to return to the same environment.

Nursing care

Sometimes the nurse feels that a patient who is described as having a sociopathic personality is a criminal and should be excluded from all ward and hospital activities. Or she may believe that he does not require hospitalization and may disregard the need to establish firm, consistent limits. Either of these extremes in attitude will prove to be unsound if the nurse follows them in giving care to such a patient.

Since the patient with antisocial attitudes is often attractive, above average in intelligence, and an interesting conversationalist, the nurse should avoid allowing the patient to gain control of the situation. It is helpful to remember that these individuals are usually clever and frequently use extremely poor judgment. They are likely to be troublemakers among other patients and have been known to organize psychotic individuals into helping them accomplish antisocial plans.

Although the nurse can be most effective if she uses a helpful, friendly approach in her dealings with the patient with antisocial attitudes, she needs to be constantly alert to the possibility of his attempting to control the situation. The nursing personnel, with the aid of the physician in charge, should identify attitudes they believe will be most effective in dealing with this patient and should list the responsibilities that he will be expected to fulfill. When these decisions

have been made, it is of primary importance for the nursing personnel to be consistent in carrying them out and in holding the patient to his obligations.

These patients should not be scolded or lectured. Such an approach is never helpful and will serve only to make the patient angry. Since it is thought that these individuals learn little from experience, punishing them accomplishes nothing. Limits must be set upon their behavior, since they frequently indulge in temper tantrums or destructive activities to achieve their objectives. The nurse who is confronted by such a behavior problem should call for enough help to control the patient and to stop the destruction he is causing. Patients do not respond to reasoning during an episode of explosive behavior.

When the patient is demonstrating antisocial behavior it is important for the nurse to treat him in such a manner that he will know that she wants to help him even though she cannot allow him to continue the behavior he is exhibiting.

Organizing the hospital day. Patients with antisocial attitudes need a variety of challenging activities throughout the day. They are likely to plead for special privileges, but the nurse should be cautious about granting such requests, since these individuals may not be reliable. They, like all other patients, should be rewarded for acceptable behavior with praise and recognition. If possible these patients should be placed in situations where they can obtain socially acceptable satisfactions. Thus success in some type of industrial therapy is ideal for them. It is essential to hold these patients to the responsibilities expected of them, since they are likely to cooperate only at their own convenience.

Since many of these patients lack a well-developed social conscience, they usually function poorly in group activities. However, insofar as possible it is suggested that they be helped to accept a role in some of the group functions in which other patients are participating.

Patients with antisocial attitudes vary greatly in emotional needs and personality limitations. Their care in the psychiatric hospital should be designed to help them with their individual problems and to make it possible for them to cultivate a more socially acceptable approach to living.

Nurses misjudge this group of patients more often than any other with whom they come in contact. Inexperienced nurses are likely to feel that the hospital is holding a perfectly normal person without justification. It would be well for all nurses to remember that it is almost unheard of for a psychiatric hospital to keep a patient who does not need the specialized types of care it offers.

Case history

The following story was adapted from a recent newspaper* account of the antisocial behavior of young adolescent youth:

A 15-year-old youth was arrested for breaking into and robbing eighteen Catholic churches. In addition to these robberies he admitted burglarizing several homes in the area of the city in which he lived.

*Philadelphia Bulletin, Sept. 23, 1969.

This boy had been abandoned on the steps of a large hospital when he was an infant. He was found by a kindly nurse's aide who took him to her home and cared for him. She was a member of a Catholic church and chose to name the boy after the priest of the church she attended. After ten years the foster mother reported that "he went bad" and was sent to a Youth Study Center where psychiatric help and rehabilitation were attempted. The child never returned to live with his foster mother. Instead he lived with anyone who would offer him bed and board for a few days. He was arrested at the office of a community organization, which he said was his home. At that time he had several thousand dollars in a paper bag hidden among his possessions.

Although no other information was available, his story demonstrates rather clearly many of the characteristics of an individual who because of his behavior is said to possess an antisocial personality. Although we know nothing about his foster mother or the relationship that she estabilshed with him, we can be sure that until he was ten years old he was taken to church regularly and taught the basic beliefs of the church. It is interesting to speculate about why he turned against the church with which he was affiliated. It is possible that the church symbolized his foster mother and her teachings, which he rejected. It is safe to suggest that in some way he was unconsciously striking out against his foster mother when he attacked the church that she respected and loved.

Certainly this boy failed to develop a socialized superego. Thus his behavior was dominated by instinctual demands that included the amassing of money, which is symbolic of power. Money also made it possible for him to indulge many of his phantasies. It is not possible to know what ego identity this adolescent had developed, but we do know that he failed to develop a constructive identity and had not incorporated socially useful controls. Like other individuals who are said to possess antisocial personalities, he seemed incapable of conforming to social or legal standards. Even though he was treated at the Youth Study Center he did not profit by this experience and thus can be said not to be able to profit by experience. He appeared to have no sense of responsibility.

The situation demonstrates the reason why for many years such behavior was thought to result from a constitutional defect within the makeup of the individual. Antisocial behavior is usually exhibited early in life. It is difficult to identify a reasonable explanaton for its occurrence. This boy was abandoned by his own parents. To some this may suggest that they too were lacking in the ability to accept responsibility and to conform to social or legal standards. Some people might conclude that this young man inherited a defective personality. However, current theories of personality development would not support this belief. Instead, the search for the basic problem would focus upon the relationship that existed in the family situation where this young man lived during his first ten years.

It can readily be seen that treatment of this boy was challenging, since his conflict obviously lay in the emotional and volitional areas of life. His antisocial personality developed very early and progressed rapidly. Certainly, institutionalization was indicated.

A friendly, accepting, human environment is the only type of situation in which personality defects can be corrected. However, at the same time, such an individual requires firm, consistent, reasonable controls. The treatment goals would include helping this young man to accept and utilize more socially approved behavior in relation to other people and society's institutions. Success in achieving these goals is problematic at best and depends upon the ability of the treatment team to identify and work with the healthy aspects of the individual's personality.

PATIENTS WHOSE BEHAVIOR IS CLASSIFIED AS DYSSOCIAL REACTION

There are a group of individuals who, in contrast to the patients with antisocial personalities, develop warm relationships and strong loyalties with other people, especially people of their own ethnic or cultural group. However, these individuals are antisocial in their orientation and may actually carry out criminal activities. Today this phenomena can be observed among the adolescents who have developed strong feelings of loyalty to the other members of the gang to which they belong. In such a situation the gang behavior may be culturally and environmentally determined. Members of the gang may be helped to redirect their loyalties if they can be removed from the environment that reinforces the gang behavior.

On the other hand there are adults whose behavior falls within the category of dyssocial reaction who lack moral responsibility and who deal in excessive rationalization about their antisocial conduct. Many of the individuals in this group are professional criminals.

SEXUAL DEVIATION

According to the psychoanalytical explanation, perversions are the result of failure to outgrow some infantile or preadolescent manner of obtaining sexual pleasure. The sexually perverted individual is one who continues to get sexual relief by immature methods throughout adult life.

The normal development of sexual life in the human being is a slow and complex psychobiological process. As Freud has postulated, the sexual instinct passes through several stages of growth, and an arrest or fixation at immature levels may cause serious distortions of the total personality.

The various sexual perversions are, therefore, malconditionings or incomplete expressions of the psychological accompaniments of sexual activity. Apart from the explanations offered by the psychoanalysts, little is known as to the etiology of most deviations in sexual behavior. In general, society looks with antipathy and disfavor upon individuals who practice sexual perversions and in some instances offers violent resentment. Although the legal attitudes toward sexual deviation are becoming more rational, there are laws on the statute books to punish sex offenders, many of whom are unfortunate victims of a distorted psychosexual development. These legal implications are probably based on mid-Victorian attitudes and a failure to understand the origin of sexual deviations. They may also be related to society's concern about a threat to normal propagation and successful survival of the race. Sex variants tend to repeat their particular perversion even after experiencing cruel, inhuman punishment and suffering.

Behavior characteristics

As more psychological understanding of the personalities of individuals who have failed to achieve a mature psychosexual development is achieved, there is a growing belief on the part of specialists that the psychopathology underlying their problems is basically psychoneurotic. Usually sexual deviation is only one manifestation of a deep-seated personality disorder of long duration. All individuals who utilize a perverted outlet to release sexual tension exhibit a pattern of behavior that is repeated compulsively without reason or logic. It is not a substitute for normal heterosexual relations but is carried on to meet a specific unconscious need, which the individual himself does not understand.

The following is an example of such behavior. A respected middle-aged married citizen of a small midwestern town was arrested for voyeurism or for being a Peeping Tom. He admitted that for most of his life he had been peeping at night into the bedroom windows of his neighbors. Unfortunately he was not apprehended for many years, and when he was finally caught, the anger of the townspeople was so great that he and his family were forced to leave the community.

In addition to voyeurism, some of the other sexual perversions include pedophilia, fetishism, transvestism, and exhibitionism. A brief explanation of each follows.

Pedophilia is the technical word used to describe adult males who demonstrate a pathological sexual interest in children. This situation usually occurs when the adult feels inadequate sexually and is afraid to approach an adult female for fear of being rejected or of being sexually inadequate. Thus the individual approaches a child sexually in the unconscious hope that he will be accepted by a less discriminating person. His behavior is apt to frighten the child who usually cries out for help. The cry frightens the offender who may flee. Unfortunately some offenders have injured or killed the child to keep from being apprehended.

Fetishism occurs in men who may unconsciously fear genital heterosexual contact due to castration fears that developed early in life. For these men sexual feeling is attached to some inanimate object that may have belonged to a woman for whom the individual once developed admiration, or the object may simply have a female association. The fetish may be a glove, a shoe, a girdle, or some other very personal feminine object. Since contact with the object usually leads to orgasm, the use of the fetish is a substitute for genital heterosexuality.

Transvestism occurs when an individual has an unconscious urge to dress in the clothing of the opposite sex. In some men this urge is one of several manifestations of a profound personality disturbance involving homosexuality with a paranoid ideation.

Exhibitionism occurs when the male has an uncontrollable urge to exhibit the genitalia to others, usually females. This symptom is thought to occur in males who are defending themselves against guilt and fear of punishment arising out of unconscious incestuous wishes. Thus the male exhibits the penis to reassure himself that it is still intact and that he has not been punished for his incestuous desires. Exhibition of the genitals may also serve to demonstrate sexually aggressive feelings toward all women.

Homosexuality

Although there are a variety of sexual perversions, the one that receives the most attention in our modern culture is homosexuality. It involves sexual attachment and love for a person of the same sex. There is a wide range of homosexual behavior in both men and women. According to the statistics revealed by the armed services, draft, and induction boards, it occurs frequently.

The basic cause of this emotional problem is thought to lie in the early childhood experiences of the individual. It is essentially an arrest in the individual's psychosexual development. Homosexuality is often attributed to excessive domination by the parent of the opposite sex or by fixation on siblings of the same sex. In extreme forms, the evidence of homosexuality is clearly shown in the tendency to take on the manners, the dress, and the vocational interests that normally belong to the opposite sex. This is, however, not a universal rule, and milder degrees of homosexuality are intermixed with manifestations of natural heterosexuality. In the homosexual male, effeminacy of the body may or may not be in evidence, and frequently the physique may be definitely athletic and suggestive of normal masculinity.

When confronted by a situation where denied homosexual longings can no longer be repressed or when the individual is threatened by open exposure of his psychosexual defects, homosexual men whose abnormal sexual desires are latent may react violently with behavior described as *homosexual panic*. This reaction may take on the proportions of a true psychosis. However, it is usually of short duration unless it appears as a prelude to schizophrenia. Homosexual panic occurs in the individual whose homosexual desires are latent. It often occurs when the individual is compelled to live in intimate relation with a large group of the same or of the opposite sex.

Changing attitudes toward sexual deviation

The individual who has failed to reach psychosexual maturity and who satisfies his sexual impulses by utilizing one of the sexual perversions is said to be a sexual psychopath or sexual deviate. Historically, some nations have looked upon sexual deviation entirely as a moral and legal problem. Partially because of their heritage of the English moral code, Canada and the United States adopted this attitude. Recently there have been some suggestions that a beginning understanding of the psychological causes of sexual deviation is developing. Some positive changes in attitude can be observed in the treatment of these individuals by the courts, professional people, and the law enforcement officers. Today there seems to be a beginning recognition of the fact that sexual deviates suffer from a serious personality defect due to an arrest in psychosexual development. This deviation probably came about through no fault of theirs but rather because of faulty parent-child relationships. Specifically, sons may unconsciously identify with the female role when brought up by overprotective mothers, or in homes where there is no father, or in situations where the father is an awesome, threatening figure. Thus these boys may grow up rejecting the

male role and feeling emotionally like women.

At least one nation, Great Britain, has adopted laws that permit homosexual activity between consenting adults. Many experts believe that adult homosexuals should not be hounded by the police and punished by jail sentences as some states in the United States have permitted in the past. Everyone agrees that children and adolescents should be safeguarded against seduction by a sexual deviate. Many of the laws relating to homosexuality were originally enacted as a safeguard. The entire legal question about sexual deviation is currently being reviewed in many nations. Certainly this is a difficult question that needs rethinking in the United States.

Prevention and treatment

Sexual deviation is difficult to treat successfully because the problem arises out of a faulty personality structure. By the time an individual comes to the attention of professional workers who can provide treatment, the personality structure has been patterned in a defective manner. The individual expresses sexual impulses in a deviant way because his psychosexual development has been arrested or has regressed to an immature level. Thus sexually deviated behavior is a deeply ingrained part of the individuals personality. In addition he has little understanding of it, and since it temporarily relieves his sexual tensions, he is often loathe or unable to substitute more mature behavior.

The only treatment method now available that can assist the individual to make such a profound alteration in his personality adaptation is psychoanalysis. This treatment is expensive, involves a great deal of time and personal commitment on the part of both the patient and the psychiatrist, and is available to a limited number of people. Success is entirely dependent upon the cooperation of the individual seeking help. Although sexual deviates are interested in avoiding involvement with the legal authorities, they are not always interested in profoundly altering their sexual behavior.

If competent psychiatric treatment is available, if the sexually deviated individual is highly motivated to change his lifelong pattern of adaptation, and if he is prepared to continue therapy for a prolonged period of time, some positive changes in sexual behavior may be achieved.

Unfortunately, in some states sexually deviant individuals who are taken into custody by law enforcement officers are required by the court to seek psychiatric help. Occasionally they are sentenced to spend a specific length of time in a center where psychiatric treatment is provided. Such court action is an attempt to utilize current knowledge concerning the psychological causes of sexual deviation. However, this approach usually does not achieve positive results for the individual or for society.

Many sexual deviates are sentenced to prison terms because some aspect of their behavior is considered damaging to the morals of others. Prison environments have a negative influence on these individuals. In spite of this, it is sometimes necessary to confine some of them to corrective institutions if they have committed serious social offenses.

When an individual who is a sexual de-

viant requests psychiatric help and willingly accepts hospitalization, it is thought to be therapeutically valuable to admit him to a psychiatric treatment situation. In this way the patient's therapist can supervise his environment and plan to meet his needs. Another advantage of hospitalization is that it removes the patient from the environment in which sexual deviation was his mode of expression. In time, with competent psychiatric help the individual may be able to redirect his sexual and aggressive drives so that his personal and social functioning may be improved.

Sexual deviation, like all human problems with a psychological origin, should be prevented so that treatment will be unnecessary. The first step in prevention is effective sexual education for all children. Currently, much discussion is being carried on throughout the United States concerning sex education. The arguments focus upon who should provide it and where it should be given. Some lay people are attacking the efforts that have been made in some schools to provide adequate sex education. The schools introduced this instruction because there was evidence that sex education was not being adequately provided elsewhere. Certainly children require accurate and complete sexual information if they are to develop wholesome, mature attitudes. Most authorities agree that such information can be taught most effectively in schools by individuals who are educationally prepared to provide such information. Most people also agree that this teaching should be reinforced and elaborated by the parents in the home.

Not only is adequate sex education essential, but also it is necessary to provide positive parent-child relationships and a healthy family environment in the early formative years in order for children to achieve mature psychosexual development. Because children identify sexual roles at an early age, they need the presence of both parents in the home in order that they may establish an identification with the parent of the same sex. Thus the family pattern established in homes is crucial to the healthy emotional development of children. During their formative years they need guidance from wise parents in redirecting aggressive impulses into constructive and socially acceptable channels.

It would be helpful if early identification and corrective experiences could be provided for children who seem to be developing social reactions that vary greatly from those expected from others of their peer group.

Nursing care

When an individual suffers from arrested psychosexual development, his total personality is affected. Thus the nurse can expect immature behavior in many areas from an individual who utilizes a sexually deviant means of expressing sexual needs. He may sulk, demand special attention, display many dependent needs, utilize provocative behavior, blame others for his situation, or become sarcastic and hostile toward the hospital staff.

The wise nurse will seek guidance from the psychiatrist in relation to the most appropriate ways to deal with the behavior such a patient is presenting. Certainly the nurse should avoid identifying with the patient or reenforcing his negative behav-

ior by giving nonverbal approval to it.

Sometimes nurses behave as if the patient who has a history of sexual deviation is a social outcast. When individuals harbor such feelings, they inevitably treat the patient in a cold, unfriendly manner. Such feelings on the part of a member of the professional treatment team tends to destroy much of the therapeutic effect the group is attempting to achieve. Such attitudes suggest that the individual holding them fails to realize that the sexually deviant person is not entirely responsible for his problem.

Sexually deviant individuals, like all other patients, deserve a friendly, accepting climate where they are treated with respect and consideration. In addition they require the establishment of firm limits that are fairly and consistently enforced. Since the nurse has a good deal of responsibility for developing the climate in the treatment situation, her understanding of the patient's problem and her attitude toward him is of major importance. The patient needs to have a well-planned schedule of daily activities available so that he can avoid lethargy and boredom. He needs help in becoming an active participant in some aspects of the planned schedule of activities.

Case history

The patient, a young man, 20 years of age, was admitted to a psychiatric treatment center because of a handwashing compulsion, feelings of unreality, and because he feared that he would kill his mother.

He was an unplanned baby, born after his parents had been married for 12 years. His father frankly stated that he wanted a girl and paid no attention to the child until he was old enough to walk. The child never seemed content in his mother's arms and pushed her breast away from the first time it was offered to him. As he grew older he bit and scratched her.

When the patient was 5 years old his father died. He became overly attached to his mother and shared her bed until he was 11 years old. During these years he would scream for his mother if she were out of sight. He frequently called out to her "Mama are you all right"?

His mother began drinking heavily after the father's death and often relegated his care to a neighbor woman. At age 11 his care became more than the mother could manage, and she sent him to live at a boy's boarding school. This decision made him desperately unhappy, and he pled with her not to send him away. During these years he was sent to a boy's camp during the summer months. This was seen by him as banishment and made him desperately unhappy. He especially disliked the camp because he did poorly in all sports. About the time he was in the eighth grade his mother became interested in remarrying. He told her that he would kill himself if she did.

As he grew older his relationship with his mother became progressively more strained. When he was 16, in the hope of improving the situation, his mother allowed him to remain at home and attend high school. Instead of responding to this decision with pleasure, his anger toward his mother increased, and he began calling her a liar and other derogatory names.

During his sixteenth year he had his first homosexual experience, during which he participated in anal intercourse as the passive partner. After this first experience he participated frequently in homosexual relations. This activity caused him to feel ashamed, guilty, and angry. The handwashing compulsion as a ritualistic protection against his bad thoughts and deeds developed soon after

he bagan engaging in mutual masturbation and anal intercourse. It relieved his anxiety and guilt feelings.

In studying this young man's life history it seems clear that he spent his years at home seeking closeness from his mother. After his father's death he became very good and docile in the hope of winning his mother's acceptance and love. Until puberty this boy dedicated himself to being his mother's "good little girl." At puberty his behavior changed because he was in great conflict. His conflict appeared to be based upon his fear of behaving like a man sexually and being punished for being sexually dangerous to women (especially his mother) or renouncing his masculinity and being humiliated by being treated like a woman (when he accepts the role of passive partner during anal intercourse with a man). His conflict between his fear of injuring someone if he behaves like a man and of acting like a woman and being humiliated resulted in a complete inability to make decisions or to function in any situation. The handwashing ritual like all symptoms fulfilled an important purpose in his life. In addition to relieving tension it kept his hands free from harming others.

This young man lost his father at the age of 5 years, which is a crucial time in a child's life. It is not unusual for children of that age to phantasize that they were responsible for the loss of the absent parent. During his formative years he slept with his mother. Undoubtedly his close contact with his mother aroused sexual feelings and gave rise to sexual phantasies. When he was banished at 11 years of age to the boarding school he undoubtedly felt that it was a punishment because of his "bad" thoughts (sexual thoughts). He had no male parent with whom to identify and after whom to pattern his behavior. An attempt to adapt by accepting the feminine role resulted in guilt and frustration.

Obviously this patient's basic personality development was defective, and homosexuality was only one of several pathological symptoms that he developed. In evaluating his future it is unrealistic to expect psychiatric help to provide him with a well-integrated personality. Psychotherapy can give him some palliative relief from some of his most painful symptoms and help him cope more effectively with his emotional problems.

PROBLEMS OF ALCOHOL AND DRUG ADDICTION

There are many chemical substances that, when taken internally, cause abnormal mental reactions. Not all of them are taken intentionally. Some are given as medication to which there is an individual sensitivity, and still others may be absorbed slowly without the knowledge of the individual. Examples of the latter form of poisoning are lead and manganese encountered in industry and the inhalation of exhaust fumes from automobiles. When excessive amounts of many drugs are absorbed or allowed to accumulate slowly in the blood, delirium, loss of memory, and stupor may result.

Far more common are the mental reactions caused by the intentional and habitual use of drugs, such as alcohol, barbiturates, bromides, and morphine, which deaden the senses and provide a temporary escape from anxiety.

ALCOHOLISM

People whose intake of alcoholic beverages is so great that it interferes markedly with their work performance and their functioning as responsible citizens are referred to as alcoholics.

Alcoholism may take many forms and has many causes. One individual may be a chronic alcoholic, which means that he drinks excessively and is incapacitated most of the time. Another person may be referred to as a periodic or cyclic alcoholic, which means that he drinks excessively during certain periods of his life but during other periods may not drink at all. A third type of alcoholism is exhibited by an individual who drinks large quantities of alcohol daily over a period of years. At first he may not seem to be seriously affected by this overindulgence. Slowly and insidiously, physical, mental, and emotional deterioration occurs. Eventually this person may be described as suffering from alcoholic deterioration. No matter what type of alcoholism is being considered, the problem is thought to have its basis in some emotional conflict, frustration, or overwhelming feeling of inadequacy. Alcohol makes it possible for the individual to escape temporarily from overwhelming emotional or social problems.

In general, those individuals who take alcohol to excess do so because they are unhappy, distraught, and maladjusted and because alcohol furnishes them a temporary release from the stresses of living. Most alcoholics are fundamentally unstable, sensitive, self-indulgent people, and many of them are suffering from a poorly developed sexuality. Drink not only offers a surcease from their feelings of inferiority but also provides an occasion for conviviality and sympathy and provides them with a temporary and false sense of ease and security. Inhibitions are weakened, and repressed desires may be freely expressed. Thus the individual's ethical and moral sense is eventually blunted. The alcoholic lives at a level of responsibility where high social adaptation is not possible. Excessive alcoholic intake sometimes precipitates a psychotic reaction. Its effects are not uniform and may bring to the surface many different reactions, some of these apparently determined by racial, social, and temperamental factors that vary with each individual.

Understanding the alcoholic patient

Each alcoholic is a unique individual with problems that are characteristically his own. Consequently, the treatment and nursing care of the alcoholic patient begins with understanding his personality and the problems from which he has a need to escape. Many alcoholic patients use alcohol in somewhat the same way that psychotic individuals use psychotic symptoms. That is, alcoholics escape from reality through alcohol, whereas some psychotic patients escape from reality through the use of their symptoms. When some alcoholics are deprived of alcohol, they may substitute psychotic symptoms such as withdrawal from reality, depression, or a paranoid reaction.

Sometimes alcohol is used to cover psychotic or neurotic symptoms. Thus some people who are labeled as alcoholics are actually suffering from a depression or anxiety state. Such patients are clearly in need of the care and treatment usually provided in a psychiatric hospital.

Many alcoholics are described as having oral personalities. This means that they are emotionally immature and are fixated at a very early stage of emotional development. This early stage of emotional development is called the oral-dependent period and is characterized by infantile emotional reactions. Such individuals get many of their emotional satisfactions from the intake of food and fluids by mouth. They are not emotionally mature enough to function as independent adults and unconsciously want to be dependent upon a strong person, much as they once were upon a mother figure. Such emotionally immature adults are extremely difficult to help because they have faulty personality structures and a limited amount of ego strength. For this reason some psychiatrists are reluctant to accept alcoholics for treatment. Some authorities believe that a patient with a weak ego structure is unable to relate positively to another person and thus will be unable to profit from psychotherapy. Some psychiatric treatment centers have adopted a policy of refusing admission to alcoholics because experience has shown that many of them respond poorly to treatment. However, some centers have concentrated on the treatment of the alcoholic patient. Alcoholism is such a serious social and health problem that the United States Public Health Service is encouraging the establishment of centers to study and treat alcoholism.

Treatment

Several treatments have been developed in an attempt to help alcoholics function without alcohol. One of these is called the aversion treatment. This treatment consists of allowing the patient to drink a good deal of his favorite alcoholic beverage, after which an emetic drug is administered. In a few minutes the patient becomes acutely nauseated and spends approximately an hour vomiting and retching. This treatment is administered two or three times a week until the patient develops such an aversion to alcohol that he begins to gag at the sight of the alcoholic beverage toward which the aversion has been developed. This treatment does not help the patient solve any of his basic emotional problems, although some psychiatrists have combined the treatment with psychotherapy. The aversion treatment does keep some patients away from alcohol for several months, and a few are able to give it up permanently. Many patients substitute some other emotional support for alcohol and frequently begin the use of drugs, particularly the barbiturates, after giving up the use of alcohol.

A drug, disulfiram (Antabuse), which was developed a few years ago, has been used successfully to treat some alcoholics. It functions something like the aversion treatment in that the patient who takes a specific amount of Antabuse daily will become nauseated when he takes even a small amount of alcohol. This drug is helpful as long as the patient is in the hospital under close supervision and takes the drug regularly. Away from the hospital some alcoholics stop taking the drug. The drug is considered to be dangerous in some instances, and a few patients have suffered untoward reactions from it.

Although alcoholism is one of the major mental health problems in our nation today, few specific ways of helping alcoholic patients have been identified.

Every alcoholic drinks for a reason. That reason is fundamentally an inability to adjust to certain demands of normal living or an attempt to cope with a basic defect in personality development. Occasionally this disorder can be rectified, and the necessity for alcohol is no longer present.

Hence, the primary treatment of the alcoholic is to aid the patient in coping with life's responsibilities without having to resort to the use of alcohol as a defense. This generally means a long period of reeducation. The success of this reeducation depends to a large extent on the patient's personal motivation.

Rehabilitation
of the alcoholic patient

The magnitude of the problem of alcoholism in the United States is demonstrated by the fact that it has now become the fourth largest health problem. Today it follows cardiovascular disease, cancer, and mental illness in the list of health problems as set forth by the United States Public Health Service. Rehabilitation of individuals who suffer from this condition is difficult and often inadequate. This situation exists primarily because only a few communities have recognized and accepted full responsibility for offering aid to patients with this problem.

As a result of shortsightedness on the part of many communities, there are a limited number of facilities for treating persons who suffer from alcoholism. This is remarkable in view of the fact that some authorities believe that there are between 4 and 5 million alcoholics or problem drinkers in the United States. Of these problem drinkers it is estimated that about 700,000 are women.

The stigma attached to alcoholism has been one of the chief causes for the attitude of disinterest toward the problem. Until recently this disinterest has blocked the way toward a more adequate approach to the treatment and rehabilitation of individuals suffering from alcoholism.

For generations both professional and lay people in our nation have dismissed the alcoholic as a person for whom little could be done, since they believed that he possessed an inadequate personality and was socially and morally incapable of giving up the habit and assuming a more responsible way of life. Alcoholism, like mental illness, has been one of the human problems to which many taboos have been attached. Thus both these tragic social and health problems failed to receive serious scientific attention until recently. Today there is more professional help available for persons who are mentally ill than for those who suffer from alcoholism.

Actually, the problems of mental illness and alcoholism are not so unrelated as they appear to be at first glance. Recently much has been written and said about alcoholism being a disease. This designation is probably not entirely accurate. One authority has made the following statement:

"There is no creditable evidence that alcoholism is a disease *entity* in the sense that it has a single specific cause such as a vitamin deficiency, a hormone disturbance, or a defective hereditary background, although these conditions may coexist in the alcoholic person just as they do in other persons. The purpose of promoting the idea that alcoholism is a disease is to remove it from the category of punishable crimes and to place it in the health field, where it can be treated by medical measures. To understand the alcoholic, we must look behind the symptoms to see what kind of a person he is; we must avoid the fallacy of treating the disease and overlooking the person. Alcoholism is more accurately thought of as a behavioral syndrome in which the drinking is symptomatic of physiological, psychological, social, and economic stresses on the individual."*

The first step in rehabilitating the alcoholic is to discover the reasons that underlie his personal problem. Hand in hand with this task is the task of encouraging the patient to accept the fact that he is an alcoholic, that he is unable to control his life without the help alcohol provides, and that he needs assistance to cope with this problem. Discovering the reasons that underlie the patient's need for alcohol frequently requires the combined work of a team of professional workers, including the social worker, the psychologist, the psychiatrist, and the nurse. Each alcoholic is an individual with a severe personality dysfunction caused by problems that are uniquely his own. Thus it becomes necessary to know a great deal about the patient's family relationships, his psychological makeup, and his emotional health before a decision can be made concerning the treatment and rehabilitation methods appropriate for him.

Significant help for the alcoholic requires some outside intervention to enable him to establish an emotional reorientation to the world. He must be helped to shift his emotional tensions and pressures in such a way as to achieve satisfactions from life without having to seek release of tensions from alcohol.

This formula for helping the alcoholic is deceptively simple. In reality it is extremely difficult to assist an individual to

---

*From Lewis, John A.: Alcoholism, Amer. J. Nurs. **56**:433, April, 1956.

establish an emotional reorientation to the world. To date, few psychiatrists or rehabilitative institutions have been successful in helping alcoholics achieve these goals. Part of the reason for the difficulties that have been experienced in helping alcoholics has to do with the fact that many alcoholics are emotionally immature and have strong unconscious dependency needs. These needs to be dependent upon a strong person, as they once were upon a mother figure, may be met by some of the situations that are precipitated by alcoholism.

An individual who has been an alcoholic for several years has usually developed a sense of worthlessness, a deep sense of guilt, and a feeling of hopelessness. Alcoholic persons present a professional staff with tremendous personality problems to be solved. In the past, many psychiatric hospitals and psychiatrists have refused to accept alcoholic patients for treatment on the basis that there were other patients who needed help and for whom their services could be more effectively used.

A perceptible change in the attitude of both lay and professional people toward the problem of alcoholism has been noticeable during the last decade. There has been an increase in clinics in this country, which have as their major purpose the treating of alcoholics. More hospitals of a general nature have designated beds for use by patients who are suffering from alcoholism. Within the last few years many statewide conferences that focused upon the problems of prevention and treatment of alcoholism have been held. These conferences were organized in the hope that the public health agencies might take the lead in solving this national problem.

Industrial management and alcoholics themselves have created two strong national forces that have provided much of the impetus for this change in attitude. Industry has come to recognize alcoholism as one of the primary reasons for the loss of man-hours on the production line. This loss of the worker's time and efficiency has become such a significant factor in the economic health of the nation that the leaders in industry have begun to seek answers to the problem through the medical services that industry normally provides. Thus industrial physicians and nurses have been alerted to their role in the prevention and treatment of alcoholism. Clinics have been developed to cope with the problems of these patients. Some industries have added psychiatrists to their medical staffs. Help has been sought from members of Alcoholics Anonymous. This organization has provided the second great impetus in this country to better understanding, treatment, and rehabilitation for alcoholics.

Alcoholics Anonymous was founded in 1935 by two alcoholics and admits to membership only individuals who are themselves alcoholics. It has had a dramatic development and today numbers more than 160,000 members throughout the world. Alcoholics Anonymous offers the alcoholic answers to his emotional needs because it utilizes the psychological principles that have been recognized as being effective in solving problems related to personality defects. Recently it has added two affiliated groups. One is for the teenaged children of alcoholics and the other is for their wives.

Because membership is limited to individuals who themselves have been unable to control the problem of alcohol, members have a good deal of sympathy, patience, and understanding for each other. They work in teams of two or three and call upon known alcoholics who are in need of help. Through the program of the organization they are able to meet the alcoholic's dependent needs by seeking him out, encouraging him, helping him find a job, accompanying him to meetings of the organization, and giving him a sense of personal value and worth. Membership requires that each individual admit that he is powerless over alcohol and is in need of help from a power greater than himself. He searches out his own past errors and, having admitted them to another human being, undertakes to make amends for them. He strives to follow a simple code of living without drinking that eventually becomes a philosophy of life. The organizational meetings include testimonials by the members concerning their struggles with alcohol and their eventual triumph.

Alcoholics Anonymous offers a new experience in group participation and the use of group support. Thus it is that this organization is able to assist its members to develop a new emotional orientation toward life and to begin to meet the problems of life without the aid of alcohol. Many physicians refer alcoholic patients to this organization for help. Most social agencies work closely with Alcoholics Anonymous, and it is generally accepted as the most helpful approach available at this time to the problem of alcoholism. The following life story of one member will serve to point up the effectiveness of the work of this group.

Case report

Mr. White, a successful shoe salesman 34 years of age, was the father of four children, who ranged in age from 10 to 2 years, when his wife was killed in an automobile accident while on her way to a club meeting with two other women. When this tragedy struck the White family, they were living in a modest home they had started to purchase. Mrs. White's parents lived in the same neighborhood and were able to help with the care of the children. However, Mr. White was responsible for their total care after he came home from work each evening and all day on Saturday and Sunday. In addition, he found that he had to plan meals, direct the housekeeper who came in for a few hours each day, and make many decisions about the care of the home and the children that were entirely new to him. Mr. White missed the golf games he had formerly enjoyed on Sunday afternoons. In many ways he felt overwhelmed by the responsibility of being both mother and father to a family of four children. He felt lost without the advice and counsel he had grown to seek and expect from his wife.

In spite of his fears, he planned ways to make it possible for him to carry this added responsibility. At first neighbors and fellow workers were concerned and asked often about how things were going. Occasionally someone invited the family out for a meal so that once in a while he was relieved of the monotony of preparing the evening meal. However, in a few months people began to take his tragic plight for granted and no longer seemed concerned about him or his family.

It was about six months after the death of Mrs. White that he began stopping in for a drink after work. Soon he found that the companionship in the bar was so pleasant that he lingered longer than he should and drank more than he had intended. Frequently the children were crying when he arrived home because they were hungry and there was no one at home to prepare the evening meal. The 10-year-old daughter did all she could and eventually began assuming the responsibility for cooking supper. This made it possible for Mr. White to spend many more evenings away from home and frequently to return inebriated. Soon his paycheck began to dwindle. He no longer worked efficiently, and his commissions decreased. Eventually he was told that he need not report for work. Things grew progressively worse for the White family. After Mr. White lost his job, the unpaid grocery bills began to accumulate. The housekeeper stopped coming. Mr. White drank more and more to ease his anxiety and his feelings of guilt.

Two members of Alcoholics Anonymous knocked on the front door one evening when Mr. White was lying on the couch sleeping off the latest bottle of whiskey and the children were finishing a meager supper of cereal and milk. When the knock came, the 10-year-old daughter opened the door somewhat fearfully. She answered the questions about the grocery bills and her father's job. The visitors explained that they planned to find a home for the children until Mr. White was well enough to care for them. They told her that they were planning to place her father in a hospital for a few days until he felt like working. These plans were carried out. The children were placed in a foster home, and Mr. White was admitted to a general hospital in which Alcoholics Anonymous maintained a unit for the use of their members who were in need of physical care. He remained in the hospital for two weeks. During this time he received vitamin therapy and the rest and normal diet he needed. Members of Alcoholics Anonymous visited him regularly and discussed his problems. They talked about the ways in which the organization could help him. When he was ready to leave the hospital, friends from Alcohol Anonymous helped him find a job, and for a few days they accompanied him to and from work. They also began taking him to the organizational meetings where he became interested in other men who needed help with problems much like his own. As time went on, Mr. White was able to reestablish his home and to resume the care of his children. Eventually he remarried and was able to establish a home from which he received the emotional satisfactions that he needed. Thus he was helped to give up alcohol permanently.

The story of Mr. White is an example of how a new force (Alcoholics Anonymous) entered the life of an individual in trouble and, by utilizing the efforts of its members, effected a shift in the emotional tensions and pressures in his life. This shift resulted in the eventual reestablishment of Mr. White's emotional equilibrium and his complete rehabilitation.

DRUG ADDICTION AND INTOXICATION

According to John E. Ingersoll, director of the U. S. Bureau of Narcotics and Dangerous Drugs, the "abuse and misuse of narcotics and dangerous drugs has reached epidemic proportions in this country. A significant segment of the American community is involved in at least the occasional use of drugs. This constitutes a serious threat to our national health."*

The use of drugs, especially by adolescents, has become so prevalent and of such concern to the nation that articles are featured on the subject in almost every newspaper and magazine. *Time* magazine of September 26, 1969, used its cover story to focus attention upon this national prob-

---

*From Lewis, Claude: Philadelphia Bulletin, Sept. 17, 1969.

lem. In that article the author stated that "drug use reflects shifts in adult American values as well as persistent unwillingness of youth to accept the straight world. . . . Essential to any intelligent public approach to drugs is the realization that they are not an isolated phenomenon but a product of a complex often frustrating society."*

In mid-September 1969, the Senate Committee on Juvenile Delinquency began hearings to consider new legislation on drugs. Many authorities believe that the legal approach to the drug problem in the United States should be revised. Unfortunately, there seems to have been little carry-over learning from the experience the nation had with the Volstead Act in the early 1920's when an attempt was made to outlaw alcoholic beverages. It seems clear that a repeat of that period of disregard for the law will be experienced if an attempt is made to stop the flow of marijuana into the United States through the enactment of laws.

Dr. Stanley Yolles, director of the National Institute of Mental Health, estimates that between 12 and 20 million people in the United States have used marijuana at least once and that 50% of the students on college campuses located on the east and west coasts have tried marijuana at least once. These comments testify to the widespread concern currently being expressed in the communication media throughout the nation concerning the use of drugs in the United States.

Professor Hardin Jones of the Donner Laboratory at the University of California in Berkeley estimates that the consumption of drugs is rising in the United States at the rate of 7% a month.†

Most of the users of drugs do not come to the attention of physicians or nurses. Those who require treatment are usually individuals who have taken drugs because of unresolved childhood conflicts, depressed feelings, seriously disturbed basic personalities, or other unresolved psychiatric disorders. Their treatment is focused not only upon helping them cope with the drug problem but also upon resolving their basic personality disturbance.

Morphine or morphine derivatives

The habitual use of morphine or one of the morphine derivatives or pharmacological substitutes (heroin, codeine, Dilaudid, Metopon, or Demerol) is generally found in individuals who are unstable, emotionally immature, and lacking in the capacity to face reality. Very few of them have actually acquired the habit from thoughtless overmedication by a physician, although many addicts claim this to be the cause of their problem. Addicts usually resort to skillful lying and other clever forms of deceit to conceal the habit from others and to obtain the drug through illegal channels.

The victim of opiate or heroin addiction must live close to his source of supply, which means that he is compelled to associate with the people who smuggle it into the country and who sell the drug. The drug produces a temporary state of well-being, troubles appear to be trifling

---

*From Pop drugs; the high as a way of life, TIME, Sept. 26, 1969.
†Buckley, William F., Jr.: Philadelphia Bulletin, Sept. 28, 1969.

and remote, and there is a comfortable sense of complete relaxation. Ever increasing amounts are necessary to produce this exhilaration, so that the chronic morphine or heroin addict may require as much as 15 to 20 grains daily. Unfortunately, when the effects wear off and sufficient amounts are not immediately available, certain *withdrawal symptoms* promptly appear. Tears, sneezing, coryza, yawning, great irritability, and restlessness become quickly evident. Within 24 hours this is followed by abdominal cramps, vomiting, and diarrhea. To these distressing symptoms are added headache, sweating, and pains in the muscles and joints of the lower extremities. Finally, on the third day of abstinence the nervous irritability is so pronounced that the patient becomes hysterical, noisy, and threatening; he frequently throws and destroys objects within his reach. Within a week, however, all these painful withdrawal reactions disappear.

Most addicts are undernourished, either because they have anorexia or because they have insufficient funds to purchase enough food. Opiate or heroin addiction does not cause mental deterioration, but the treatment addicts receive from society causes them to deteriorate socially. Contrary to general opinion, the addict is not a fiend or a criminal. He is, in fact, an inadequate immature individual who shrinks from authority and commits a minor offense only to obtain money to buy the drug. Whenever an addict obtains an adequate dose, he may expose his addiction with an abnormal euphoria and contentment or even a sleepy languor. The pupils may show a telltale "pinpoint" constriction, and in most instances the arms and thighs are scarred or pigmented by the hypodermic needle.

Withdrawal of morphine, its derivatives, or synthetic substitutes

It is absolutely necessary to treat the addict in a closed institution in order to prevent the concealed continuance of the habit. Gradual withdrawal of the drug with palliative treatment of the withdrawal symptoms is thought to be the most effective measure. On the first day the patient should receive about 2 or 3 grains, which is approximately the amount necessary to allay the worst of the withdrawal pains. On the second and third days the dose should be reduced to 1 grain, giving $\frac{1}{4}$ grain every 4 hours. On the fourth day $\frac{1}{6}$ grain of morphine should be allowed four times a day; on the fifth day this should be reduced to $\frac{1}{8}$ grain. A hypodermic of sterile water should be injected on the day following. The patient should not be informed as to the dosage given at any time.

Withdrawal of morphine or its derivatives has been made more humane through the use of the drug methadone, which suppresses the withdrawal symptoms. The use of methadone has been a somewhat controversial method of treating drug addiction. This is partially due to the fact that methadone has been declared to be a narcotic by the Federal Bureau of Narcotics and as such has been declared illegal. Thus its procurement has been difficult. However, some authorities believe that the use of methadone with former heroin addicts holds the best hope for halting their criminal activities and for making them self-supporting citizens.

It has been used successfully with large groups of heroin addicts in two large eastern cities.

In the use of methadone the addict loses his dependency upon morphine or one of its derivatives by becoming addicted to the "substitute" methadone. The addict then requires regular doses of methadone daily.

This treatment has at least two advantages. It is relatively inexpensive. An individual can be maintained on methadone for a few cents a day. A second advantage is that an individual who is on methadone does not lose his ability to function normally. He can usually hold a job and function as a responsible citizen.

Chlorpromazine has been helpful in relieving tension states that occur when narcotics are being withdrawn. Severe withdrawal symptoms can be avoided with proper medical management.

Heroin addiction

Although heroin, a morphine derivative, is hazardous, it is the addict's drug of choice in the United States. This is probably because it is more easily obtained in this country than is morphine, and it is more potent than other narcotics. Heroin can produce the same terrifying withdrawal symptoms that may be suffered by patients who are being withdrawn from morphine. Like morphine, heroin causes the patient to feel what he describes as "normal," which means that his basic needs feel as if they have been met. Under the influence of heroin he feels sexually satisfied, full of food, free from anxiety and pain, and is not concerned with a feeling that he should fulfill aggres-

sive strivings. The need to continue this satisfied state drives heroin addicts to commit a variety of crimes to support their habit, which becomes increasingly and exorbitantly expensive.

Outcome of opiate or heroin addiction

Unless the opiate addict is highly motivated to give up the habit, he is likely to return to it after reduction treatment. Sooner or later most of them gravitate into the habit of seeking their former associations, of visiting old haunts, and finding life more tolerable by resuming the drug and the artificial sense of security it affords.

Barbituric acid intoxication

There are many preparations of barbituric acid, of which barbital (Veronal) is the most frequently employed. Most of the barbiturates tend to accumulate slowly in the tissues, particularly when taken for the relief of emotional tension or insomnia or when administered to control a noisy, psychotic patient. These drugs are frequently taken in enormous single doses by unstable people with the intent of committing suicide.

Early stages of intoxication are initiated by muscular incoordination with ataxia, dizziness, nystagmus, slurred speech, and a silly, sluggish mentality. The patient acquires many bruises by falling or stumbling against walls and furniture. In more profound barbituric acid intoxication, there are varying degrees of stupor, speech is incoherent, memory is defective, and hallucinations may appear. When aroused, the patient is usually very irritable and resistive. He presents the symptoms of a patient suffering from delirium. Recovery may be slow and may leave in its wake a mild degree of permanent dementia.

Treatment

Treatment consists of withdrawal of the drug. Prolonged bed rest, saline cathartics, and a high-calorie diet are the best restorative measures.

In cases of deep coma, hypotension, shallow breathing, and subnormal temperature, more drastic measures must be taken. Artificial respiration and hemodialysis by the artificial kidney are effective means of clearing barbiturates from the blood.

A new antidote for barbiturate intoxication is Megimide (β-ethyl-β-methylglutarimide), which is given intravenously in 50 mg. doses at intervals of 3 to 5 minutes until the return of muscle tone and pharyngeal and laryngeal reflexes. This drug is also useful in terminating barbiturate anesthesia.

Amphetamines

Amphetamines are called speed in the language of the modern drug users and are the most widely used of the really dangerous drugs. They are drugs that have been legitimately used in small doses under medical supervision to treat depression and curb appetite. They are known medically as Methedrine or Dexedrine. Individuals who take these drugs solely to become "high" take from six to two hundred times the daily dose usually prescribed by a physician. The effect of such large doses is to elevate the blood pressure, sometimes to dangerous levels. Such large doses have been known to cause immediate death. This fact accounts for the current saying among drug users that speed kills.

Individuals who use the amphetamines feel that these drugs sharpen their physical and sexual reactions and increase their confidence. Thus a period of frantic activity results from the ingestion of large amounts of one of the amphetamines. This is followed by a great letdown in which the fatigue and depression are so tremendous that the addict is apt to seek release by taking the drug again. Chronic use can lead to a schizophrenic-like psychosis or massive, irreparable brain damage that may result in death.

LSD or lysergic acid diethylamide

LSD is a drug that was originally used for research into the etiology of schizophrenia. Ingestion of reasonably small doses of LSD produce temporary hallucinations and other schizophrenic-like symptoms. Mescaline and psilocybin are related substances found in nature. Mescaline is an alkaloid derived from a plant that grows wild in the southwestern part of the United States and in Mexico.

LSD is referred to as acid by members of the subculture of drug addicts. It is 4,000 times as strong by weight as mescaline. The user experiences waves of color, and vibrations seem to pass through the head. Reality gives way to intense hallucinations. Individuals have been injured because LSD causes them to imagine that they can fly or achieve other miraculous

197

stunts. Users take massive doses that sometimes bring to the surface long repressed mental conflicts and psychotic reactions, which may continue even when the drug wears off.

Marijuana intoxication

Until recently, marijuana was an easily obtained and relatively inexpensive drug. It comes from the cannabis indica plant, which grows wild in Mexico and is easily cultivated in the United States. It is usually absorbed into the body through the smoking of cigarettes called "reefers."

Inhalation causes a state of exhilaration or euphoria. Under its influence the victim feels light in body, as if he were floating through space, and the general behavior is not unlike a mild mania. Marijuana is not an aphrodisiac, but it can lower inhibitions and intensify sexual pleasure. It seems to make many users temporarily passive, in contrast to alcohol, which frequently releases aggression. Marijuana affects the individual's sense of time but not his motor and perceptual skills. Users become psychologically dependent upon it but not addicted in the sense that one becomes addicted to morphine.

Currently a great deal of attention is being given to marijuana by the government because its use by college students has risen dramatically, as a substitute for more dangerous drugs and for alcohol. Official arguments have been carried on in the press concerning the relative dangers of marijuana and the appropriate penalties that should be levied against people who use it. Unfortunately, there is little actual research upon which to base a scientific, unbiased judgment concerning the immediate dangers of smoking marijuana or the eventual outcome of long-term use of this drug. Certainly the present laws controlling its use are inequitable, as well as widely unenforceable.

Some drug addicts who have been able to give up the habit, like cured alcoholics, have developed a method for helping others suffering from addiction. In many large cities there are institutions that are much like half-way houses. They are usually under the direction of a trained professional worker, who may have one or two other professionally trained people to assist him. Most of the therapy as well as the other work required to keep the place functioning is done by the addicts who are there to be helped or by those who have been helped and who stay on to make a contribution to the work.

In these situations, addicts who sincerely want to get rid of the drug habit live with other people struggling with similar problems. The house is usually organized along the lines of communal living, with each person accepting a share of the work necessary to keep the house liveable and to produce the meals. Several group sessions are carried on each week, during which members of the group are supportive to each other but very straightforward in demanding that the group members face their rationalizations, evasions, personal problems, and social deceptions. If a member returns to drugs he is expected to leave the group. This realistic but supportive approach has apparently helped many addicts to give up drugs and return to school or to a job.

Case history

The 24-year-old patient began using marijuana and then heroin when he was a junior in high school. This occurred when his 14-year-old girl friend refused to date him any longer. About the same time he was sent by his mother who lived in New York City to attend high school in a distant southern city because his parents were getting a divorce.

According to the patient, marijuana made him feel excited, stimulated, and happy. Everything seemed more pleasant, and he enjoyed his daydreams. He was also sexually stimulated by the drug. About the same time, the patient tried taking barbiturates, which made him sleepy. Because he did not enjoy their effect, he did not continue them. He got drunk a few times, but alcohol failed to produce the calmness and contentment he was seeking. Since marijuana did not completely fill the bill either, he tried heroin. At the time the patient first began using heroin he was convinced that his willpower would be great enough to keep him away from the drug when he wanted to be free of it.

He first took heroin in the vein. Among addicts this method is referred to as the "main line" method. He described feeling a "flash," which was accompanied by a flush of blood from the abdomen to the head and a feeling of "happiness." Although the "flash" passed away, a constant feeling of euphoria remained. For the first time in his life the patient experienced a feeling of deep contentment. He said, "It didn't affect my intellect, only my emotions. I was happy and content." From that time on the patient took heroin to assist him in facing any situation that caused him to be tense or anxious. Heroin helped him feel independent of his mother and reduced his nervousness when he was out with a girl. Heroin lessened his sexual desire and made it impossible for him to reach a sexual climax.

After the patient discovered the contentment heroin could achieve for him, he became involved in crimes to support his drug habit. As his need for larger and larger quantities of heroin grew and his habit became more costly, his crimes became more frequent and more serious. His mother repeatedly intervened to keep him out of jail by paying his fines. He entered several colleges but because of his drug habit was never able to stay in any of them for more than one semester.

Finally the patient tried to withdraw himself from heroin. He thought he could achieve this alone, since he had been withdrawn twice before in treatment centers. Of course he was not able to accomplish his goal, and finally at 24 years of age signed himself into a psychiatric treatment center in the hope of getting rid of the drug habit so that he could return to college. He had set for himself the goal of becoming an engineer.

The patient was extremely hostile toward his mother and referred to her as a physical woman but not a mother. The reasons for his hostility seemed obvious when reviewing the family history. His parents were married when the mother was 16 years old. The patient was their first child, and his mother reminded him frequently that his birth had been traumatic for her. During the patient's formative years his father suffered from tuberculosis and spent many months in a tuberculosis sanitarium. When the patient was 3 years old his mother focused much attention during his bath upon his genital hygiene. As he grew older she allowed him to observe her dressing and bathing but scolded him if he evidenced interest in her body. He began heterosexual experiences at the age of 16 years and homosexual activity at age 18.

This patient was highly intelligent and tested in the superior range on an intelligence test. When he became motivated to give up drugs, his only hope for achieving a more socially productive adaptation lay in long-term psychotherapy. It was obvious that his psychosexual development had been defective because of his rejecting, seductive mother and the frequent absence of a father figure from the home. His original experimentation with drugs and alcohol and sex may have been an expression of rebellion against an ambivalent mother who banished him in high school but who intervened on his behalf with the police.

Rehabilitation of the patient addicted to drugs

For many years the national government has maintained one treatment center at Lexington, Kentucky. It is now called the National Institute of Mental Health Clinical Research Center. In such a specialized hospital everything possible is done to help addicts break their habit and become useful, productive citizens. Many addicts have been treated at Lexington several times. Unfortunately, the personality of some drug addicts is so faulty that they are not able to function without the emotional support the drug provides.

Drug addiction is increasing in this country. Many communities have organized facilities for treating patients who suffer from this problem. As in all situations that involve the emotional life of the patient, it is necessary to discover why this kind of emotional support is needed and then attempt to supply the support in more positive ways, while at the same time helping the patient to give up the drug.

Some authorities believe that a more realistic approach to the problem of drug addiction would be to supply each addict with a minimal weekly supply of the drug to which he is addicted. This practice, it is argued, would make the illegal traffic in drugs unprofitable. It is thought that this practice of supplying a small amount of the drug to the addict each week would aid in cutting down the crimes that addicts now commit to obtain drugs. It would make it possible for the addict to purchase adequate food and maintain his physical health at an optimum level instead of denying himself food in order to purchase the drug, as he frequently does at the present time.

Much more study and research must be done on drug addiction before a more effective approach to treatment and rehabilitation can be made.

NURSING CARE FOR PATIENTS WHO USE ALCOHOL AND DRUGS

Unfortunately patients who use alcohol and drugs are rejected by society, and many nurses carry this cultural attitude with them as they perform their professional activities. Patients who rely upon the emotional support of external factors such as alcohol and drugs are unquestionably emotionally inadequate, fearful, lonely people who are in desperate need of help. The subtle rejection, which a nurse cannot help but convey to a patient when she actually believes that he is unworthy, simply reinforces his low self-esteem. Thus it would be better for a nurse to be reassigned to a different kind of responsibility if she finds that she is incapable of wholeheartedly accepting the alcoholic or addicted patient and of providing a positive attitude of understanding and genuine interest in him.

Both the alcoholic and the addicted patient require a controlled environment in which certain limits are maintained. If they are to profit from hospitalization they must remain in the institution and free from alcohol or drugs. This sometimes requires great emphasis on enforcing protective rules and regulations.

These patients are almost universally in need of good physical care and nutritional buildup when they come to the hospital. As soon as possible they should be encouraged to participate in the planned activities provided in the hospital. Direct comments about their problems should be avoided. The principles of effective nursing care apply in dealing with these patients as with all other physically and emotionally ill individuals. Their ability to effectively utilize the therapeutic activities in the hospital is in direct relation to their personal motivation to be helped to give up alcohol or drugs.

IMPORTANT CONCEPTS

1. Patients with a personality disorder often reveal the existence of inner conflicts and difficulty by a lifelong pattern of repetitive disturbances in social and sexual adaptation.
2. Patients with an antisocial personality seem incapable of conforming to social or legal standards of living and lack a sense of responsibility.
3. The defect from which patients with an antisocial personality suffer lies in the emotional and volitional aspects of their personalities.
4. Individuals with an antisocial personality are thought to have failed to develop a constructive identity or to evolve socially useful adaptations

and controls and are dominated by the primitive demands of the id.

5. Individuals with an antisocial personality are treated most successfully within an institution that provides an organized, structured, controlled environment.
6. Treatment goals for patients with antisocial personality traits include helping them to accept more socially approved attitudes and standards in their relationships with other people.
7. Patients with antisocial personalities should be rewarded with praise and recognition for acceptable behavior.
8. Sexual perversions develop as a result of a failure to outgrow infantile or preadolescent ways of obtaining sexual pleasure.
9. Usually sexual deviation is only one manifestation of a deep-seated personality disorder of long duration.
10. Sexual deviation is difficult to treat successfully because the problem arises out of a faulty personality structure.
11. Successful psychotherapeutic treatment for the sexually deviant individual requires a competent psychiatrist, a highly motivated patient, and a long period of time for treatment.
12. No matter what type of alcoholism is being considered, the problem is thought to have its basis in some emotional conflict, frustration, or overwhelming feeling of inadequacy.
13. The treatment and nursing care of the alcoholic patient begins with understanding his personality and the problems from which he has a need to escape.
14. The primary treatment of the alco-

holic is to aid him in meeting life's responsibilities without utilizing alcohol as a defense. This generally means a long period of reeducation.

15. Morphine or heroin addiction does not cause mental deterioration as does alcohol, but the treatment that addicts receive from society causes them to deteriorate socially.

16. It is absolutely necessary to treat morphine or heroin addicts in a closed institution in order to prevent concealed continuation of the habit.

17. Unfortunately, many nurses approach the treatment of the alcoholic or addicted patient with the same rejection that is meted out to them by society in general.

18. These patients are almost universally in need of physical rehabilitation and a nutritional regimen designed to restore their physical stamina.

19. The permanent rehabilitation of alcoholic and addicted patients is largely influenced by their personal motivation.

SUGGESTED SOURCES OF ADDITIONAL INFORMATION

Brody, E. B.: Border line state, character disorder and psychotic manifestations; some conceptual formulations, Psychiatry 23:75-80, 1960.

Burton, Genevieve: An alcoholic in the family, Nurs. Outlook 12:30-33, May, 1964.

Cleckley, Hervey: The mask of sanity, ed. 3, St. Louis, 1955, The C. V. Mosby Co.

Cohen, Felix: Alcoholic Anonymous principles and the treatment of emotional illness, Ment. Hyg. 48:621-626, 1964.

Doyle, Thomas L.: Homosexuality and its treatment, Nurs. Outlook 15:38-40, Aug., 1967.

Gelber, Ida: The addict and his drugs, Amer. J. Nurs. 63:52-56, July, 1963.

Klimenko, Antonia: Multi family therapy in the rehabilitation of drug addicts, Perspect. Psychiat. Care 6:220-223, 1968.

Kolb, Lawrence C.: Noyes' modern clinical psychiatry, ed. 7, Philadelphia, 1968, W. B. Saunders Co., pp. 193-210; 501-515; 516-525.

Lewis, John A.: Alcoholism, Amer. J. Nurs. 56:433-435, April, 1956.

Muhlenkamp, Ann F.: Personality characteristics of drug addicts, Perspect. Psychiat. Care 5:213-217, 1968.

Osnos, Robert: A community counseling center for addicts, Nurs. Outlook 13:38-40, Nov., 1965.

Parry, Allen: Alcoholism, Amer. J. Nurs. 65:111-115, March, 1965.

Price, Gladys M.: Alcoholism—a family, community, and nursing problem, Amer. J. Nurs. 67:1022-1025, May, 1967.

Quiras, Alyce: Adjusting nursing techniques to the treatment of alcoholic patients, Nurs. Outlook, 5:276-279, May, 1957.

Rohde, Ildaura Murillo: The addict as an inpatient, Amer. J. Nurs. 63:61-68, July, 1963.

Rohde, Ildaura Murillo: Panic in the street, Nurs. Outlook 13:45-47, Nov., 1965.

Sankot, Margaret, and Smith, David E.: Drug problems in the Haight-Ashbury, Amer. J. Nurs. 68:1686-1688, Aug., 1968.

Taylor, Susan D.: Addicts as patients, Nurs. Outlook 13:41-44, Nov., 1965.

Thompson, George N.: Acute and chronic alcoholic conditions. In Arieti, Silvano, editor: American handbook of psychiatry, vol. 2, New York, 1959, Basic Books, Inc., Publishers, pp. 1203-1221.

CHAPTER SIXTEEN

Behavior disorders occurring
as a result of aging

Acceptance of the challenges presented by the period in life known as old age is highly individual. Just as different individuals respond in a variety of ways to the problems and opportunities presented by adolescence, so do they cope with old age in highly diversified ways.

Old age is not a precise term. It refers to the natural process through which there is a gradual lessening of mental acuity, a narrowing of social interests, and a limitation of physical activity. It comes to some individuals much earlier than to others. Although many people are highly productive and intellectually capable throughout an extremely long life, the usual time at which old age is generally thought to begin is 65 years, the age at which retirement frequently occurs.

For many people this is a period of personal fulfillment, with time available to enjoy the leisure-time activities that had to be forsaken during an earlier and busier period. Individuals who were self-reliant, psychologically independent, and who utilized their resources to accumulate wisdom, frequently welcome this period of life as one of continued contemplation and personal development.

Improved health care and prosthetic aids ensure an increasing number of elderly people an opportunity to enjoy the years after retirement.

Except in social situations, nurses infrequently come in contact with aged individuals who continue to maintain an independent, productive existence, even though their numbers are steadily increasing. Instead, nurses usually find that the aged patients who require their professional help and understanding are suffering from physical and emotional problems. Thus the remainder of this chapter focuses upon some of these problems.

Elderly people are not highly adaptable to new ideas or changes in the routine of their daily lives. Old age is usually associated with many bodily infirmities—bones lose their dense structure, muscles become hypertonic, and internal organs undergo a gradual atrophy. Joints are less flexible; tremor is often present; and vision may become slowly clouded by cataract formation.

The brain of elderly persons frequently becomes smaller; there is always some atrophy, and abnormal deposits of iron are scattered through the nerve cells. Peculiar formations called senile plaques are characteristic, and arteriosclerosis is always a concomitant condition. Inability to solve personal problems seems to be the crucial factor that leads to confusion and irritability in the aging person. Arguments over property, fear of poverty, and unhappy situations between parents and children are psychological reasons for the development of senile agitation in many patients. Blindness, loss of hearing, a paralytic stroke, or some painful affliction such as carcinoma, chronic infections, and failing circulation are equally responsible as causative factors.

When a man or woman develops a senile mental disease, he or she brings into it all the personality attributes and defects that have existed throughout his or her life. In addition, these qualities of personality have become more pronounced or exaggerated.

Simple deterioration

Simple deterioration is the most common form of senile psychosis. This is a gradual and orderly progress toward dementia, with the following outstanding symptoms: (1) loss of memory for recent events—the happenings of today are hazy, whereas minute details of events of early life are readily recalled; (2) lack of impressibility—important events are no longer significant if they do not touch directly upon the life of the patient; (3) tendency to reminisce—dwelling on the life and achievements of early years, with a desire to recount them frequently; (4) intolerance of change—an alteration in routine is likely to precipitate tension and irritability; (5) disorientation—the year is frequently forgotten and then the day of the month, but the day of the week, which more directly dictates the routine of the patient's life, is generally retained; (6) restlessness—a desire to be up and about, to travel from relative to relative, sometimes resulting in the individual's getting lost; (7) insomnia—a tendency to get up in the late hours of the night or early morning and to putter aimlessly about the house; (8) failure of judgment—an aversion to taking on new responsibilities and a tendency to withdraw into apathy and indifference.

Superimposed upon this picture of simple and progressive senile dementia there occur other symptoms that justify additional classification. These include the delirious and confused types, depressed and agitated types, paranoid types, and presbyophrenic type. The descriptive name is dictated by the outstanding and characteristic behavior of patients suffering from each condition.

ROLE OF THE NURSE IN GIVING CARE TO AGING PATIENTS

With the increasing number of persons in our population who have lived beyond the age of 60 years, society is confronted with a challenging problem of caring for large numbers of aged people who have become incapacitated physically and mentally. The members of the nursing profession have a responsibility to assist aging persons to be as happy, physically well, and constructively occupied as it is possible for them to be.

Symptoms of senile psychosis may appear in some persons as early as the middle fifties, whereas some very elderly persons may be without mental symptoms. This marked individual variation in the ability to function effectively during the declining years appears to be significantly related to the type of personality the patient has developed throughout life. The range and type of intellectual interests the person has cultivated seem to have a real bearing upon how long and how effectively he can function without developing the characteristic symptoms of senility. These include irritability, confusion, memory loss, and a tendency to reminisce. It is interesting to note that people who have developed broad interests, who have engaged in some type of intellectual work during the productive years, and who have been well adjusted are much more likely to avoid senile deterioration than are individuals who have earned a living primarily through the use of their hands.

Consequently it seems logical to conclude that the prevention of psychiatric problems in the later years of life is largely dependent upon the personality pattern developed during the productive years. It follows that the cultivation of many interests, particularly those in which intellectualization is required, and the development of a well-adjusted personality is one effective way to avoid senile deterioration.

Old age is a problem period for many people. The person who is growing old is often lonely, since he usually has outlived many of his friends. Frequently economic insecurity is the source of much anxiety. Fear of becoming a burden upon others is a common source of worry. Many aged persons are not able to solve these problems successfully and cope with them by responding with various types of unusual behavior, depending on the underlying personality pattern of the individual.

The nurse who successfully cares for aged, senile patients needs to have a genuine interest in and love for people. It is essential that she be patient, tactful, genuinely warm and friendly, and thoughtfully sympathetic. It is important that the nurse be able to gain personal satisfaction from the knowledge that she is contributing to the happiness of her patients without finding it necessary to see great progress made in their physical improvement.

Some aged patients need institutional care

Elderly people become easily confused by environmental changes and are usually much happier, more easily cared for, and less likely to become disoriented if they can remain in a situation with which they are familiar. However, some senescent individuals present such difficult behavior problems that they are in danger of injury in the relatively unsafe atmosphere of the ordinary house. It may become necessary to place them in an institution equipped to give them more carefully supervised care than is possible in a home. Unhappily, in some instances the only institution available for such a patient is a psychiatric hospital, although this is usually not an ideal place for the elderly person who has developed some mental symptoms.

Providing the patient with a safe environment

Careful planning is necessary before a hospital ward or a home is safe for an aged person, whose sight may be dimmed, whose balance is unsteady, and whose footsteps are unsure. Ramps should replace stairways, since stairs present a serious hazard to the aged. Highly polished floors and small rugs should be avoided. The glider chair should replace the rocking chair. All small, low footstools and tables should be discarded so that the patient will not trip and fall over them. Handrails placed along the corridors and in the bathroom will make it possible for patients whose gait is unsteady to travel about safely, although unattended.

The aged patient should always be helped into and out of the bathtub, since bathing is probably the most hazardous of all procedures in the daily care. It is thought by many that shower baths are to be preferred for elderly people, since they are in some ways less dangerous to the patient.

The high hospital type of bed should be replaced by the low one so that the elderly patient can get into and out of bed without the danger of falling.

Physical needs of the aged patient

In developing a plan of nursing care for any patient it is essential to secure his active cooperation. He should be a respected collaborator rather than a silent recipient of care.

The daily bath is usually considered to be of great importance. However, frequent baths for the aged patient should be avoided because of the drying effects that too much soap and water have upon the parchmentlike skin of the elderly person. Unless the patient is incontinent or careless with regard to excreta, twice a week is as often as a complete bath should be given to the aged person.

Aged patients may need help in dressing, and the nurse should be sure they are warmly clothed. Since such people often suffer from impaired circulation, it is always wise to have sweaters easily available for them.

Avoid sedating the patient with any of the barbiturate drugs, since the cumulative effect of barbituric acid often results in a delirious reaction. Most physicians feel that an ataractic is a more acceptable drug for use with the aged patient than are any of the barbiturates.

Frequent rest periods for the elderly person are necessary, but confining the aged patient to bed unless he is actually physically ill carries serious consequences for him. Most physicians encourage the nurse to help the aged patient who is physically ill and confined to bed to sit upon the side of the bed several times a day. This procedure is designed to increase the circulation and to encourage deep breathing, thereby avoiding respiratory infections.

It is important to keep up the nutritional intake of the aged patient, but it is usually a mistake to attempt to introduce new foods. Insofar as possible, elderly people should be served those foods with which they are familiar and should be allowed to eat them in whatever order they choose.

Some nurses assume responsibility for feeding the patient when the procedure becomes time consuming because of the tremulous, halting attempts the aged person makes to feed himself. It is of great psychological importance to help these patients do as much for themselves as possible. If the nurse in her need to keep the patient tidy or to hurry the feeding process begins to spoon-feed him, she has done a great deal toward reducing him to the psychological level of an infant. He will either rebel and become angry or accept the feeding and become completely dependent upon the nurse. This dependency is likely to carry over into many other aspects of his physical care, and soon the nurse will find that she must carry out all the responsibility for the physical care of the aged patient.

One of the most important principles underlying the care of the aged is the importance of securing the patient's active cooperation in doing as much as possible for himself within the limitations of his physical and mental health. Unless his cooperation is secured, he is likely to resist any treatment provided for him. The nurse should be on hand to assist, encourage, and direct the patient, but she should encourage him to do what he can for himself.

Ventilation is a point upon which the nurse and the aging person often disagree. Many nurses believe that fresh air is essential and thus insist upon opening the window in the room where the patient sleeps. It is unfortunate when the nurse imposes upon the patient her own attitudes or beliefs. Most elderly people require more heat than do the young or middle-aged. Often they are unpleasantly cold at a temperature at which others are comfortable. Nursing care for aging people must be designed to meet the individual needs of the person for whom it is planned.

Complaints about bowel function are commonly expressed by older patients. Most physicians believe that mild laxatives are probably the most effective answer to this probem. The nurse needs to adopt a sympathetic attitude toward this type of complaint and to realize that older patients do frequently develop annoying or painful bowel symptoms.

Keeping the aged patient happy

The goal for the care of the aging patient is to maintain him on as happy and productive a level as possible for as long as possible. The first task is to keep the patient happy. This involves helping him to feel respected, wanted, and useful. The nurse can help him to feel wanted by giving him attention and praise. If it is indicated, she can encourage the relatives to visit frequently and to bring suitable gifts. She can help the patient feel that he belongs by designating a bed, table, chair, and place in the dining room for his use alone. She can try to organize the routine of the ward so that as many as possible of the patient's personal likes and dislikes are respected. She can accept his unusual behavior with understanding.

The patient can be helped to feel useful by encouraging him to care for his own personal needs insofar as this is medically sound. Occupational therapy may be helpful in giving the patient a feeling of being of some value. This therapy should be selected from the standpoint of the patient's interests, abilities, and physical health. Many aging people have manual skills that can be revived and which may actually prove to be of financial worth to the individual.

Recreational activities are significant in keeping elderly people happy and should be selected because they appeal to the aged and are within their physical ability to perform.

Nursing care of the senile patient who is psychotic

Nursing care for the aging patient who is psychotic makes use of all the principles of care that have been discussed in relation to the care of any aged person. The nurse's approach will be modified somewhat, depending on the particular psychotic behavior pattern exhibited by the patient.

IMPORTANT CONCEPTS

1. For some individuals old age is a time of rewarding contemplation and fulfillment.
2. It is essential to secure the patient's

active cooperation in any treatment provided for him.

3. Inability to solve personal problems seems to be a crucial factor in the development of confusion and irritability in the aging person.

4. When an elderly person develops a senile mental disease, he brings into it all the personality attributes and defects that have developed throughout his life and that have frequently become more pronounced or exaggerated.

5. It seems logical to conclude that the prevention of psychiatric problems in the later years of life is largely dependent upon the individual personality pattern developed earlier in life.

6. Aged patients should be encouraged to do as much as possible for themselves within the limitations of their physical and mental health.

7. The goal for the care of the aging patient is to maintain him on as happy and productive a level as possible for as long as possible.

SUGGESTED SOURCES OF ADDITIONAL INFORMATION

Austin, Catherine L.: The basic six needs of the aging, Nurs. Outlook 7:138-141, March, 1959.

Burnside, Irene M.: Group work among the aged, Nurs. Outlook 17:68-71, June, 1969.

Burnside, Irene M.: Sensory stimulation: an adjunct to group work with the disabled aged, Ment. Hyg. 53:381-388, 1969.

Busse, E. W.: Some emotional complications of chronic disease, Gerontologist 2:153-156, 1962.

Charles, Don C.: Outstanding characteristics of older patients, Amer. J. Nurs. 11:80-83, Nov., 1961.

Cowdrey, E. V.: Care of the geriatric patient, ed. 3, St. Louis, 1968, The C. V. Mosby Co.

Crate, Marjorie A.: Nursing functions in adaptation to chronic illness, Amer. J. Nurs. 65:72-76, Oct., 1965.

Cumming, Elaine, and Henry, W. E.: Growing old: the process of disengagement, New York, 1961, Basic Books, Inc., Publishers.

Davis, Robert W.: Psychologic aspects of geriatric nursing, Amer. J. Nurs. 68:802-804, April, 1968.

Evans, Frances Monet Carter: Visiting older people: a learning experience, Nurs. Outlook 17:20-22, March, 1969.

Goldfarb, Alvin I.: Responsibilities to our aged, Amer. J. Nurs. 11:78-82, Nov., 1964.

Hall, Bernard H.: The mental health of older citizens, Nurs. Outlook 4:206-208, April, 1956.

Hulicka, Irene M.: Fostering self-respect in aged patients, Amer. J. Nurs. 3:84-89, March, 1964.

Lidz, Theodore: The person—his development throughout the life cycle, New York, 1968, Basic Books, Inc., Publishers, pp. 476-495.

Linden, Maurice E.: The emotional problems of aging, Nurs. Outlook 11:47-50, Nov., 1964.

McCown, Pauline P., and Wurm, Elizabeth: Orienting the disoriented, Amer. J. Nurs. 4:118-119, April, 1965.

Mead, Margaret: The right to die, Nurs. Outlook 16:20-21, Oct., 1968.

Monteiro, Lois A.: Hip fracture; a sociologist's viewpoint, Amer. J. Nurs. 67:1207-1210, June, 1967.

Noles, Eva M.: Nursing a geriatric patient, Amer. J. Nurs. 1:73-74, Jan., 1963.

Patrick, Maxine Lambrecht: Care of the confused elderly patient, Amer. J. Nurs. 67:2536-2539, Dec., 1967.

Rautman, Arthur L.: Role reversal in geriatrics, Ment. Hyg. 46:116-120, 1962.

Selye, Hans: Stress of life, New York, 1958, McGraw-Hill Book Co.

Sink, Susan Mary: Remotivation: toward reality for the aged, Nurs. Outlook 14:26-28, Aug., 1966.

Soller, Genevieve R.: The aging patient, Amer. J. Nurs. 11:114-117, Nov., 1962.

Tannenbaum, David E.: Loneliness in the aged, Ment. Hyg. 51:91-99, 1967.

Thompson, Prescott W.: Let's take a good look at the aging, Amer. J. Nurs. 3:76-79, March, 1961.

Tibbitts, Clark: Social change, aging and public health nursing, Nurs. Outlook 6:144-147, March, 1958.

Wayne, George J.: The psychiatric problems of the elderly patient, Ment. Hyg. 44:257-268, 1960.

Wolff, Kurt: Geriatric psychiatry, Springfield, Ill., 1963, Charles C Thomas, Publisher.

Yalom, Irvin D., and Terrazas, Florence: Group therapy for psychotic elderly patients, Amer. J. Nurs. 68:1690-1694, Aug., 1968.

CHAPTER SEVENTEEN

Contributions of nursing to specific psychiatric therapies utilized in the treatment of mentally ill patients

Down through the ages man has searched for treatments with which to solve the problem of mental illness—a problem that has been present among a few members of the human family since the beginning of time. Treatment has ranged from trephining the skull, which was used by prehistoric man, to soft music and beautiful surroundings, which were used by the ancient Greeks. Floggings, purgings, and starvation were used in more recent times. A variety of primitive shock treatments have been used in past centuries. These have included throwing patients into a pit filled with snakes and ducking them in ice-cold water. Benjamin Rush, who was America's first psychiatrist, lived between the years of 1745 and 1813. He worked at Pennsylvania Hospital in Philadelphia and devised an instrument, the gyrator, for the treatment of mental illness. It employed a system of centrifugal action to whirl the patient about to increase the flow of blood to his brain. About 1792 Dr. Rush invented the tranquilizer, a type of restraint, and the ducking stool.

Many of these strenuous attempts to restore a patient's normal behavior were based on the belief that he had lost his senses as a result of an emotional crisis and that restoration would be achieved when he experienced another equally disturbing event. Tranquility for emotionally disturbed patients has always been one of the goals of treatment and remains one of the goals today.

In more modern times the cold, wet sheet pack and the continuous tub bath were used in attempts to help the patients achieve more tranquil emotional states. The individual reactions to these measures varied widely. They have been largely replaced by the newer psychopharmacological agents that were introduced in the United States in 1953 on a research basis. Use of these drugs in the treatment of mental illness has had a dramatic effect on the care of emotionally ill patients and on the national attitude toward all aspects of mental illness. Some authorities believe that the more positive attitudes toward mental illness that have been generated by the new drugs are as significant in the care and treatment of mentally ill patients as the action of the drugs.

ATARACTICS OR TRANQUILIZING DRUGS*

Although much is still to be learned about the psychological effect of the ataractic drugs, they appear to modify certain aspects of mental and emotional illness without stupefying the patient. Many of these drugs have the advantage of producing tranquilization and therefore are technically called ataractics. This tranquilizing action appears to be as effective for patients suffering from a psychotic reaction as it is for patients who respond with neurotic behavior. It appears that the more acute the psychotic reaction, the more dramatic the patient's response to the drug will be.

In some manner tranquilizers affect cer-

*For a list of the tranquilizers, minimum and maximum dosage, use, side effects, and precautions see Tables 1 and 3 in Appendix B.

tain portions of the brain, particularly the hypothalamus and the reticular formation, in which are centered the patterns for alarm, for fight, and for flight. The chief action of the tranquilizers appears to be a depression of both sympathetic and parasympathetic centers in the areas that deal with the organism's response to alarm with a consequent toning down of emotional overactivity.

The phenothiazines

The phenothiazines are probably the most powerful of all the ataractics. They have a positive effect on excited, overactive, assaultive behavior. There are several drugs in this group and new ones are constantly being placed on the market. It is impossible to anticipate accurately the future of this aspect of psychiatric treatment. It is possible that the field may be narrowed to a few drugs that will be used more or less universally. It is possible that much more effective and specific drugs will be developed.

Chlorpromazine (Thorazine). Chlorpromazine is probably the most popular and useful of all the tranquilizers. It exerts a unique, selective, inhibiting action on the functions of the central nervous system and is highly effective in controlling anxiety, agitation, apprehension, hostility, confusion, and delirium. It is practically a specific in abating the symptoms of patients suffering from the manic phase of manic-depressive psychosis and in reducing the excitement in disturbed schizophrenic patients.

Agitated and anxious patients usually become calm when given chlorproma-zine. The usual dose is an intramuscular injection of 50 mg. of chlorpromazine on the first day. The dosage may be increased daily by 50 mg. until 150 mg. per day is reached. The patient's intelligence, memory, and judgment remain intact and may be strikingly improved in individuals who suffer from an acute psychotic disturbance. After receiving chlorpromazine, patients are usually able to follow hospital routine, participate in planned social activities, and establish relationships with other people so that the nurse and physician have an opportunity to establish a psychotherapeutic relationship with them. Most patients receive the drug by mouth. The usual regimen is 100 to 300 mg. of chlorpromazine three times a day for a period of two or three months.

Chlorpromazine is not so effective in the treatment of patients who are depressed but who are not agitated. It may produce symptoms of depression in some patients. It may also produce tremor and symptoms of parkinsonism. These symptoms quickly subside when the medication is withdrawn. Jaundice and liver involvement, the most striking side effects, are uncommon but may appear within a week or two after the administration of chlorpromazine, irrespective of dosage. Lowered blood pressure is a very common complication and may produce giddiness and light-headedness. Leukopenia, dermatitis, and gastric distress may be encountered as side effects. All these conditions disappear when the drug is withdrawn.

Promazine hydrochloride (Sparine). Promazine hydrochloride is believed to have fewer side effects than chlorpromazine. Such symptoms as falling blood pressure and mental depression usually do not occur when this drug is used. It has been particularly useful for treatment of the toxic effects of acute alcoholism and drug addiction. The drug can be given intravenously in 50 to 100 mg. initial doses and may be followed by oral administration of 25 to 200 mg. at 4-hour intervals.

Prochlorperazine (Compazine). Prochlorperazine is highly effective in treating a wide variety of mental and emotional conditions, such as anxiety, senile agitation, and postalcoholic states. Like all phenothiazines, it has demonstrated antiemetic activity in such conditions as pregnancy, postoperative states, duodenal ulcer, and migraine and tension headaches. It should be given only in dosages of 5 mg. three or four times a day.

Perphenazine (Trilafon). Given in doses of 4 to 8 mg., perphenazine is another fairly typical phenothiazine, having all the properties common to this class of drugs.

Reserpine

Reserpine is one of many natural complex chemicals found in the juices of an Indian shrub called snakeroot (*Rauwolfia serpentina*). In 1952 Swiss chemists isolated an alkaloid that had all the medicinal properties of the whole root but that was concentrated 500 times. They called this alkaloid reserpine. The drug was introduced into American hospitals on a research basis in 1953 about the same time as was chlorpromazine. Its effects are remarkably similar to those of chlor-

promazine, although they differ in detail.

Reserpine may aggravate or even precipitate a depression. This undesirable reaction should be guarded against, and the drug should be withdrawn when signs of depression are observed. Reserpine depresses the blood pressure more effectively than any of the other tranquilizing drugs. This may account for the inertia, lethargy, or the depressed feelings from which the patients who are taking reserpine may suffer. It reduces the heart rate, which may be a desirable effect in many patients. A common annoying complication is nasal congestion or stuffiness.

Reserpine, like chlorpromazine, has been found valuable in the treatment of tense, hostile, aggressive, overactive patients. Improvement is generally evident in from four to eleven days after the drug has been started.

Meprobamate

Meprobamate is marketed under the familiar trade names Miltown and Equanil. It is a simple compound and has three distinct pharmacological properties: a muscle relaxant action, an anticonvulsant action, and a pronounced tranquilizing effect. It differs from other tranquilizing drugs in both the simplicity of its chemical structure and its mode of action. The drug does not affect autonomic functions. Meprobamate has proved to be of particular value in treating patients who suffer from anxiety and tension states and related conditions, such as tension headache, sleeplessness, and menstrual stress. The muscle-relaxant properties of the drug are of value in the treatment of cervical myositis, acute and chronic low back pain, various osteoarthritic conditions, and cerebral palsy.

Side effects from meprobamate occur rarely. Some patients complain of drowsiness when they begin taking the drug. This often passes away in a week or so if the medication is continued. A few cases of allergic skin reactions have occurred, but very few cases of blood changes or liver or kidney damage have been reported. Meprobamate can be used with patients undergoing electroconvulsive treatment and does not precipitate depression. The average dose is a 400 mg. tablet given three or four times daily.

ANTIDEPRESSANTS *

Various preparations are utilized to modify depressive states in patients suffering from both psychotic and psychoneurotic states. The most popular are combinations of dextroamphetamine sulfate and a quick-acting barbiturate such as pentobarbital sodium or amobarbital. Two examples of this combination are Dexamyl and Desbutal. These preparations give the patient in mild depression a feeling of energy and well-being. They tend to restore mental alertness and to revive normal interest.

There are many drugs called antidepressants on the market today, but it is difficult to establish their efficacy because of the lack of effective controls and unconscious and situational factors involved in every case of depression.

Methylphenidate (Ritalin). Methylphen-idate is a new synthetic cortical stimulant. It arouses apathetic, depressed, and retarded patients to a more normal level of mental and physical activity. It improves withdrawn, regressed, senile behavior patterns.

Methylphenidate overcomes the lethargy induced by large doses of tranquilizing agents such as reserpine, chlorpromazine, and promazine. It also counteracts the oversedation induced by barbiturates, anticonvulsants, and other drugs.

THE NURSE AND THE NEW PSYCHOPHARMACOLOGICAL AGENTS

The widespread use of the psychopharmacological agents in the treatment of mental illness has greatly influenced the role of the nurse in psychiatric settings. Because of the large number of medications to be given, many nurses find themselves fulfilling only one aspect of the many-faceted role of the nurse. It is not unusual for a nurse to spend the largest part of her time on duty pouring and dispensing drugs. This is especially discouraging in view of current thinking regarding the effectiveness of the drugs. Most authorities agree that the new drugs do not cure mental illness or solve the patient's basic emotional problems. Instead, the drugs relieve tension and provide varying degrees of symptomatic relief from the disabilities of mental illness. Because the acute symptoms are alleviated, many physicians, nurses, and families are encouraged to believe that the patient is basically changed when his improve-

---

*For a list of the antidepressants, minimum and maximum dosage, use, and side effects and precautions, see Tables 4 and 5 in Appendix B.

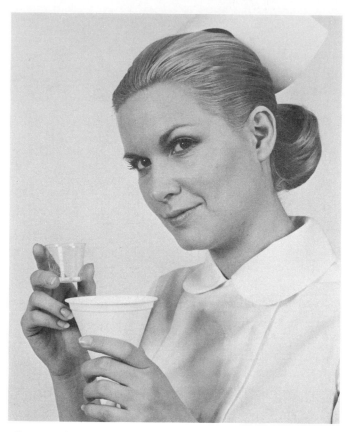

FIG. 18. *The nurse's responsibilities and opportunities have increased with the advent of the psychopharmacological agents.*

ment is actually temporary and superficial.

Mentally ill patients are frequently too ill to be left with the responsibility of remembering to take their medications or of accurately reporting the amount taken. This should be a responsibility of the nurse, in most cases.

The nurse's responsibilities and opportunities have increased with the advent of new drugs. She must know the therapeutic dosage and action of each drug and the specific untoward reactions that may be expected.

The safety of the patient requires that he be observed closely and his response to the medication be recorded accurately. His physical well-being depends upon the nurse's being vigilant in observing him in

relation to untoward reactions to the drug. Her records guide the physician in his decisions about future dosage and change in medication.

The nurse must do far more than administer drugs and observe the patient's response if she is to meet the needs of the mentally ill patient. The attitude and approach used by the nurse as she dispenses medications are thought to be almost as significant in the patient's therapy as the actual drug itself. When drugs are administered to a crowd of patients without individualizing the approach to each patient, much of the possible therapeutic effect of the drug may be lost.

Because of the effectiveness of the drugs, nursing staffs in psychiatric hospitals have been relieved of much of the problem of coping with destructive, uncontrolled behavior that once took so much of their time. Today the usual patient who is receiving one of the tranquilizing drugs is able to assume much of the responsibility for his own physical care. This provides the nurse with an apportunity to utilize her skills in communicating, listening, giving emotional support, and helping the patient become involved in the social and recreational activities provided in the hospital.

ELECTROCONVULSIVE THERAPY

Electroconvulsive therapy is one of the most convenient and practical forms of somatic therapy. It was introduced in 1938 by two Italian clinicians, Ugo Cerletti and Bini, who had done ample experimentation on dogs before they applied this treatment to human beings. Although its use has been replaced to a limited extent by psychopharmacological therapy, it is still used with excellent results in the treatment of agitated and retarded depressions and to a lesser degree in the treatment of overactivity.

Electroconvulsive therapy is a relatively safe procedure in that it has few contraindications. It can be given to most elderly patients with greater safety than many other somatic therapies. Hypertensive cardiorenal disease, active tuberculosis, acute infections, and severe debility are contraindications to its use.

Electroconvulsive therapy is a fairly simple procedure to administer. It consists of producing a typical grand mal convulsion by applying controlled electric current. The current enters the patient's frontal lobe through electrodes placed on his temples. Two or three treatments are given each week until approximately twenty have been given. Breakfast is not served to the patient until after the treatment is over. Continuation of treatments is dependent to some extent on the patient's response to the therapy.

Preparation of patient

When electroconvulsive therapy is to be initiated, it is the responsibility of the physician to discuss the treatment plans with the patient, to order the routine x-ray examinations and laboratory work before the treatment is begun, and to obtain the signed treatment permit from the relatives. The nurse is also involved in preparing the patient for the procedure. Sometimes the patient has not understood the physician's explanation when the treatment was discussed and does not understand why breakfast is withheld or why he is not allowed to get dressed in the morning. The nurse may discover that the patient is frightened at the thought of receiving treatment and refuses to leave the ward. She is then confronted with the responsibility of reassuring the patient and helping him to accept treatment.

Nurses should avoid using the words electric shock when talking about this therapy within the hearing of patients. It is much better to refer to it simply as the treatment when discussing it with patients. The words electric shock may be frightening to a confused person and may suggest electrocution.

When reassuring the patient and encouraging him to cooperate with treatment plans, the nurse can say honestly that there will be no pain connected with the treatment and that the patient will remember nothing except a desire to sleep. It may be helpful to promise to accompany the patient and to stay with him throughout the experience. If this promise is made, the nurse must actually carry it out. It may also be reassuring to the patient when he learns that there will be a doctor and other nurses with him during the actual treatment.

Sometimes the nurse is not able to reassure or convince the patient to accept the treatment. At this point the doctor should be called. If he is unsuccessful in convincing the patient and still believes that treatment is essential, enough help should be summoned to make it possible to transport the patient safely from the ward to the therapy room. After the first few electroconvulsive treatments, many patients accept the treatment without question. However, because this treatment disturbs the memory, patients do not remember having had the experience and usually require encouragement before each time it is given.

Before the therapy is given, the patient should be toileted. If this is not done, the patient is inevitably incontinent during the treatment. Temperature, pulse, respirations, and blood pressure should be checked before the patient is allowed to go to the therapy room. If any of these findings are unusual, the doctor should be notified. The treatment is usually cancelled for patients who have signs of physical illness.

Because some patients do not react to electroconvulsive therapy with a convulsion after having received sedatives, most physicians request that sedatives be withheld for 24 hours before treatment.

An airway is placed in the patient's mouth and one of the muscle-relaxing drugs is usually injected before the treatment is started. Oxygen is usually kept on hand in case the patient has respiratory difficulty after the treatment has been given. During and following the treatment the care of the patient is the same as that provided for any unconscious patient who has just had a convulsive seizure.

Untoward reactions

Respiratory arrest appears to be one of the pronounced untoward reactions to electroshock. Artificial respiration given immediately after the electroconvulsive therapy will stimulate respiration and will reduce the period of apnea. The head should be moved from side to side while the jaws are held in a fixed position.

Dislocation of the jaw is another problem that may follow this treatment. The jaw can be reduced by downward pressure on the molars and upward pressure on the chin.

Occasionally electroconvulsive therapy is followed by a period of extreme excitement. An intravenous injection of 2 to 3 grains of Amytal sodium will promote a restful period of sleep after the treatment.

After five or six treatments, patients frequently complain of confusion and loss of memory, particularly for recent events. This situation puzzles and perplexes the patient. He may fear that his memory will not return. Relatives are likely to express concern about this development unless the treatment has been carefully explained to them before it was undertaken. They should be prepared to expect such unusual developments and to understand that the symptoms will clear up completely after the series of treatments has been concluded. They should be reassured that there will be no permanent untoward aftereffects from the treatments.

Therapeutic effect

In the treatment of depressions, particularly midlife depression, improvement begins early and is usually noted after the first two or three treatments. Recovery usually occurs after a series of six to ten convulsive treatments. Electroconvulsive therapy is discontinued when the patient attains a feeling of well-being, is no longer preoccupied with morbid thoughts, and is free of agitation. If symptoms reappear, a second series of treatments is given. As with any other form of somatic treatment, when the patient's emotional tone improves, an excellent opportunity is provided for the physician as well as for the nurse to establish a therapeutic relationship with the patient and to help him solve emotional problems that contributed to the mental illness.

The nurse's responsibility

Although very little is known about how electroconvulsive therapy achieves its results, it seems to break through the psychotic process and releases the patient to become more accessible to other people. Thus after the patient has received a series of treatments it is frequently possible for the nurse to develop a relationship with the patient and to begin to help

him become an active participant in the hospital environment.

Immediately following the treatment the patient should not be left alone until the nurse is positive that the respirations and pulse are within normal limits and that the patient is sleeping. Because some patients become very confused and overactive following electroconvulsive therapy it is wise to use a recovery room in which several patients can remain under the watchful eye of one member of the nursing staff until they are awake and have fully regained contact with the environment. As an additional precaution many hospitals have added side rails to the beds.

Many authorities believe that one of the chief values of electroconvulsive therapy is that patients become more accessible to psychotherapy following its use, and thus they may be helped to begin socializing with others and taking part in other therapeutic activities afforded by the hospital.

The nurse has not fulfilled her responsibility to the patient when she is sure that he has recovered physically from the treatment. She should be alert to the importance of planning recreational activities for patients who are receiving electroconvulsive treatments and of helping them focus their attention upon the environment rather than upon their own problems.

Some psychiatrists segregate patients who are receiving electroconvulsive therapy and concentrate on helping them to develop relationships with other people and to involve themselves with their environment. This is done with the cooperative planning of the occupational therapist, the recreational therapist, the nurses, and other hospital workers involved in the patients' care. Such plans usually include filling the days and evenings with a variety of interesting activities designed to help patients to express themselves, to gain personal satisfaction, and to function as members of a group. The nurse's role is to develop a positive relationship with these patients, to encourage them to participate in the planned activities, and to be an understanding and resourceful companion.

OBSERVATION OF PATIENT BEHAVIOR

One of the most significant aspects of the nurse's responsibility in the care of mentally ill patients is accurately observing and recording patient behavior. Recording information that contributes to better understanding of the patient on the part of the professional team requires three abilities: (1) the nurse must be alert enough to observe behavior; (2) she must have enough knowledge of human behavior to understand what she is observing; and (3) she must know how to record meaningfully what she observes. It is to be hoped and expected that the nurse is skillful at recording information by the time she is ready for an experience in psychiatric nursing. However, her previous clinical experience in nursing may not have helped her understand how or what to observe about the behavior of the mentally ill patient. Every aspect of the patient's day is worthy of comment in the recorded observations if the behavior involved is unusual or contributes something unique to understanding the total personality of the patient. In recording

the behavior of the mentally ill patient, emphasis is placed on direct quotations from conversations the nurse may hold with the patient or may overhear the patient having with another person. As the nurse learns to understand more about the meaning of human behavior and learns to know the patient as an individual, she will become more skillful in recognizing significant behavior.

The observer needs to be alert to the patient's facial expression, voice quality, neatness and appropriateness of dress and grooming, participation in ward activities, response to other patients and to the nurse herself, ability to follow ward routine, response to the dining room situation, reaction to therapeutic interviews with the psychiatrist, response to visitors, and many other aspects of the 24-hour living situation.

It is suggested that the patient's behavior be described rather than labeled. Instead of recording that a patient is hallucinating, it is more meaningful to record exactly what was observed. The following is an example of this type of recording. "Stood near the ventilator for 10 minutes with hand cupped around ear as if trying to hear better. Carried on an animated conversation. Although no other person was present, the patient could be heard saying 'How dare you call me those names! You are a liar!'"

Instead of recording that the patient is disoriented and misidentifies people, it would be more meaningful to record the following: "Mr. J. greeted the nurse by saying 'Good morning, Mary. Have you cooked breakfast yet?' In the afternoon he asked 'When are we going to have breakfast?' Patient believes that nurse is his wife, and he is not able to differentiate between morning and afternoon."

OCCUPATIONAL THERAPY

The modern psychiatric hospital usually possesses a well-equipped occupational therapy department where skillful, well-prepared therapists help the patient develop an interest in one of several available and appropriate activities. The therapist correlates the patient's activity in the occuaptional therapy department with the physician's total goals for therapy. Her approach to the patient is highly individual and is based on her knowledge of him as a person and his emotional needs. Occupational therapy encourages the patient to become involved in some activity, which may reestablish old skills and knowledge or initiate new abilities that can serve as a hobby or as a basis for developing other more challenging interests. It also serves to develop the patient's self-esteem and self-confidence and eventually may contribute much toward helping him feel capable of coping with life outside the hospital.

The nurse's role

The nurse can be influential in helping the patient to become interested in participating in occupational therapy sessions if she has an understanding of the opportunities that are offered there and the importance of helping the patient reestablish interest in accomplishing something through his own efforts. She may be the first person to learn that the patient has an old, partially forgotten interest that may be rekindled and used therapeutically with the help of the occupational therapist. The nurse may be the one who helps the patient maintain an interest in occupational therapy activities when he seems to be losing his initial enthusiasm. The nurse and the occupational therapist are often the only persons from whom the patient receives encouragement for the work he accomplishes. It is important that the nurse and the occupational therapist share knowledge and information about the patients with whom they work jointly, since they can be mutually helpful.

The nurse may be even more helpful in the area of occupational therapy for those patients who are not well enough to leave the psychiatric unit to participate in the activities of the occuaptional therapy department. For these patients she may be able to provide simple activities that do not require elaborate equipment. Knitting, crocheting, and embroidering are activities that may be provided for female patients if it is possible to supervise them adequately. The needles used in these familiar handcrafts may be too hazardous to be used by a few patients. Some types of artwork may be successfully introduced to patients in psychiatric units. Selected ward tasks may be appropriate if the patient enjoys the work and if it provides an opportunity for him to relate to at least one other person.

The walls of some hospital units have been decorated by artistically gifted patients at the suggestion of the nurse. The walls of one psychiatric hospital were beautifully covered with murals done by the patients under the direction of one of them who was a professional artist. Patients also enjoy decorating the hospital unit for holidays. This can provide much

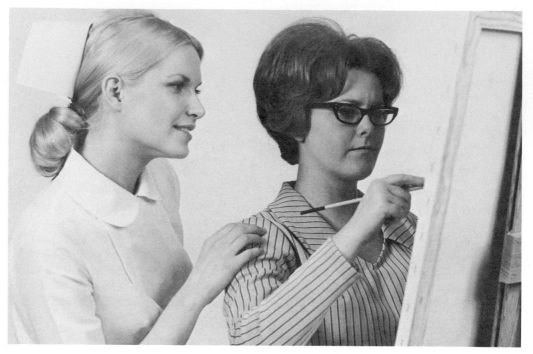

FIG. 19. *The nurse helps patients reestablish new interests by participating with them in occupational therapy.*

pleasure, initiate a mutually helpful working relationship among patients, and serve to interest patients in participating more formally in occupational therapy activities. The nurse is usually an intimate part of these ward activities and has an opportunity to give guidance, encouragement, and support to those who are participating.

RECREATIONAL THERAPY

Many psychiatric hospitals are not yet fortunate enough to have a recreational therapist on the staff. In such situations the nurse may find that it is important to contribute a good deal of time and thought to helping the staff work out recreational activities with patients. If the recreation is to meet patients' needs, they must be actively involved in planning and initiating the activities.

If the nurse is imaginative she will find that many recreational activities do not require a great deal of equipment and can be carried on without much expense. Recreation must meet the needs of the group for which it is intended. Consequently, a group of teen-aged patients will be interested in a much different type of recreation than will adult patients. Patients beyond 60 years of age will probably want to plan activities that differ from those planned by the other two groups. Young patients will be interested in activities that provide opportunities to get rid of excess energy and to express their interest in the opposite sex. Thus dancing and sports will be among the recreational activities that they enjoy. Older patients enjoy dancing but to somewhat different music. They also like card games and may enjoy a bridge tournament.

Recreation, like occupational therapy, must be included in the life of patients if they are to be helped to develop an interest in reestablishing a balanced life away from the hospital. The nurse may be the key figure in providing this aspect of their daily lives.

MUSIC THERAPY

Some psychiatric situations are fortunate to have a trained worker available who is able to assist patients to rekindle an old interest or develop a new interest in music. Since music provides an avenue for expressing feelings, it is uniquely helpful to patients, especially those who find self-expression difficult. Musical activity can provide an excellent focus for group experience and group cooperation.

In situations where there is a music therapist available, patients usually have the opportunity to participate in the hospital orchestra, band, or chorus. These groups provide music for various special occasions. Participating with a mutually cooperative group gives the members a sense of being a contributing member of the hospital community as well as providing them with a great deal of personal pleasure. The nurse's role in music therapy is that of giving encouragement, praising those who have participated musically, assisting individual patients to sustain an initial interest, and providing emotional support to a patient whose interest in music is just beginning to emerge.

IMPORTANT CONCEPTS

1. Use of psychopharmacological agents in the treatment of mental illness has had a dramatic effect on the care of patients in psychiatric hospitals in this country and on the national attitude toward all aspects of mental illness.

2. Some authorities believe that the more positive attitude toward mental illness that has been generated by the tranquilizing agents is as significant in the care and treatment of mentally ill patients as the action of the drugs.

3. In some manner tranquilizing drugs affect certain portions of the brain, particularly the hypothalamus and the reticular formation in which are centered the patterns for alarm, for fight, and for flight.

4. The phenothiazine family of drugs, the most important of which is chlorpromazine (Thorazine), has a positive effect on excited, overactive, assaultive behavior.

5. Authorities agree that the psychopharmacological agents do not cure mental illness or solve the patient's basic emotional problems but relieve tension and provide varying degrees of symptomatic relief.

6. The attitude and approach used by the nurse as she dispenses medications is thought to be almost as significant in the patient's therapy as the actual drug the patient receives.

7. Because of the effectiveness of the psychopharmacological agents, nursing staffs in psychiatric hospitals have been relieved of coping with destructive, uncontrolled behavior, which once took up a great deal of their time. The nurse is now able to utilize her psychiatric nursing skills in relating to patients and helping them to become involved in the social and recreational activities provided in the hospital.

8. Electroconvulsive therapy has been replaced to a limited extent by psychopharmacological therapy, but it is still used with excellent results in the treatment of agitated and retarded depressions and to a lesser degree in the treatment of overactivity.

9. After five or six electroconvulsive treatments, patients frequently complain of confusion and loss of memory, particularly for recent events. The nurse can reassure them that their memory will return unimpaired after the series of treatments has been completed.

10. Although very little is known about how electroconvulsive therapy achieves its result, it seems to break through the psychotic process and allows the patient to become more accessible to other people. This gives the nurse an opportunity to develop a therapeutic relationship with the patient.

11. Occupational therapy encourages the patient to develop an interest, which may reestablish old skills and knowledge or may initiate new abilities that can serve as a hobby or as a basis for developing other more challenging interests. It also serves to develop the patient's self-esteem and self-confidence.

12. If the nurse fully understands the opportunities provided by occupational therapy and the importance of helping the patient to accomplish something through his own efforts, she can be influential in initiating the patient's participation in the activities of this department.

13. The nurse is usually an intimate part of occupational activities that are carried on within the psychiatric unit. She has an opportunity to give guidance, encouragement, and support to those who are participating.

14. Patients must be actively involved in planning and initiating recreational activities if needs are to be met.

15. Recreation, like occupational therapy, must be included in the life of patients if they are to develop an interest in reestablishing a balanced life away from the hospital.

16. It is more meaningful if the nurse describes rather than labels patient behavior.

SUGGESTED SOURCES OF ADDITIONAL INFORMATION

Ayd, Frank J.: The chemical assault on mental illness; the major tranquilizers, Amer. J. Nurs. **65**:70-78, April, 1965.

Ayd, Frank J.: The minor tranquilizers, Amer. J. Nurs. **65**:89-94, May, 1965.

Ayd, Frank J.: The antidepressants, Amer. J. Nurs. **65**:78-84, June, 1965.

Beavers, Stacie Virginia: Music therapy, Amer. J. Nurs. **69**:89-92, Jan, 1969.

Berblinger, Klaus W.: The influence of personalities on drug therapy, Amer. J. Nurs. **59**:1130-1132, Aug., 1959.

Bross, Robert B.: The modern mood-changing drugs, Amer. J. Nurs. **57**:1142-1143; 1146-1147, Sept., 1957.

Lynn, Frances H., and Friedhoff, Arnold J.: The patient on a tranquilizing regimen, Amer. J. Nurs. **60**:234-240, Feb., 1960.

Maloney, Elizabeth M.: The fears and feelings of the patient on electroconvulsive therapy, Amer. J. Nurs. **58**:560-562, April, 1958.

Maloney, Elizabeth M., and Johannesen, Lucile: How the tranquilizers affect nursing practice, Amer. J. Nurs. **57**:1144-1146, Sept., 1957.

CHAPTER EIGHTEEN

Behavior disturbances in children and adolescents due to alterations in normal patterns of personality growth and development

Child psychiatry is recognized as an area of specialization in both medicine and nursing. Thus it deserves more attention than can possibly be provided in a textbook devoted primarily to the field of adult psychiatric nursing. Although many of the basic principles useful in understanding and dealing with emotional problems of adults apply to emotionally disturbed children, there are special problems and concerns in this aspect of psychiatry that require additional knowledge and training. There is even less agreement among authorities concerning the cause, prevention, and treatment of behavior disturbances found in children than there is concerning similar problems involving adults. Certainly an understanding of normal personality growth and development is essential before beginning a study of behavior disturbances in children. Thus it is suggested that before reading any further the student review Chapter 2, which deals with personality development.

HISTORICAL BACKGROUND

Interest in child psychiatry has developed rapidly in the last half century. Before 1920 many authorities believed that mental illness was limited to adults. The occasional mentally ill child who came to the attention of physicians was thought to be a clinical curiosity. There is no mention of children in the classic treatise on psychiatry by Emil Kraepelin, a famous German psychiatrist. This book was published in Leipzig in 1904 and is studied even today. In 1912, Boston Psychopathic Hospital, now Massachusetts Mental Health Center, became the first psychiatric hospital in the United States to accept children in an outpatient clinic. The first written report concerning the existence of childhood schizophrenia was published by H. W. Potter in the American Journal of Psychiatry in 1933. Although this article precipitated much controversy among psychiatrists, the entity of schizophrenic reaction–childhood type is almost universally accepted today.*

EXTENT OF THE PROBLEM

A report prepared for presentation to the U. S. Congress in 1969 by the Joint Commission on Mental Health of Children stated that mental illness among children has risen 150% in the last ten years. The executive director of the National Committee Against Mental Illness, Michael Gorman, estimated that the nation had 4 million emotionally disturbed children in 1969. Added to the gloomy picture of the care given disturbed children and adolescents in the United States was the fact that fifteen states had no public or private facilities for treating mentally troubled juveniles, and another twenty-four states had no public institutions to care for children from low- and middle-income groups who were in need of institutional care.

---

*Langdell, John L.: Family treatment of childhood schizophrenia, Ment. Hyg. 51:387-392, 1967.

CAUSATIVE FACTORS INVOLVED IN THE PROBLEM

Some authorities believe that the rapid rise of emotional disturbances among children and adolescents is related in some way to the fundamental problems and insecurities that have developed in many American homes in the twentieth century. Others go so far as to suggest that the phenomenal rise in emotional illness among children may indicate that there is a breakdown in the structure of the American family, the basic unit in this culture. Certainly the current high divorce rate, with the resultant loss of one parent or the sharing by the children of the homes of two parents; the changing roles of the sexes, with the loss of a clear demarcation between the responsibilities of mother and father; the rise of the institution of baby-sitting, in which children are frequently cared for by a variety of individuals, many of whom are minimally competent to deal with children; the emphasis upon materialistic goals in this culture; and the relative relaxation of moral and religious standards are all factors that may provide many children with home lives that seem unsafe and insecure to them.

Other possible causative factors cannot be ignored in considering the cause of emotional disturbances among children. Some of these may be the increase of children in the total population, which could result in a larger number of emotionally disturbed individuals even if the percentage remained constant. Another factor may be the greater demands put upon children by members of a sophisticated and technologically oriented society. A third may be minimal brain injury occurring at birth, which may go undetected and unrecognized but which may profoundly affect behavior.

Childhood emotional disturbances are not distinct and well-defined clinical entities, and there is no universal agreement as to their cause. However, in studies on both emotionally well and emotionally ill children there is much to suggest that an emotionally healthy climate within the family is essential if children are to develop into mentally healthy individuals. Thus it seems reasonable to look to the early parent-child relationships, especially the quality of mothering that the child receives, for cues to why some children fail to achieve the psychosocial maturational levels usually achieved by mentally well children or why they fail to react socially to other people in the way most children respond.

Among the most important abilities children learn as a result of their earliest experiences with a mothering person is a trusting attitude toward others and toward the environment. This ability to trust is a basic ingredient in the development of a well-integrated personality. It develops as a result of the way in which the mothering person responds to the infant's very earliest need for food, comfort, cuddling, and attention. The responses experienced by the infant to these needs establish the basis for the mother-child relationship, which is profoundly influential in the child's total personality development. If the ability to trust does not develop, it is reasonable to conclude that all was not well in the very earliest experiences with which the child was involved. Unless the child is handled with patience and love, the habit-training period is another time in the growth of the child that is potentially fraught with emotional problems. At this time the child learns that refusing to cooperate in the toilet-training efforts of his parents provides him with a powerful method for controlling the situation. If the parents respond with rigid and harsh treatment to the child's first experiment in exerting his own will, a situation involving conflict is apt to arise. The child will react in his own unique way, but the possibilities include rebellion or overconformity.

Likewise, as the child develops physically, emotionally, and intellectually, he advances from one phase of psychosexual development to another. More is expected of the child in each phase. Each phase presents the child with potential emotional difficulties somewhat unique to the phase through which he is passing. The key to the situation and to successful personality development is found in the relationships the child and the parents are able to develop and maintain and the effectiveness with which the child is guided through each of the several phases of development.

UNDERSTANDING PARENTS OF DISTURBED CHILDREN

Because parents, especially mothers, have been intimately involved in the development of the emotional difficulties of children, nurses and physicians sometimes feel that they are to blame for the child's condition. This feeling is expressed in attitude more often than many professional workers realize. Parents usually feel guilty and apologetic in the face of the many searching questions that are asked when they seek professional assistance for their disturbed child. These feelings on the part of parents are understandable. However, professional workers could be much more helpful if they approached the parents with the understanding that within their limitations most parents do the best they can in accepting the responsibilities of child rearing. Parents usually strive to be successful in rearing healthy children even though their personality structures and emotional conflicts may not always permit success. In addition, it is well known that parents respond differently to individual children, so that one child may thrive in a home under one type of parental supervision and another child may not be able to tolerate the situation. An individual child may not be temperamentally able to develop a normal, healthy personality in a given situation with parents possessed of unique dispositions.

By the time parents have sought professional help for an emotionally disturbed child, the interpersonal interactions between the parents and the child probably have been unsatisfactory and unresolved for some time. Thus the parents are understandably distressed by the situation and require the same support and understanding that is provided for individuals undergoing excessive stress in any situation.

Because "the psychological fate of the child is to a considerable extent determined by the emotional health of the parents and by the complex forces interacting within the family group,"* the parents are usually involved in the total treat-

---

*From Kolb, Lawrence C.: Noyes' modern clinical psychiatry, ed. 7, Philadelphia, 1968, W. B. Saunders Co., p. 528.

ment program for the disturbed child. Most authorities agree that this is required if effective help is to be provided. Improvement in the child's behavior may depend upon alterations in the parents' attitudes and approaches. Thus parents are usually included in the treatment plan as much as the child and may be seen by the same psychiatrist or by a second psychiatrist or a psychiatric social worker who works for the collective good of the family. Whatever decisions are made about the final treatment plans, the parents are usually as much a recipient of psychotherapeutic help as the child himself.

IDENTIFYING PERSONALITY DISORDERS AMONG CHILDREN

It is sometimes more difficult to identify personality disorders among children than among adults because children are actively involved in a dynamic growth process that produces constantly changing behavior. Although children may not be able to complete each developmental task successfully, their behavior like that of normal children shows rapid modifications.

When children are slow to walk or talk or to develop any of the other physical, intellectual, or social achievements upon which the judgment of normal development is based, the advice of a pediatrician should be sought. If the child's development continues to lag, professional help should be requested from a child psychiatrist. Evaluation of slow or normal

developmental progress should be based upon a thorough study of the child and his family. A developmental history is required as well as a complete physical and psychological examination. An understanding of the parents' attitude toward their life together and toward their child should be acquired through an in-depth study of the family. Some evaluation of the response of the child to his parents is important. The information required to understand the essential difficulties involved in the development of the emotionally disturbed child's reactions may include the shared knowledge of the parents, other key relatives, neighbors, teachers, the family physician, and so on.

CLASSIFICATION *

As has been stated earlier there is little agreement among child psychiatrists concerning the nomenclature appropriate for identifying the types of disturbances from which children suffer. Because the child is easily influenced by all types of environmental changes and has a poor tolerance for variations in his emotional climate, the behavior disorders of childhood have been classified under the title of transient situational personality disorders.

Transient situational personality disorders

Habit disturbances, which include such behavior as nail biting, thumb sucking,

---

*The diagnostic categories and explanation have been taken from Ulett, G. A., and Goodrich, D. W.: A synopsis of contemporary psychiatry, ed. 4, St. Louis, 1969, The C. V. Mosby Co. pp. 201-202.

enuresis, soiling, masturbation, and tantrums, is the first subheading under this general topic. These words are all descriptive of behavior usually utilized by a child to express unmet needs or unconscious unmet strivings. Thus some of these habits are developed by the child in an attempt to comfort or reassure himself in tense, lonely, or frightening situations. Others are used to express rebellion or anger at parental figures and their handling of the situation.

Children are rarely admitted for institutional care because of one of the above behaviors and can usually be treated while remaining in their homes. However, one or more of these expressions of unmet needs are usually present in children who do require institutional care.

A second group of behaviors called *conduct disturbances* include truancy, stealing, destructiveness, cruelty, sexual offenses, and the use of alcohol. Although these behaviors usually appear in older children, they are also expressions of unmet needs, anxiety and tension, or of anger and rebellion. Children who utilize one or more of these behaviors usually have a distorted perception of the world and have experienced unsatisfactory family relationships throughout their total personality development. As in other childhood disturbances, a complete understanding of the child and his family is required before treatment is attempted. These behavior disturbances are apt to be the expressions of a severely disturbed child and often require long-term treatment, including hospitalization.

A third group of problem behaviors utilized by some children comes under the heading of *neurotic traits*. These be-

haviors include tics, habit spasms, somnambulism, stammering, overactivity, and phobias. Like the others that have been discussed, they are defenses against anxiety. Some of them, especially tics and stuttering, may be examples of conversion.

Personality growth disturbances

Another group of childhood disturbances, categorized under the title of personality growth disturbances, includes problems in personality growth that interfere with school or social adjustment. Illustrations include the overconforming child who is not able to relate on a child's level to other children, the child with an educational disability including a reading disability, and the intelligent child who because of the need to utilize patterns of withdrawal gives the appearance of being feeble minded.

Psychophysiological disorders

Psychophysiological disorders include feeding difficulties (chronic anorexia, food faddism, recurrent vomiting, obesity), difficulties of coordination (writing dysfunctions), respiratory dysfunctions (asthma, rhinitis), neurodermatitis, enuresis, lower bowel dysfunctions (colitis, constipation), and so on. Each of the psychophysiological disorders mentioned above presents a complex of symptoms that originally were utilized by the child to defend against unbearable tension resulting from some interpersonal conflict, usually existing within the family. Successful treatment of the problem depends upon being able to identify the conflict and assist the child to resolve it. If the situation has continued over a long period of time as so often happens in asthma, enuresis, colitis, or anorexia the behavior becomes progressively more complex, and the relationship to the original conflict becomes somewhat obscure. All the conditions mentioned under the heading of psychophysiological disorders are difficult to treat and require close collaboration between the pediatrician, the child psychiatrist, and the psychiatric social worker who deals with the family situation. The emotional conflict underlying any one of these disorders is usually of long standing and is deeply significant to the child. Thus treatment may require hospitalization to interrupt the hostile relationship the child has developed in the home situation and until some resolution of the underlying problem can be effected.

Psychoneuroses

Children sometimes respond to an unfavorable emotional climate by developing psychoneurotic reactions not unlike those observed among adults. These may include phobias, anxiety states, hysterical symptoms, or depressive states. Neurotic symptoms unique to very young children have been described by both Spitz and Bowlby, who observed chronic withdrawal and depression on the part of children who were removed from the mothering person and placed in an institution.

Psychoses

Childhood schizophrenia will be dealt with in detail in this part of the chapter because the behavior of a majority of the disturbed children with whom students

of nursing become acquainted is classified under this heading.

Childhood schizophrenia is thought to develop as a result of the interaction between a constitutionally susceptible child and an environmental situation psychologically not compatible for the child. It is considered by authorities to be an emotional disturbance of psychotic proportions observed in the behavior of a child who has not yet reached puberty. It is more accurately described in terms of patterns of behavior rather than as an illness with clearly defined diagnostic boundaries. Children who have experienced some organic brain damage or sensory deprivations are thought to develop childhood schizophrenia more readily than children without one of these physical problems. However, it frequently occurs in children who apparently have not been subjected to any damaging physical insults.

Although children afflicted with childhood schizophrenia exhibit a broad spectrum of behavior patterns, most of them present some or all the following behaviors: autistic withdrawal, failure to develop language or to use communicative speech, failure to develop according to the normally expected psychosexual pattern, use of repetitive mannerisms, impairment of ego functioning, failure to develop a clearly defined body image, lack of sexual identity, and inability to perceive time and space accurately. The older the child is when he develops schizophrenic behavior, the more nearly the symptoms approximate those found among adult schizophrenic patients.

Under the broad category of childhood schizophrenia there are two fairly clearly identified patterns of behavior that carry the descriptive names of *early infantile autism* and *symbiotic infantile psychotic syndrome*. Early infantile autism was first described in 1943 by Dr. Leo Kanner, a psychiatrist at Johns Hopkins University. Symbiotic infantile syndrome was first described by Dr. Margaret S. Mahler in 1956. Although both these clinical entities were controversial when introduced, they are fairly widely accepted today. Children suffering from either of these are withdrawn from reality and have a severe disturbance of their self-identity.

These two syndromes are clearly related to the early mothering experiences the child has received. Infantile autism is usually recognized by the age of 1 year and not later than the second year. It occurs more frequently in boys than in girls. The child is thought to be fixated at, or regressed to, the earliest developmental period of his life when he has not yet differentiated the mother's body, the breast or bottle, and the blanket and other inanimate objects in his immediate world from himself. Thus the mother is not a representative of the outside world to the child and apparently has not been perceived as an entity. Since the child has not been able to utilize the mother in relating to the world, he seems incapable of forming a relationship with any person and thus is emotionally unresponsive to human contact. Bruno Bettelheim, famous child psychoanalyst, accepts the theory that the basic cause of the autistic child's problem is parental rejection.

Many autistic children come from homes where the parents are highly intelligent and economically and professionally successful. Their lives seem to be focused upon achieving recognition in the areas of their scientific and academic interests. The family life is such that little genuine mothering is provided for the child. In reporting the child's problems the parents usually comment that he does not talk and is obsessively attached to some inanimate object such as a doll or teddy bear. He usually plays alone with this inanimate object for hours. He may display temper tantrums if his environment is altered in the slightest way. Thus he creates a small world restricted to himself. Although his parents sometimes seek professional help because they believe he is mentally retarded, the autistic child frequently displays flashes of intelligence. He seems devoid of emotional ties and appears to have chosen to utilize autism as a psychotic defense against the outside environment, which demands some emotional response he is incapable of making.

In large institutions where many children are hospitalized it is not unusual to observe units that house twenty to forty autistic children, all under the age of 10 years. Most of them are nonverbal or communicate through the use of a functional sign language. They appear to live in an emotional vacuum. Many of these children resort to aggressive hurting acts directed toward themselves. These acts may include head banging, hand biting, or other behavior that is self-mutilating. Some of these children appear to be acutely unhappy and cry pitifully. Many of them exhibit temper outbursts or other frantic behavior. This behavior, which is almost incomprehensible to adults, appears to help the child gain some concept of his body and its boundaries and thus achieve some sense of identity. Heroic steps are sometimes necessary to safeguard these children against their own self-destructive behavior. These steps may include protective clothing such as football helmets and so on.

The child who displays behavior classified as the symbiotic infantile psychotic syndrome apparently was able to progress somewhat farther toward achieving normal personality development than did the autistic child. He is thought to have progressed to the maturational level at which he was able to recognize his mother as a separate individual differentiated from himself. At this point he was able to make use of his mother to satisfy his needs. Unfortunately, for reasons which are not clearly understood, the symbiotic child was unable to continue the process of separation from the mother when he reached the age where the development of some autonomous functions were expected. As he developed physically, his emotional ability to differentiate himself from his mother became less and less effective until he was confronted with a situation that demanded a level of adjustment greater than he was able to achieve.

Such a situation is thought to have been the precipitating factor in the child's psychotic break but was not the cause. Separation of the child from the mother may occur when she must be hospitalized, when he must be enrolled in a nursery school, when he is hospitalized, or when a sibling is introduced into the family. Any one of these real life events may cause the child to panic and break with reality because of the threatened loss of the oneness with the mother, which the child has not been able to abandon.

The symptoms of symbiotic infantile psychotic syndrome are usually recognized by the parents between the second and the fifth year. The child often appears agitated, has temper tantrums, seems to be panic stricken, hallucinates, and distorts reality in a bizarre way. For these children reality is unbearable, and thus autistic withdrawal becomes a defensive maneuver.

TREATMENT

General goals of treatment for all emotionally ill children include providing opportunities to develop a more accurate concept of self, to develop more appropriate object relationships, and to work through or relive those phases of psychosexual development that were missing, distorted, negatively experienced, or hurriedly passed through.

The symbiotic psychotic child may profit by the special therapeutic environment provided by institutions such as a school for disturbed children. Substitutes for the unhealthy symbiotic relationship with the mother should be provided for the child.

Although the autistic child rejects contacts with others, it is thought that he may profit from individual psychotherapy because his greatest task is to learn to relate to others. Since he avoids bodily contact, cuddling or holding such a child it not helpful and may actually repel him. His attention and interest must be obtained through the use of other methods that will be pleasantly stimulating. One such method may be provided through the use of music.

The problem of the autistic child was brought to the attention of the general public in an article that appeared in Time magazine on August 1, 1969. This article reported the annual 1969 meeting of the National Society for Autistic Children, which was founded in 1965 by parents of autistic children. According to this report, the use of the principles of reinforcement therapy (operant conditioning—see Chapter 19) produced favorable results in altering the behavior of the autistic child. The therapist rewards the child with praise and candy when a specific aspect of his behavior is considered normal for his age. After many weeks or months of repeating the reward-praise reinforcement of normal behavior, the child's autistic behavior may be replaced by the more normal behavior that has been reinforced. A part of reinforcement therapy may include negative reinforcement if the child reverts to autistic behavior. The therapist may reproach the child with a forceful "NO!" or even punish the child in order to negatively discourage autistic behavior.

Instead of placing the child in an institution for treatment, some children are treated while remaining in the home. This plan may be less disturbing to both the parents and the child. If this is to be the treatment plan, it is absolutely essential that the psychiatrist develop a close working relationship with the parents, especially the mother. He will require some feedback about the child's behavior at home. In addition, in helping the child to relive some phases of psychosexual development, his behavior may regress. He may revert to taking milk from a bottle or to soiling himself. Thus the mother must understand the treatment approach and why regressed behavior may occur.

Equally as important are the changes that need to be made in the attitude of the mother toward the child, which may be achieved if she works with the psychiatrist in attempting to alter these problems.

Play therapy

Play therapy is almost universally employed in the treatment of emotionally disturbed children. Its use is based upon the knowledge that play is the medium through which children normally express themselves. Psychiatrists utilize the child's play as a means of gaining insight into his unconscious feelings and attitudes about life as he is experiencing it. Thus the psychiatrist furnishes the therapy room with a variety of toys and other equipment from which the child may choose those things with which he wishes to play. The psychiatrist remains in the playroom with the child. He spends time in getting acquainted with the child and in developing a relationship of trust. He observes the child carefully and listens attentively to the child's comments. If he and the child have developed a relationship of trust, the psychiatrist may ask the child to tell him something about the meaning of the play in which he is engaging. Usually a complete dollhouse and a family of dolls are part of the equipment in a play therapy room. This equipment is purposefully included because the way the child plays with the family of dolls provides insights into the relationships the child is experiencing with the members of his own family. Since the child's emotional life revolves around the members of his family, these insights are significant.

When children are questioned about spanking or punishing one of the child dolls excessively, one learns much about the punishment the child has experienced or phantasizes that he should have experienced. Children sometimes try to destroy an offending child-doll or one of the adult members of the doll family. When asked to talk about these occurrences, the child may explain some of his unconscious fears or his feelings toward a sibling or a parent. Thus play therapy helps the psychiatrist and the child to communicate with one another. Even when the child is essentially nonverbal, much can be learned from observing the child at play.

Finger painting and other forms of art work may be utilized in therapy. This type of activity may appeal more to some children than does playing with toys. This is especially true in the case of an older child. Much can be learned from the child's choice of color, from the choice of topic to be featured in the art work, and from the story the child may tell about the painting when it has been completed. Finger painting is one of the substitute activities that may be provided for children who have not successfully passed through the habit-training aspect of psychosexual development.

Nursing care of the disturbed child

Providing therapeutic nursing care for disturbed children is one of the most challenging tasks a nurse can undertake. The behavior of emotionally ill children is frequently more baffling and more difficult to understand than the behavior of emotionally ill adults. If the care provided for disturbed children is to be therapeutic it must be based upon the individual needs of the child. The nurse, like all other individuals working with disturbed children, will find it necessary to study the child and the symptoms he displays in order to identify his immediate needs and to respond to them in a realistic and helpful way. Thus, in so doing, an attempt is made to offer the child experiences that can correct, in some measure, the negative experiences that have been a part of his life.

Since many of these children are highly sensitive to their environment and the people who make up the environment, nurses and child care workers need to examine their feelings, attitudes, and behavior in an attempt to understand their own reactions to the child. In this way they can modify their behavior for the benefit of the child. A good rule to follow in dealing with the behavior of disturbed children is to look for the cues the child is expressing through his behavior and to respond naturally and appropriately.

Disturbed children require attention and guidance in the same areas of personal care that mothers usually provide for children who live at home. Thus the nurse working with disturbed children will need to involve herself actively in the child's bathing, toileting, feeding, dressing, and play activities. In addition, these children require organization and supervision in a variety of play activities, protection from some potentially dangerous situations, and at times may require appropriate punishment. Like normal children, each disturbed child is unique and occasionally requires special understanding and attention. It is a demanding task to respond as a wise adult to all the situations that may arise from the activities of daily living. The cooperation of all the nurses and other child care workers involved in the situation is required to assist each child to express his needs and find satisfying ways of meeting those needs.

Sometimes disturbed children, like all children, need to be held, cuddled, rocked, or comforted. Such an activity is clearly a part of the role of the nurse and requires a good deal of knowledge, sensitivity, and mature judgment to realize when and how much of such gratification is therapeutic for each child.

When hospitalization is recommended for disturbed children it is done in the hope that the climate of the institution will provide greater opportunities for ego development than can be provided in their homes. Thus the goal for every hospitalized child is the development of a climate that will encourage the adaptive aspects of the child's ego, so that he will experiment with methods for coping with the environment and for developing more effective ways of dealing with people.

Disturbed children are frequently unclear about simple aspects of reality and need to have repeated clarification about these confusions. Thus the nurse-child interactions should logically focus upon the reality of the situation, with emphasis being placed upon verbal communication about reality matters.

Inappropriate response to environmental stimuli is a frequent problem for the disturbed child. The nurse needs to help the child recognize more appropriate responses to stimuli. Opportunities should be provided for him to utilize these new responses.

Special emphasis should be placed upon communicating verbally and nonverbally with the autistic child even though his response may be unintelligible to the nurse. Most mothers talk to their very young children even though the children cannot respond due to the fact that they have not yet achieved a language. Likewise, talking to the autistic child about the environment and the happenings of the day may be helpful even though he does not appear to respond. A soft, warm voice, a friendly facial expression, and other nonverbal ways of responding positively to the autistic child may be effective in communicating genuine concern and interest to him. It has been suggested that the child's attention should be "engaged by consciously echoing and imitating his vocal and motor behavior. Eventually, through imitation and identification the child is led to more advanced communication and relatedness."*

The symbiotic child needs help in gradually developing independence. Opportunities should be provided through which the child can learn to recognize himself as an independent person apart from his mother. He needs to be encouraged and supported whenever he attempts to perform any aspect of his own daily physical care such as dressing or feeding himself.

Consistency in dealing with all children is of major importance. This is especially

---

*From Spurgeon, Ruth: Nursing the autistic child, Amer. J. Nurs. **67:**1418, July, 1967.

true in the care of disturbed children. When several people are involved in providing care for children in an institution, consistency is difficult to achieve but is nonetheless important. Assuring a consistent approach depends upon adequate communication between all people involved. Thus frequent staff meetings between the nurses, physicians, and the child care workers are essential. Every adult involved must understand what approach is being made to each child, why it has been adopted, and what it is expected to achieve. Repeated clarification of the treatment goals for each child is essential. Each worker must have frequent opportunities to share with the group his personal experiences in caring for the child. Thus all workers will be equally aware of the child's progress, and inconsistencies in the treatment approach can be eliminated.

Disturbed children sometimes become hyperactive and exhibit destructive behavior. It may be necessary to restrain these children to avoid injury to themselves or to others. Restraint can best be accomplished by holding the child firmly until the outburst has subsided. Assuring the child that the staff is not frightened by his behavior may be reassuring to him because the child may fear his own angry feelings. It may also be reassuring to the child to tell him that he will not be allowed to hurt himself or other people.

The nurse frequently has an opportunity to talk with the parents of disturbed children when they return the child after a day at home or have been visiting the child in the institution. Most parents of disturbed children are themselves working with a psychotherapist and thus have opportunities to discuss their concerns and anxieties. However, the nurse is the most available professional person to whom they can turn to share the most recent concerns that may have arisen or to ask advice about some aspect of behavior the child has developed. The nurse's interest in their child and in their concerns and her willingness to listen to their fears and doubts are therapeutic for the parents.

ADOLESCENT TURMOIL

Adolescence is the term applied to the complex period of life between the ages of 12 and 21 years when many emotional and personal crises occur. During this period the individual exerts a great deal of effort to control impulses and desires that come about as a result of his biological maturation. In addition, the adolescent strives to become independent and to be emancipated from his parents. Thus he is torn between his devotion to his family and his need to depend upon them, and his conscious and unconscious need to reject him.

The adolescent is constantly carrying on an intrapsychic struggle as he attempts to develop a new psychological equilibrium. The outcome of this struggle depends to a large extent upon his successful achievement of the developmental tasks that must be accomplished during the earlier years of life. The strength of the individual's early ego development is tested during the adolescent years.

Adolescence is a period when individuals normally experience fluctuations in behavior, instability of emotional equilibrium, and rapid changes in mood. Unfortunately a few adolescents actually become mentally ill and develop the characteristic symptomatic behavior of schizophrenia, including bizarre ideation, hallucinations, withdrawal, ideas of reference, and feelings of unreality. Schizophrenia occurs more frequently during the adolescent years than in any other period of life because of the uncertainty and emotional turmoil that exists at that time.

Adolescents may also develop any one of the several neuroses that have been described elsewhere in this text. Treatment of major emotional problems among adolescents requires the use of the same psychiatric skills as those used for adults who suffer from these illnesses.

The diagnosis of *adolescent turmoil state* may be assigned to young people who are admitted to a psychiatric hospital in an emotionally disturbed state during which their behavior is indistinguishable from that usually observed during a true psychotic episode. The adolescent patient may hallucinate or be highly suspicious. However, in an adolescent turmoil the symptoms prove to be temporary, and the situation clears after a few weeks of hospitalization. Thus the term adolescent turmoil suggests that the patient has reacted to an emotionally stressful situation with behavior that bordered upon being psychotic. The neutral environment of the hospital diminished the emotional stress that was upsetting the individual and helped him to gain control and to reconstitute his personality. Such a situation is thought to have been caused by the inability of the individual's ego to cope with the conflicting social and personal pressures which are present in the lives of all adolescents.

Treatment of adolescent turmoil requires collaboration between the psychiatrist, the nurse, the family, and the social worker in identifying the patient's problem and in helping him to cope with it.

The environment in the hospital should be consistent, secure, and supportive to help the patient avoid greater personality disintegration. Adolescents require a steady, constant, understanding relationship with adults. Such a relationship is especially important between nurses and adolescents in psychiatric hospitals. Young patients are in contact with nurses for many hours each day and may respond to them as they have responded to parents or teachers in the past. Nurses must be familiar with the normal behavior of adolescents before attempting to work with disturbed individuals in this age group.

IMPORTANT CONCEPTS

1. Child psychiatry is recognized as an area of specialization in both medicine and nursing.
2. There is even less agreement among authorities concerning the cause, prevention, and treatment of childhood behavior disturbances than there is concerning similar problems among adults.
3. Understanding normal personality growth and development is essential before one can understand emotionally disturbed children.
4. Before 1920 many authorities believed that mental illness was limited to adults.
5. Mental illness among children has in-

creased dramatically during the last ten years.

6. The cause of the great increase in emotional disturbances among children is obscure but is probably related to some of the basic problems in the culture.

7. Childhood emotional disturbances are not distinct and well-defined clinical entities, and there is no universal agreement as to their cause.

8. An emotionally healthy climate within the family is essential if children are to develop into mentally healthy individuals.

9. The ability to trust is a basis ingredient in the development of a well-integrated personality and is learned by infants as a result of their earliest mothering experiences.

10. Each phase in the course of psychosexual development presents the child with more pressure to conform and thus more opportunity to develop emotional difficulties.

11. Parents respond differently to individual children, so that one child may thrive in a home where a second child may be unable to tolerate the situation.

12. Improvement in the child's behavior may depend upon alterations in the parents' attitudes and approaches. Thus parents are usually provided with psychotherapeutic help at the same time that the child is being treated.

13. Evaluation of slow or normal developmental progress should be based upon a thorough study of the child and his family.

14. Much of the disturbed behavior adopted by children is an attempt by the child to comfort or reassure himself in tense, lonely, or frightening situations and to defend against anxiety.

15. Childhood schizophrenia is thought to develop as a result of the interaction between a constitutionally susceptible child and an environmental situation psychologically not compatible for the child.

16. Most children afflicted with childhood schizophrenia present one or all the following symptoms: autistic withdrawal, failure to develop language or to use communicative speech, failure to develop according to the normally expected psychosexual pattern, use of repetitive mannerisms, impairment of ego functioning, failure to develop a clearly defined body image, lack of sexual identity, and inability to perceive time and space accurately.

17. Early infantile autism and symbiotic infantile psychotic syndrome are two fairly clearly identified aspects of childhood schizophrenia and are clearly related to the early mothering experiences received by the child.

18. Because learning to relate to others is the greatest task of the autistic child, he is thought to be able to profit from individual psychotherapy.

19. The symbiotic psychotic child may profit from the special therapeutic environment provided by schools for disturbed children, especially if substitutes for the unhealthy symbiotic relationship with the mother are made available to the child.

20. General goals of treatment for all emotionally ill children include pro-

viding opportunities to develop a more accurate self-concept, to develop more appropriate object relationships, and to work through or relive phases of psychosexual development that were imperfectly experienced.

21. Play therapy is used as a means of gaining insight into the child's unconscious feelings and attitudes and as a means of communicating with the child.

22. If the care provided for disturbed children is to be therapeutic it must be based upon the individual needs of the child.

23. Nurses and child care workers need to examine their feelings, attitudes, and behavior in an attempt to understand and modify their behavior for the benefit of the child.

24. Disturbed children require attention and guidance in the same areas of personal care as mothers usually provide for children at home.

25. Sometimes disturbed children, like all children, need to be held, cuddled, rocked, or comforted.

26. Nurse-child interactions should focus upon the reality of the situation, with emphasis on communication about reality matters.

27. The symbiotic child needs help in gradually developing independence.

28. Consistency in dealing with all children is of major importance and is crucial in dealing with emotionally disturbed children.

29. The young person who is suffering from an adolescent turmoil is reacting to an emotionally stressful situation with behavior that borders on being psychotic.

SUGGESTED SOURCES OF ADDITIONAL INFORMATION

Ackerman, Nathan W.: Child and family psychiatry today: a new look at some old problems, Ment. Hyg. 47:540-545, 1963.

Axline, Virginia M.: Dibs—in search of self, Boston, 1964, Houghton Mifflin Co.

Boatman, M. J., Paynter, J., and Parsons, C.: Nursing in hospital psychiatric therapy for psychotic children, Amer. J. Orthopsychiat. 32:808-817, 1962.

Bowlby, John: Maternal care and mental health, ed. 2, World Health Organization Monograph Series No. 2, Geneva, 1905, World Health Organization.

Bowlby, John. Separation anxiety; a critical review of the literature, J. Child Psychol. Psychiat. 1:251-269, 1961.

Caplan, Gerald: Prevention of mental disorders in children: initial explorations, New York, 1961, Basic Books, Inc., Publishers.

Christ, Adolph E., and others: Nurse-patient group contact on a child psychiatric day care unit, Nurs. Outlook 15:44-47, Aug., 1967.

Christ, Adolph E., and others: Role of the nurse in child psychiatry, Nurs. Outlook 13:30-32, Jan., 1965.

Dittman, Laura L.: A child's sense of trust, Amer. J. Nurs. 66:91-93, Jan., 1966.

Galdston, Iago: The American family in crisis, Ment. Hyg. 42:229-236, 1958.

Kanner, L.: Child psychiatry, ed. 3, Springfield, Ill., 1957, Charles C Thomas, Publishers.

Kolb, Lawrence C.: Noyes' modern clinical psychiatry, ed. 7, Philadelphia, 1968, W. B. Saunders Co.

Kraft, Ivor: Preventing ill health in early childhood, Ment. Hyg. 48:413-423, 1964.

Langdell, John I.: Family treatment of childhood schizophrenia, Ment. Hyg. 51:387-392, 1967.

Mahler, M. S.: On child psychosis and schizophrenia. Autistic and symbiotic infantile psychoses in the psychoanalytic study of the child, New York, 1952, International Universities Press., vol. 7, pp. 286-305.

Peet, Doris Stephenson: Children reborn, Amer. J. Nurs. **64**:102-106, Feb., 1964.

Redl, Fritz: Controls from within, Glencoe, Ill. 1952, The Free Press.

Redl, Fritz, and Wineman, D.: Children who hate, Glencoe, Ill. 1951, The Free Press.

Spitz, René A.: Hospitalism. An inquiry into the genesis of psychiatric conditions in early childhood in psychoanalytic study of the child, New York, 1945, International Universities Press, vol. 1, p. 53.

Spurgeon, Roberta K.: Nursing the autistic child, Amer. J. Nurs. **67**:1416-1419, July, 1967.

Szurek, S. A.: Dynamics of staff interaction in hospital psychiatric treatment of children, Amer. J. Orthopsychiat. **17**:652-664, 1947.

CHAPTER NINETEEN

Patients whose behavior is related to faulty intellectual development

A grasp of several areas of scientific knowledge is required to develop an adequate understanding of the cause and prevention of mental retardation and the treatment of individuals who are mentally retarded. Understanding the broad scope of this problem may encompass aspects of one or more of the following areas of learning: medicine, sociology, psychometric testing, genetics, nutrition, psychiatry, neurophysiology, education, and community planning. Effective prevention and treatment of mental retardation require a multifaceted approach directed toward correcting many inequities in the living situation of several million citizens. Thus adequate discussion of mental retardation requires more attention than is possible in one chapter of this text.

Some experts suggest that such a large and important social problem should not be introduced if adequate attention cannot be provided for it. Others point out that mentally retarded individuals frequently require psychiatric help and are sometimes housed in institutions that have been organized for the care and treatment of the mentally ill. These facts suggest that a textbook of psychiatric nursing should include some of the essential information about the cause, prevention, and treatment of mental retardation. It also seems clear that information about mental deficiency should be included in the pediatric nursing course, since problems related to it are usually identified during the individual's early childhood.

DEFINITION OF MENTAL RETARDATION

The words mental retardation are used to describe a condition in which the individual's intellectual and social development have been partially or completely arrested in the early years of life. If the intellectual development has been relatively normal before adolescence and stops sometime after its onset, some designation other than mental retardation is appropriate.*

There is little agreement about the appropriate terminology by which to designate these individuals. The American Psychiatric Association recommends the designation of mental deficiency, and the American Association on Mental Retardation prefers mental retardation. The older terms idiot, imbecile, and moron are used infrequently today.

CAUSES OF MENTAL RETARDATION†

Although the cause of mental retardation is unknown in approximately 75% of the individuals diagnosed as being mentally deficient, some specific conditions are known to be accompanied by or result in mental retardation.

There are some known inherited abnormalities of brain development due to specific metabolic defects that result in mental retardation. Some of these diagnostic entities fall under the heading of *lipoidoses* and include the following:

1. Amaurotic familial idiocy or Tay-

---

*Jervis, George A.: Factors in mental retardation, Children 1:207, 1954.
†Adapted from Kolb, Lawrence C.: Noyes' clinical psychiatry, ed. 7, Philadelphia, 1968, W. B. Saunders Co., pp. 302-323.

Sachs disease results from the accumulation of ganglioside in the central nervous system. The disease is transmitted by a single recessive gene. The child becomes progressively more apathetic and develops muscular weakness. Death usually occurs before the age of 3 years.

2. Niemann-Pick disease results from deposits of sphingomyelin in the nervous system as well as in the reticuloendothelial system. This condition is transmitted as a recessive gene and manifests itself symptomatically by the time the child is 6 months old. This condition is accompanied by spasticity, abnormal movements, tremor, and convulsions. The child becomes progressively more disabled, with an intellectual retrogression. Death usually occurs by the third year.

3. Gaucher's disease presents a clinical picture much like that seen in Niemann-Pick disease, with the child suffering a rapid downhill course.

4. Metachromatic leukodystrophy results in a progressive impairment of the brain function, with resulting death by the age of 6 years.

Another inherited abnormality that results in defective brain development is due to specific metabolic defects in relation to the utilization of amino acids. This condition is called *phenylketonuria* and is due to a disturbance in protein metabolism. It is inherited from parents carrying a recessive gene. Unless it is treated very early in the child's life, severe mental retardation occurs, with tremors, cortical atrophy of the frontal lobe, dwarfism, and failure to develop speech. The treatment is to restrict phenylalanine in the diet, which requires a special formula for the infant.

Galactosemia is an abnormality in carbohydrate metabolism inherited as a recessive trait. It produces a profound disturbance in growth and development and leads to mental retardation unless recognized and treated early. The treatment is to eliminate milk and substitute soybean or casein hydrolysate substitutes.

Gargoylism or *Hurler's disease* is probably due to a generalized enzymopathy resulting from the deposit of a mucopolysaccharide in almost all organs and connective tissue of the body. The child develops a stunted body, a protruding forehead, a saddle nose, coarse features, and other grotesque bone changes as well as mental retardation. Death usually occurs before the age of 16 years.

Mongolism or *Down's disease* is a condition carried as a recessive gene. The child is born with the somatic cells having forty-seven chromosomes instead of the normal forty-six. The abnormality is found within the twenty-first chromosome. It is estimated that from three to four infants out of each 1,000 are born with mongoloid features. Five to ten percent of these children actually suffer with the severe symptoms of Down's syndrome. These children develop an intellectual capacity that rarely exceeds 50 and often is as low as 15 or 20. There is no specific treatment for this condition.

A few children develop mental deficiency because of an unfavorable condition that existed during fetal life. Some of the conditions that may result in defective infants include (1) eclampsia, (2) RH blood incompatibility, (3) toxic drugs in the mother's blood, (4) rubella infection early in the life of the fetus, and (5) syphilis infection.

Environmental or traumatic factors during or after birth may result in the development of a mentally-retarded infant. The situations that may result in a defective child include (1) difficult labor resulting in cerebral trauma, (2) brain damage at birth due to hemorrhage into the brain tissue or anoxemia of the brain, (3) encephalitis caused by a virus from one of the early childhood diseases such as measles, scarlet fever, or chicken pox, and (4) prematurity, which increases the infant's vulnerability to all events.

At least two endocrine disorders result in mental retardation unless replacement therapy is introduced very early in the child's first year. These conditions are *cretinism,* which is caused by hypothyroidism, and *Fröhlich's syndrome,* which is a result of a pituitary gland dysfunction.

Only about 25% of all the mental retardation in this country has been caused by the several possible factors just discussed.

A few children appear to be mentally defective but are able to achieve at a normal level on intelligence tests. Such a situation, in which the child has an apparent inability to cope with learning situations, lacks interest in his environment, and fails to respond appropriately in social situations, is thought to be due to a long-standing emotional deprivation. It may be that the child has been so emotional and culturally deprived within the family and school that to a large extent he has ceased to involve himself intellectually or socially with his environment.

The cause of mental retardation in the majority of the individuals who are diagnosed as being retarded is obscure. It occurs much more often among children born into families who are described as living in poverty than among families who have an adequate financial income. In such families, because of financial limitations, prenatal care is frequently poor or entirely absent, inadequate nutrition is often the rule, and infants are apt to receive a limited amount of handling, cuddling, and intellectual stimulation from overworked mothers who have too many children and too many responsibilities. Thus authorities believe that the prevention of mental retardation among children of socially and financially-deprived families requires a total effort from government and social agencies to provide the conditions necessary for the normal growth and development of children. This means that mothers must have adequate prenatal and obstetrical care. Adequate care during this period is the first step in preventing abnormal fetal development and prematurity, which frequently result in faulty intellectual development.

Better housing is essential. More opportunities must be provided for children to engage in intellectually stimulating play activities. More adequate diets for these families are necessary to ensure the physical health of children and make it possible for them to participate in family and community activities. Parents need to be helped to understand the psychological and social requirements of their children and how these essential aspects of normal development can be supplied. More adequate educational programs are necessary and must be available for children at an earlier age if those who are potentially capable at birth of developing into intellectually and socially effective individuals are to achieve at their highest possible level.

IDENTIFICATION OF
MENTAL RETARDATION

The diagnosis of mental retardation should be made only after a multifaceted assessment of the individual has been carried out. This should include a study of his physical, social, cultural, educational, vocational, and emotional capacity. However, the determination of mental retardation leans heavily upon the results of a battery of psychometric tests from which a definitive score is derived. Although authorities continue to call attention to the limitations and weaknesses of the several psychological tests currently in vogue, intelligence testing continues to be one of the major tools in categorizing individuals in relation to intellectual functioning. Such categorization is useful for many practical reasons, especially in planning educational and training programs.

A score called the intelligence quotient (I.Q.) is calculated by using a formula in which the mental age (M.A.) is divided by the chronological age (C.A.) and multiplied by 100. The mental age is determined by calculating the results of answers to questions on one of several psychometric tests. Therefore the formula is:

$$I.Q. = \frac{M.A.}{C.A.} \times 100$$

The upper age limit for the period of intellectual development is estimated to be 16 years.

Technically, individuals calculated to have an I.Q. of less than 20 are classified as idiots. Those with an I.Q. of from 20 to 49 are classified as imbeciles, and those with an I.Q. of from 50 to 69 are said to be morons. These classifications are harsh and offer little guidance in planning adequate educational or vocational programs for the individual.

Several other classifications have been suggested that may be more helpful. One classification suggested by the Committee on Mental Retardation of the U. S. Department of Health, Education and Welfare suggests the following:

LEVEL OF RETARDATION	I.Q.
Profound	Below 20
Severe	20-35
Moderate	36-52
Mild	53-68

World Health suggests

Severe subnormality	0-19
Moderate subnormality	20-49
Mild subnormality	50-69

American Psychiatric Association suggests

Severe—requires complete protective care	Below 50
Moderate—requires special training and guidance	50-70
Mild—borderline; may be trained to be economically productive in limited situations	70-85

SCOPE OF THE PROBLEM

It is estimated that there are 200,000 individuals who require institutional care in the United States because of mental retardation. It is also estimated that 225,000 retarded children are enrolled in the special classes now being offered by the public schools in this country. Some authorities estimate that about 3% of the children born each year in the United States will not achieve the intellectual development of a 12-year-old.

Most of the individuals who are mentally retarded are physically indistinguishable from the rest of the population, but they are severely limited in their ability to cope economically and socially in this highly complex society. Because of their handicaps they are mentally and emotionally vulnerable to many environmental events and constitute a high-risk group.

In February, 1962, President John F. Kennedy delivered a message to the Congress of the United States calling attention to the fact that mental retardation is a major national problem. As a result, more attention has been focused upon this problem by the government, and financial aid to the States to improve programs for the mentally retarded has been made available.

IDENTIFYING
THE NEEDS OF THE
MENTALLY RETARDED

Mentally retarded children are first of all children, with essentially the same needs as other more normal children. The difference lies in the rate at which mentally retarded children are able to achieve the levels of maturational development, their ability to grasp new ideas, their ability to handle frustration, their ability to deal with other people socially, and their educational attainment.

Likewise, mentally retarded adults have the same basic needs as do other adults. The ways in which these needs can be fulfilled are altered by the degree of the mental retardation with which the individual must cope. Mental retardation drastically effects the individual's ability to deal effectively with others in a social situation.

Most individuals with I.Q. ratings of less than 25 are too retarded to benefit from educational programs on even the most simple level. These individuals require personal care not unlike that provided for infants. They also need to be safeguarded against ordinary physical danger.

Those with I.Q. ratings of 25 to 50 are usually able to benefit from habit training and with repetitive, patient teaching can master simple motor skills. Thus individuals in this group can be expected to learn to toilet themselves, keep themselves clean, and feed themselves.

The group whose I.Q. ratings range from 50 to 70 are classified as educable and, in addition to those things expected of the group discussed above, can profit from a simple educational program. Some of these individuals can be taught to perform uncomplicated tasks through which they may become economically useful. A general guiding principle in dealing with all mentally retarded individuals is to encourage the utilization of their intellectual abilities at the highest possible level but at the same time to avoid pressuring them to achieve at a level that is clearly beyond their capacities.

The individual's level of mental retardation dictates to a large extent where he can be cared for most effectively and the program from which he can receive the greatest benefit. All programs of care should be highly individual. The goal of treatment for each mentally retarded individual should be to assist him to achieve at the highest level of intellectual and social functioning possible for him.

IMPORTANCE OF PARENT-CHILD
RELATIONSHIP

Because mentally retarded children have essentially the same emotional needs as do other children, they too need the experience of a warm parent-child relationship. Retarded children have a greater chance of developing their intellectual and social potential if they are nurtured within a family, at least during the preschool years. No longer is institutional placement considered the only solution for a family when a child has been diagnosed as being mentally retarded.

When the child reaches school age, it may become apparent that the best possible plan for him is to live at an institution among other children with whom he can compete successfully. Even if the child spends most of the week at a special school, it is important for him to return to his family for weekend visits and on holidays. This is the ideal solution if the family is warm, accepting, and loving toward the child.

Parents need help in accepting a mentally retarded child and in providing the affection, security, and approval all children require if they are to develop a stable personality. Unfortunately, parents may feel ashamed of a retarded child and develop a sense of failure in relation to him. The child may be rejected, emotionally deprived, and coerced to achieve beyond his abilities.

Parents, especially mothers who must take the major responsibility for training the child, need support and guidance if a retarded child is to be successfully reared at home. The mother needs encouragement in allowing the child to develop at his own rate without being overly protected, rejected, or forced to achieve beyond his potential. One significant way in which the public health nurse can make a contribution to improving the care of mentally retarded children is to help parents cope with their feelings and work toward meeting the needs of their children.

In spite of all efforts, there are families who cannot accept a mentally retarded child as part of the group. In such a situation a foster home placement would probably be the most appropriate solution. If this solution is not possible, institutionalization in a hospital or school designed to care for mentally retarded individuals would be the logical answer.

No matter where the child lives, he needs to be cared for by warm, friendly people who understand his handicap and who will work with him intelligently and helpfully. Mentally retarded children, like all other children, need love, respect, patience, and clearly established and sensibly enforced limits on behavior. If it is decided that the child will profit most by living in an institution, it must provide a substitute for the home and family of which he may be deprived.

Educational programs are essential parts of the daily regimen of mentally retarded individuals who live in institutions. Some of the more successful agencies operate much like boarding schools, with the curriculum including personal habit training, instruction in personal grooming and social skills, lessons in activities designed to fill leisure time hours, and help in improving interpersonal relations. In addition, those children who can profit by more formal education attend classes organized for various age and maturational levels. Educators, with special preparation in teaching the mentally retarded, guide the children in developing simple reading skills, the ability to make change, do simple sums, budget small amounts of money, and the other educational knowledge essential for independent living. Manual skills are also taught to individuals who are capable of performing them. These educational tasks must be geared to the aptitudes of the individuals involved in the program. The aim of such a program is to equip the individual with the knowledge, vocational skill, and social effectiveness required to live as independently as possible in the institution or in the community.

Some mentally retarded children who suffer from severe physical defects as well as mental deficiency may require throughout their lives the personal care usually provided for a very young child. On the other hand, some individuals who are less handicapped may become self-supporting in the community. It has been estimated that approximately one half of the mentally retarded individuals who are admitted to an institution for care and training are eventually able to live in the community.

INSTITUTIONAL REQUIREMENTS
FOR THE MENTALLY RETARDED

Many of the essential elements of an effective institution have already been mentioned. These include (1) employees who are warm, friendly, and knowledgable about the needs of the handicapped individuals with whom they work, (2) an educational program that aims to help each individual achieve his highest intellectual and social potential, and (3) the provision of a homelike atmosphere for the individual who is deprived of home and family by being institutionalized.

Thus friendly, homelike living quarters, dining rooms, and sleeping dormitories should be available. A well-developed recreational program with a variety of activities designed to appeal to many different interests, ages, and maturational levels is important. Opportunities for participation in a variety of group experiences, including musical activities, dances, sports, movies, and television viewing should be a part of the activities program. A library should be provided with colorful reading material chosen to appeal to the levels of the intellectual abilities of the individuals living at the institution.

Although many mentally retarded individuals are admitted as children, their problems frequently require long-term institutional care. Because of this, individuals may remain in the same institution for years. Thus access to a barber shop and a beauty parlor is a necessary part of the institutional offerings. Mentally retarded individuals need to be assisted to look as well groomed and attractive as possible.

Opportunities for individuals who can profit by work assignments should be available. Through appropriately assigned work, mentally retarded individuals can gain a sense of usefulness by performing meaningful tasks that make a significant contribution to the total work of the institution. Such work assignments should be rewarded appropriately with a cash payment. This does more than almost any other form of recognition to help the individual develop a sense of being useful.

TREATMENT FOR THE
MENTALLY RETARDED

Care and treatment for the mentally retarded person should be based upon an accurate evaluation of the individual's assets and capacities and the concomitant physical, emotional, and psychological problems present. Thus specific medical conditions must be treated with the appropriate therapeutic agents. Nutritional and metabolic conditions must be corrected by providing the required diet and the therapeutic measures necessary to eliminate the metabolic disequilibrium. Surgical procedures should be performed when they are indicated, especially in the case of the orthopedic deformities frequently seen in individuals who have been confined to a bed or wheelchair. Replacement therapy in such conditions as cretinism should be undertaken. All these procedures require an institutional staff of professional individuals who are capable of providing the necessary therapeutic measures. These procedures are designed to assist mentally retarded individuals to achieve the highest possible level of intellectual, physical, and social functioning.

Unfortunately, for many severely mentally retarded individuals, their ability to cope with the environment or to achieve at a higher level is not greatly improved by specific treatments. Instead, these individuals require the kind of environment that provides for their special physical and emotional needs.

Some mentally retarded individuals are aware of their limited abilities and are troubled by their inadequate coping patterns. Some realize that they are a great disappointment to their families and become guilt ridden and depressed. Many of them suffer from the same anxieties, frustrations, and psychotic symptoms found among individuals in other situations. Such emotional problems appear frequently among mentally retarded individuals and require the same kind of professional help that would be provided in other settings.

The tranquilizing drugs are useful in helping mentally retarded individuals control behavior that is disturbing to others. Chlorpromazine (Thorazine) and reserpine (Serpasil) are the drugs frequently chosen for this purpose and have proved to be helpful in quieting overactive, boisterous, excited mentally retarded individuals.

Because the occurrence of mental illness is high among mentally retarded individuals, the institution must provide some professional workers who are prepared to deal therapeutically with disturbed people. Unfortunately, many psychiatrists question the value of providing psychotherapy for such handicapped individuals. This is because they are sometimes thought to have difficulty relating to others and are limited in their ability to learn from experience. However, it has been demonstrated that selected individuals from the mentally retarded population can profit from having a therapeutic relationship with a helping person. This person may be a psychiatrist, a clinical psychologist, a psychiatric nurse, or a social worker. It is important that the therapeutic sessions be held regularly, that they focus upon reality-oriented material, that the length of the session be timed to coincide with the limited attention span of the individual, and that the helping person respect and like the retarded individual. In addition, unless the helping person is highly skilled, supervision should be sought from an experienced psychotherapist.

Group therapy is another way of providing emotional help for mentally retarded individuals. It has many of the same advantages for them as for individuals in any group therapy experience. In addition, it provides a peer group with whom the individual can relate and by whom he can feel accepted. In providing group therapy for the mentally retarded, it must be more structured than the technique usually employed, more specific limits need to be established, and the focus needs to be placed more upon action than upon ideas. A nurse with some knowledge of and experience with group therapy can make an important contribution in the field of mental retardation by providing leadership for group therapy sessions for these handicapped individuals.

Recently a technique has been introduced called *operant conditioning,* which gives promise of revolutionizing the treatment of the mentally retarded. It is a method of motivating the mentally retarded in such a way as to modify their behavior patterns in the direction of that which is considered socially desirable.

This technique is based upon B. F. Skinner's theories, developed in his book *Science and Human Behavior.** It focuses upon changing or modifying the individual's response to the environment by reinforcing certain desirable patterns of behavior or eliminating undesirable patterns. This is done by rewarding the indi-

vidual for demonstrating specific behavior patterns considered desirable. In the language of the technique, behavior patterns may be modified by operant conditioning or by operant extinction. A positive reinforcer is used to reward desirable behavior. Thus somthing that the retarded individual enjoys or that is meaningful to him is forthcoming when the approved behavior emerges. This reward can be praise, approval, food, or social privileges. Frequently candy has been used successfully as the reinforcer. It is also possible to utilize what is referred to as a negative reinforcer. A negative reinforcer might be the rewarding of desirable behavior by the removal from the environment of something the individual dislikes. Thus such actions as the extinguishing of a bright light or of a loud, unpleasant noise, or the removal of the individual from a very cold or very hot room, might be classified as negative reinforcers. The third way of reinforcing desirable behavior according to the operant conditioning technique is by the use of an adverse response to the behavior. Thus the individual would receive disapproval or punishment for the use of behavior patterns that are not considered to be acceptable or desirable.[†] In some situations punishment as a negative reinforcer has not been successful.

To utilize the operant conditioning technique successfully, the members of the institutional staff working with the individual whose behavior patterns are to be the focus of attention must agree upon the desirable behavior pattern they wish

---

*Skinner, B. F.: Science and human behavior, New York, 1953, The Macmillan Co.
†Adapted from Kalkman, Marion E.: Psychiatric nursing, ed. 3, McGraw-Hill Book Co., p.185.

to reinforce, upon the reinforcer to be used, and the way in which it is to be applied. Consistency in the approach is important.

Operant conditioning was chosen as the method of approach to a retarded, adolescent girl who soiled her bedding each night, failed to attend to her personal hygiene and grooming, and offended others because of a body odor. The hospital staff decided to encourage a dry bed, combing the hair, and bathing. Initially they focused upon keeping the bed dry. Thus the girl was rewarded with candy and with praise each morning when she was found to have a dry bed. If it was wet, no comment was made and no candy was provided. At first the bed was dry only occasionally, but after several weeks of rewarding her on the dry days, the bed remained dry most of the time. In like manner, personal grooming and bathing were encouraged and rewarded with praise and candies. After months of consistent work, this young girl was dry every night, was appropriately groomed, and no longer had an offensive odor.

As this example demonstrates, operant conditioning technique can be useful in eliminating undesirable behavior as well as motivating socially acceptable behavior. The utilization of this technique may provide the answer to the ever-present problem of setting limits for the behavior of the mentally retarded and for helping them to achieve behavior that conforms to socially acceptable standards.

NURSE'S ROLE

Mentally retarded individuals as a group are at the mercy of the people who organize and staff the institutions where they are institutionalized. Many nonprofessional workers are employed to provide the large amount of individualized personal care and supervision required by retarded individuals in every aspect of the activities of daily living. This fact presents the nurse with the opportunity to accept a major role in improving the care of the mentally retarded by teaching and directing the care given by the nonprofessional workers. Through teaching by example as well as in more formal situations, the nurse can instill positive attitudes among the workers toward their handicapped charges. She can help them understand the basic needs of handicapped individuals and develop ways of meeting those needs. She can demonstrate the importance of respecting the mentally retarded and giving them praise and encouragement. To a large extent the nurse is responsible for the psychological tone of the unit where she is employed.

The nurse's role with mentally retarded individuals also includes giving expert nursing care to retarded individuals who present challenging nursing care problems and demonstrating to less skillful workers the skills involved. She is in a position to assist in developing innovative ways of coping with some of the unique physical and emotional needs of these individuals.

The nurse works closely with the clinical psychologist in developing and carrying out decisions about the use of the techniques involved with operant conditioning. If she is prepared to do so, she should accept responsibility for providing counseling sessions for selected patients. However, because there are so many areas in which the nurse's expert knowledge and guidance are crucial in improving the care of the mentally retarded, it is necessary for her to establish priorities in relation to where her efforts could most profitably be focused to provide the greatest therapeutic impact upon the total situation.

Probably the most significant role the nurse accepts in an institution that cares for mentally retarded individuals is that of the mothering person. In this role she becomes the significant helping person in the lives of both the young children and the individuals who have been institutionalized for a longer period of time. Through her consistent presence in the situation and her conviction that mentally retarded individuals are worthwhile human beings, the nurse provides emotional support and security for these deprived individuals. There is probably no situation in which the nurse can play such a significant role in altering the situation positively than in an institution where mentally retarded individuals are cared for.

IMPORTANT CONCEPTS

1. Effective prevention and early treatment of mental retardation requires a multifaceted approach directed toward correcting many inequities in the lives of several million citizens.
2. Mentally retarded individuals frequently require psychiatric help and are sometimes hospitalized in institutions for the mentally ill.
3. Mental retardation is a condition in which the individual's intellectual and social development have been par-

tially or completely arrested in the early years of life.
4. The specific cause of mental retardation is unknown in 75% of the individuals who are diagnosed as being handicapped in this way.
5. The known causes of mental retardation include some genetically inherited conditions, a few unfavorable conditions during fetal life, a few endocrine disorders, some specific metabolic defects, and some traumatic factors that may occur after birth.
6. The prevention of mental retardation among children of socially and financially deprived families probably requires an all-out effort by government and social agencies to provide the many conditions necessary for the normal growth and development of children.
7. The diagnosis of mental retardation should be made only after a multifaceted assessment of the individual has been made.
8. Most of the individuals who are mentally retarded are physically indistinguishable from the rest of the population, but they are severely limited in their ability to cope in a highly complex society.
9. Mentally retarded children are first of all children, with essentially the same needs as more normal children.
10. Individuals with an I.Q. rating of less than 25 require complete protective care and usually do not profit by even the most simple educational program.
11. Individuals with I.Q. ratings of from 25 to 50 are usually able to benefit

from habit training and can master simple motor skills.

12. Individuals with an I.Q. of from 50 to 70 are classified as educable and can be taught to perform simple, uncomplicated tasks.

13. A guiding principle in dealing with mentally retarded individuals is to encourage the utilization of their intellectual abilities at the highest possible level but to avoid pressuring them to achieve at a level that is clearly beyond their capacities.

14. Retarded children have a greater chance of developing their intellectual and social potential if they are nurtured within a family.

15. Parents need support and guidance if a mentally retarded child is to be successfully cared for at home.

16. No matter where the retarded child lives he needs to be cared for by warm, friendly people who understand his handicap and who will work with him intelligently and helpfully.

17. The aim of the educational programs provided for mentally retarded children is to equip them to live as independently as possible in the community or if necessary in an institution.

18. Care and treatment for the mentally retarded individual should be based upon an evaluation of his assets and capacities and concomitant physical, emotional, and psychological problems.

19. Emotional problems appear frequently among mentally retarded individuals and require psychiatric help.

20. Some of the tranquilizing drugs are useful in helping mentally retarded individuals control behavior that may be disturbing to others.

21. Selected mentally retarded individuals can profit from a therapeutic relationship with a helping person.

22. The technique called operant conditioning gives promise of greatly improving the treatment of the mentally retarded by reinforcing desirable patterns of behavior or eliminating undesirable patterns.

23. To a large extent the nurse is responsible for the psychological tone of the hospital unit where she is employed.

24. Probably the most significant role the nurse accepts in an institution that cares for mentally retarded individuals is that of the mothering person.

SUGGESTED SOURCES OF ADDITIONAL INFORMATION

Barnard, Kathryn: Teaching the retarded child is a family affair, Amer. J. Nurs. **68**:305-311, Feb., 1968.

Bourgeois, Theodora L.: Reinforcement theory in teaching the mentally retarded: a token economy program, Perspect. Psychiat. Care **6**:116-126; 136, 1968.

Bowlby, John: Maternal care and mental health, Geneva, 1951, World Health Organization.

Brown, Daniel G.: Behavior modification, Perspect. Psychiat. Care **6**:224-229, 1968.

Buck, Pearl: The child who never grew, New York, 1950, The John Day Co., Inc.

Cullinane, Marie M.: The blossoming of Ruthie, Amer. J. Nurs. **68**:122-124, Jan., 1968.

Fackler, Eleanor: The crisis of institutionalizing a retarded child, Amer. J. Nurs. **68**:1508-1512, July, 1968.

Gibson, Robert: Changing concepts of mental deficiency, Ment. Hyg. 43:8-86, 1959.

Haynes, Una H.: Nursing approaches in cerebral dysfunction, Amer. J. Nurs. 68:2170-2176, Oct., 1968.

Holtgreve, Marian M.: A guide for public health nurses working with mentally retarded children, U. S. Children's Bureau publication No. 422, Washington, D. C., 1964, U. S. Government Printing Office.

Jervis, George A.: Factors in mental retardation, Children 1:207-211, 1954.

Kelman, Howard R.: A program for mentally retarded children, Children 2:10-14, 1955.

Koch, Richard, and Gilien, Nancy Ragsdale: Diagnostic experience in a clinic for retarded children, Nurs. Outlook 13:26-29, June, 1965.

Keogh, Barbara, and Legeay, Camile: Recoil from the diagnosis of mental retardation, Amer. J. Nurs. 66:778-780, April, 1966.

Lange, Silvia, and Whitney, Linda: Teaching mental retardation nursing, Nurs. Outlook 14: 58-61, April, 1966.

Legeay, Camille, and Keogh, Barbara: Impact of mental retardation on family life, Amer. J. Nurs. 66:1062-1065, May, 1966.

Patterson, Letha L.: Some pointers for professionals, Children 3:13-17, 1956.

Pattullo, Ann W., and Barnard, Kathryn E.: Teaching menstrual hygiene to the mentally retarded, Amer. J. Nurs. 68:2572-2575, Dec., 1968.

Peterson, Linda Whitney: Operant approach to observation and recording, Nurs. Outlook 15: 28-32, March, 1967.

Tarjan, George: What hospitals for the mentally retarded can achieve, Children 3:95-101, 1956.

Wright, Margaret M.: Care for the mentally retarded. Scope of the problem, Amer. J. Nurs. 63:70-74, Sept., 1963.

The nurse focuses upon psychiatric nursing in relation to its history, to the law, and to future trends

CHAPTER TWENTY

Historical review of psychiatry

In his slow development through the ages, primitive man gradually acquired a sense of compassion for his fellow creatures; he then began to recognize mental disorders and to make attempts at treating them. In the light of modern knowledge these attempts were undeniably crude and meaningless.

From the study of contemporary primitive peoples and their attitude toward mentally ill individuals, it can be safely inferred that after certain tribal rites had failed to effect a cure, the victim of mental disease in the dim past was disposed of by the simple expedient of being abandoned to shift for himself and to die quickly of starvation in a barren waste or to be devoured by animals in the wilderness. That some prehistoric peoples had, however, developed a high degree of knowledge about the brain and its functions is the conclusion of anthropologists who have studied the remains of several civilizations in both the New and the Old World. Excavations have revealed skeletons that clearly bear evidences of such successful trepanning of the skull that the subjects survived for several years. It is assumed that such operations were done to relieve headache and probably mental derangement, and that even some knowledge of asepsis may have existed in those remote days.

In recorded ancient history, such as that of the Eastern Mediterranean civilizations, there are references to mental disorders. Thus an Egyptian papyrus of 1500 B.C. contains a discourse on old age and says of it that "the heart grows heavy and remembers not yesterday." In later Egyptian civilization, particularly during the Alexandrian era, medicine developed a high status; sanatoriums known as the temples of Saturn were operated for the care of those who were mentally afflicted. The Old Testament records authentic cases of mental illness, of which King Saul offers a famous example.

The Golden Age of Greece was noted for its humane regard for the sick. The Greek physicians were poor anatomists because they deified the human body and dared not dissect it, but they were astute observers and excellent clinicians. Hippocrates (460-375? B.C.), the greatest of the old Greek physicians, knew well the symptoms of melancholia and regarded epilepsy not as the "sacred disease" but insisted that "it has a natural cause from which it originates like other afflictions." The Greeks used as hospitals temples that had an abundance of fresh air, pure water, and sunshine. These temples of Aesculapius "as often as they had patients, such as were unhinged, did make use of nothing so much for the cure of them as symphony and sweet harmony of voices." Theatricals, riding, walking, and listening to the sound of a waterfall were all recommended as methods to divert the melancholic. With this amazingly humane attitude, there were, however, instances where the treatment was not always free of its vicious aspects, since even in the best of the Greek temples, starving, chains, and flogging were advocated "because with these it was believed that when those who refused food began to eat, frequently the memory was also refreshed thereby."

There is a surprising paucity of data about the Roman era in reference to mental disease. Galen, who was actually a Greek but practiced in Rome, based his treatment on the teachings of his Greek predecessors. Other physicians of the Roman era treated mental illness by bleeding, purging, and sulfur baths.

With the collapse of Greek and Roman civilization, medicine, along with other cultural developments, suffered an almost complete eclipse. The treatment of mental illness was left to priests, and every sort of superstitious belief flourished. The insane were flogged, fettered, scourged, and starved in the belief that the devils that possessed them could be driven out by these means.

A few bright spots in this tragic picture were some monasteries or shrines where this technique of "exorcising" the evil spirit was performed by the gentle laying on of hands instead of the whip. Members of the nobility, self-appointed ascetics, and holy men of varying degrees of sincerity practiced this art, which at least had to recommend it the fact that it was not physically cruel.

Out of this tradition and belief in the "holy" or "royal touch" arose several great shrines, of which the one at Gheel in Belgium is most famous. The legend behind the beginnings of this colony is worth telling. Somewhere in the dim past there lived a king in Ireland who was married to a most beautiful woman and who became the father of an equally beautiful daughter. The good queen developed a fatal illness, and at her deathbed the daughter dedicated herself to a life of purity and service to the poor and the mentally bereft. The widowed king was beside himself with grief and announced to his subjects that he must at once be assuaged of sorrow by marrying the woman in his kingdom who most resembled the dead queen. No such paragon was found. But

the devil came and whispered to the king that there was such a woman—his own daughter. The devil spurred the king to propose marriage to the girl, but she was appropriately outraged and fled across the English Channel to Belgium. There the king overtook her and with Satan at his elbow, slew the girl and her faithful attendants. In the night an angel came, recapitated the body, and concealed it in the forest near the village of Gheel. Years later five lunatics chained together spent the night with their keepers at a small wayside shrine near this Belgian village. According to the legend all the victims recovered overnight. Here indeed must be the place where the dead girl, reincarnated as St. Dymphna, was buried, and here was the sacred spot where her cures of the insane are effected. In the fifteenth century, pilgrimages to Gheel from every part of the civilized world were organized for the mentally sick. Many of the pilgrims remained in Gheel to live with the inhabitants of the locality, and in the passing years it became the natural thing to accept them into the homes, and thus the first colony for the mentally ill, and for that matter the only one that has been consistently successful, was formed. In 1851 the Belgian government took charge of this colony of mentally ill patients. It continues to exist to the present day. Some 1,500 certified mentally ill patients live in private homes, work with the inhabitants, and suffer no particular restriction of freedom, except to refrain from visiting public places and from the use of alcohol and to report regularly to the supervising psychiatrist. In spite of the success of the Gheel colony and its great humanizing value, most attempts at duplicating it elsewhere have been complete or partial failures.

Although the treatment of the mentally ill in the Middle Ages had nothing much to recommend it, the period that followed was in some respects a great deal worse. When the church and the monastery gave up the care of the insane, it was gradually taken over by the so-called almshouse, the contract house, and the secular asylum. The more violent patients gravitated to jails and dungeons. In the sixteenth century, Henry VIII officially dedicated Bethlehem Hospital in London as a lunatic asylum. It soon became the notorious "Bedlam" whose hideous practices were immortalized by Hogarth, the famous cartoonist. There keepers were allowed to exhibit the most boisterous of the patients for two pence a look, and the more harmless inmates were forced to seek charity on the streets of London as the "Bedlam beggars" of Shakespeare's *King Lear*.

In those dark days of psychiatry, society was interested in its own self-security, not in the welfare of the insane. The almshouses were a combination of jail and asylum, and within their walls petty criminals and the insane were herded indiscriminately. In the seventeeth and eighteenth centuries the dungeons of Paris were the only places where the violently insane could be committed. Drastic purgings and bleedings were the favorite therapeutic procedures of the day, and "madshirts" and the whip were applied religiously by the cellkeepers.

Superstition about mental disease took a horrible turn in the seventeenth century. God and Satan were still thought to be engaged in a ceaseless battle for possession of one's soul. The year after the *Mayflower* sailed into Plymouth Harbor, Burton published his classic work, *Anatomy of Melancholy,* wherein he stated that "witches and magicians can cure and cause most diseases." To seek out and liquidate witches became a sacred religious duty. Twenty thousand persons were said to have been burned in Scotland alone during the seventeenth century. Small wonder that Cotton Mather precipitated the witch mania in Salem, since he was merely subscribing to the dogma of the day.

The political and social reformations in France toward the end of the eighteenth century influenced the hospitals and jails of Paris. In 1792, Philippe Pinel (1745-1826), a young physician who was medical director of the Bicêtre Asylum outside of Paris, was given permission by the Revolutionary Commune to liberate the miserable inmates of two of the largest hospitals, some of whom had been in chains for twenty years. Had his experiment proved a failure, he might well have lost his head by the guillotine. Fortunately he was right, since by his act he proved conclusively the fallacy of inhuman treatment of the insane. The reforms instituted by Pinel were continued by his pupil, Esquirol, who founded no less than ten asylums and was the first regular teacher of psychiatry. The Quakers, under the Brothers Tuke, had at this time established the York Retreat and effected the same epoch-making reforms in England.

In America, under the guidance of Benjamin Franklin, the Pennsylvania Hospital was completed in 1756. There the insane were still relegated to the cellar but at least they were assured clean bedding and warm rooms. Benjamin Rush (1745-1813), a prime humanitarian and the "father of American psychiatry," entered upon his duties at the Pennsylvania Hospital in 1783. Subscribing in part to the lunar theory of insanity and inventing an inhuman restraining device called the "tranquilizer" but at the same time insisting on more humane treatment of the mentally afflicted, he stands as a prominent transitional figure between the old era and the new.

Most of the states were still without special institutions for mentally ill persons in the first quarter of the nineteenth century. The poorhouse or almshouse was still popular, but it invariably became a catchall for all types of offenders, and the mentally ill received the brunt of its manifold evils. Most shocking to people of today was the placing of the poor and the mildly demented on the auction block, where those with the strongest backs and the weakest minds were sold to the highest bidder, the returns from the sale being assigned to the township treasury.

About 1830 a vigorous movement for the erection of suitable state hospitals spread simultaneously through several states. The excellent results obtained by a private institution such as the Hartford Retreat, founded in 1818, probably served as an object lesson. Horace Mann took an enthusiastic interest in the plight of the insane, and the advantages of a state hospital system were publicized to promote construction of such institutions. The first public psychiatric hospital in America was built in Williamsburg, Virginia in 1773. Today it is known as the Eastern Psychiatric Hospital. In 1882 a school of nursing was established near Boston at McLean

Hospital, a private hospital for the mentally ill established in 1818.

However, it remained for an asthenic, 40-year-old schoolteacher to expose to a torpid public the sins of the poorhouse. From that day in 1841 when Dorothea Lynde Dix (1802-1887) described the hoarfrost on the walls of the cells of the East Somerville jail in Massachusetts to the day when she retreated into one of the very hospitals she was instrumental in creating, she effected reforms that shook the world. She so aroused the public conscience that millions of dollars were raised to build suitable hospitals, and twenty states responded directly to her appeals. She played an important part in the founding of St. Elizabeth's Hospital in Washington, directed the opening of two large institutions in the maritime provinces of Canada, completely reformed the asylum system in Scotland and in several other foreign countries, and rounded out a most amazing career by organizing the nursing forces of the northern armies during the Civil War. A resolution presented by the United States Congress in 1901 characterized her as "among the noblest examples of humanity in all history."

By the middle of the nineteenth century the asylum, "the big house on the hill," ensconced in its landscaped park and topped by high turrets and senseless cupolas, became a familiar landmark in every state capital. In it mentally afflicted men and women lived and enjoyed a modicum of comfort and freedom from abuse. But to the general public it had a fortresslike appearance, and its occupants were a strange and foreboding lot. From this smug isolation the psychiatrist made no attempt to teach the man in the street anything to ease his fear and horror of mental disease. As a matter of fact, he could not impart much information because he had little to give. Although such matters as management, housing, and feeding of mental patients were slowly attaining decent humanitarian standards, as late as 1840 there was no clear classification of mental disorders, and a German teacher, Doctor Heinroth, was still advancing the theory that insanity and sin were identical. Not until 1845 when Griesinger published the first authentic textbook on mental disease was the position of psychiatry in relation to other medical sciences clearly defined.

Formal research into the cause and nature of nervous and mental disease gained impetus under the inspiration of Jean Charcot (1825-1893), the great French neurologist whose clinics attracted students from every country in the world. Toward the end of the nineteenth century much new knowledge was derived from the microscopic study of the brain and the introduction of laboratory methods. The development of outpatient departments for psychiatric cases dates back to 1885, when persons suffering with incipient disease were treated at the Pennsylvania Hospital and, a few months later, at Warren in the same state.

In 1883 Emil Kraepelin (1856-1926), a professor of psychiatry in Germany, published the first edition of Psychiatrie, which in English translation changed the whole view of classifications of mental disorders in America. He classified human behavior on the basis of symptomatology and offered a description of dementia praecox. Eugen Bleuler (1857-1939), a professor from Zurich, elaborated the concept of dementia praecox and expanded it into schizophrenia in 1911.

The emphasis on prevention and recognition of early stages of mental illness was not made until the turn of the present century, when Clifford Beers entered upon the scene. Having spent several years in various mental institutions as a patient, he emerged in 1907 to write his famous book *A Mind That Found Itself*. Being of a vivid, colorful temperament, he had unlimited enthusiasm, which he directed in founding the National Committee for Mental Hygiene. Under the momentum of his aggressive leadership, the movement became worldwide and now has ramifications in the form of child guidance, prison psychiatry, vocational guidance, and other practical activities that concern the normal human being as much as they do the abnormal.

Coincidentally with the mental hygiene program came the astounding contributions of Sigmund Freud (1856-1939), which revolutionized the orthodox concepts of the mind, proposed a new technique for exploring it, and brought psychiatry as a living subject to the attention of every intelligent man and woman. Psychiatry, at last, left its flying buttresses and ramparts and participated in everyday human activity.

Freud's formulations dealing with the dynamics of the unconscious mind have resulted in a deeper understanding of human behavior and a better approach to the treatment of personality problems and psychoneurotic disorders. Psychotherapy in all its many phases continues to be the core of all methods of treatment, and its techniques are being refined and improved with each succeeding year.

Along with psychotherapy, successful attacks on mental disorders have been made by means of special physical remedies, testifying to the fact that present-day psychiatry is willing to utilize any measure that offers a promise to control or to relieve, whether it be a psychological or a medical procedure.

Outstanding was the introduction of malaria and other types of fever therapy in 1917 by Wagner-Jauregg (1857-1940), a psychiatrist in Vienna. This work was indispensable in the treatment of neurosyphilis before the advent of the antibiotics. This was followed by the discovery and isolation of the various vitamin principles and their remarkable effects on delirium, and deficiency states such as alcoholism, pellagra, and polyneuritis.

During the third decade of the twentieth century came the unique shock method of treating schizophrenia with insulin, as introduced by Sakel, to be followed shortly by Meduna's treatment of mental depressions by the convulsion-producing drug pentylenetetrazol (Metrazol) and in 1938 by electroconvulsive therapy introduced by Cerletti and Bini. Finally surgery entered the psychiatric field and boldly cut into brain substance, particularly in the region of the frontal lobe, to help allay some of the worst features of otherwise hopeless agitation and deterioration. This operation, now outmoded, was called prefrontal lobotomy.

The midcentury decade brought outstanding developments that virtually made it a golden age for psychiatry. Modern technologies brought men countless conveniences, leisure, sanitation, immunity to infectious diseases, and freedom from heavy toil, but the challenging problems that remained were mental illness and the degenerative diseases. Hence there was a great resurgence of interest in mental disease. The gospel of mental health was spread over the land through every form of dissemination, including radio, television, magazines, newspapers, sermons, and lectures. The new place for the psychiatrist, the psychoanalyst, the psychologist, the nurse, and the social worker became the community clinic.

The most recent boon to psychiatry is the development of new drugs, particularly tranquilizers, with their selective action on the emotional states. The atmosphere of disturbed wards has been completely revolutionized, the morale and interest of the nurse and attendant have been vastly improved, and under the influence of the drugs the patient is more receptive to recreational, occupational, and other diversional therapies, as well as to psychotherapy.

The most recent development, referred to as community psychiatry, is moving the treatment of the patient back to his community. The focus is not solely upon the patient but upon creating a community that promotes mental health.

It is well for psychiatry to take pride in pointing to a fine record wherein a mere century has carried it out of ignorance and mysticism and out of the days when the mentally ill were whipped regularly at the full of the moon to the present era of humane treatment in modern hospitals where every facility for diagnosis and amelioration of disease is provided. In developing the curative side of psychiatry, an all-important step in advance has been the introduction of professional nurses in all psychiatric hospitals and the placing of professional nurses at the head of the nursing staffs. This system, first introduced by Dr. Samuel Hitch in 1841 at Gloucester Asylum in England, has been instrumental in improving the care of patients with mental disease, has engendered a better public attitude toward mental hospitals, and has done more than anything else to soften the atmosphere of tension and mystery that still lingers about the mentally disordered patient.

Psychiatric nursing has truly come of age. Up to 1956, responsibility for evaluation and approval of psychiatric nursing education in mental hospitals was assumed by a committee of the American Psychiatric Association. Now these duties have been assumed by the National League for Nursing. This has resulted in higher standards in nursing education and a more dignified status for the nursing profession.

SUGGESTED SOURCES OF ADDITIONAL INFORMATION

Altschule, Mark D.: Essays in the history of psychiatry, New York, 1957, Grune & Stratton, Inc.

American Psychiatric Association: One hundred years of American psychiatry, New York, 1944, Columbia University Press.

Angrist, Shirley S.: The mental hospital; its history and destiny, Perspect. Psychiat. Care 1:20-26, 1963.

Beers, Clifford: A mind that found itself, Garden City, N. J., 1936, Doubleday & Co., Inc.

Bockhoven, J. S.: Moral treatment in American psychiatry, New York, 1963, Springer Publishing Co., Inc.

Bromberg, Walter: Man above humanity, a history of psychotherapy, Philadelphia, 1954, J. B. Lippincott Co.

Deutsch, Albert: The shame of the states, New York, 1948, Harcourt, Brace & World, Inc.

Deutsch, Albert: The mentally ill in America, ed. 2, New York, 1949, Columbia University Press.

Flugel, John: A hundred years of psychology, ed. 2, London, 1951, Gerald Duckworth and Co., Ltd.

Garber, Robert S.: Two Philadelphia psychiatrists and a theory of American psychiatry, Ment. Hyg. 53:131-139, 1969.

Gorman, Mike: Every other bed, Cleveland, 1956, The World Publishing Co.

Grinker, Roy R.: Mid-century psychiatry, Springfield, Ill., 1953, Charles C Thomas, Publisher.

Jones, Ernest: Life and work of Sigmund Freud, vol. 1, New York, 1953, Basic Books, Inc., Publishers.

Lief, Alfred, editor: The commonsense psychiatry of Adolf Meyer, New York, 1948, McGraw-Hill Book Co.

Marshall, Helen E.: Dorothea Dix, Chapel Hill, N. C., 1937, University of North Carolina Press.

Moench, L. G.: Office psychiatry, Chicago, 1952, Year Book Medical Publishers, Inc.

Oberndorf, Clarence P.: A history of psychoanalysis in America, New York, 1953, Grune & Stratton, Inc.

Ray, Marie B.: Doctors of the mind, Boston, 1942, Little, Brown & Co.

Roback, A. A.: History of American psychology, New York, 1952, Library Publishers.

Thompson, Clara: Psychoanalysis; evolution and development, New York, 1950, Hermitage House.

Woodham-Smith, Cecil: Florence Nightingale, New York, 1951, McGraw-Hill Book Co.

Zilboorg, Gregory: A history of medical psychology, New York, 1941, W. W. Norton & Co., Inc.

Zilboorg, Gregory: Sigmund Freud, his exploration of the mind of man, New York, 1951, Charles Scribner's Sons.

CHAPTER TWENTY-ONE

Rehabilitation of the psychiatric patient

Until a few years ago, little thought was given to the need for rehabilitating mentally ill persons. Failure to provide adequate programs of rehabilitation was due, in part at least, to the attitude of hopelessness that was inherent in the national philosophy regarding mental illness. For decades the common attitude toward someone who had been hospitalized because of a psychiatric problem was one of pity, horror, disbelief, and pessimism. It was accepted as a fact by many people that hospitalization for a psychiatric problem meant that the patient was permanently disabled and that there was almost no hope that he might eventually return to his family and his job. Relatives usually felt that psychiatric hospitalization was a disgrace and a blot on the family honor. The fact of hospitalization for mental illness was kept secret even from close friends. As a result of such a negative attitude and the usual belief that mental illness was a hopeless problem, the public saw little reason to spend time, money, and effort in trying to restore formerly mentally ill persons to higher levels of social and economic responsibility.

Some nations in the world have been able to cope with the problem of mental illness in a more positive fashion. The community of Gheel, Belgium, has been famous for more than a century because of the universal acceptance of mentally ill patients by its residents. In that small town, generations of citizens have housed and cared for psychiatric patients as guests in their homes. Patients are free to come and go on the streets of Gheel without arousing unusual fears among the towns-people, even when their behavior is bizarre. Such a positive, accepting attitude toward mental illness is unique and has not been duplicated in the United States, although some attempts have been made to establish something like it in a few communities. Traverse City, Michigan, is one community in which a substantial beginning has been made in initiating a plan of home care for mentally ill patients. However, nowhere in the United States have the residents been able to achieve communitywide acceptance of mentally ill persons as have the residents in Gheel, Belgium. In one large Eastern city, social workers made at least one thousand telephone calls to individuals who had been suggested as persons who might be interested in participating in a program of home care for convalescing psychiatric patients. As a result of this effort, they were able to place only two patients in homes in the community.

The casualties from World War II focused the nation's attention upon the need for rehabilitating the physically handicapped. At the same time, the need to restore men who had been psychiatric casualties to the status of contributing members of society was recognized. This more positive approach toward persons who had been mentally ill and toward their need for rehabilitation came partially as a result of the comparatively high percentage of members of the armed forces who were psychiatric casualties. During and immediately following World War II popular magazines carried innumerable articles about mental illness. As a result of the nation's awareness of mental illness as a serious health problem, the national government passed the Mental Health Act in 1946. This law provided financial aid for the education of psychiatrists, psychiatric nurses, psychologists, and psychiatric social workers in the hope that a more adequate supply of such professional workers would improve the therapeutic services available to patients requiring psychiatric care. During the last two decades a beginning has been made in focusing national attention upon developing methods for preventing the occurrence of mental illness among the nation's population. Although there is much yet to be done before the prevention and treatment of mental illness is completely effective, there are reasons to hope that eventually the ever increasing numbers of hospital admissions for mental illness can be halted.

In 1955 the census of hospitalized psychiatrically ill patients in this country dropped for the first time. To be sure, the drop in the total census was not great, but this was an optimistic sign. Among other things, this points to the apparent therapeutic effects of a group of drugs introduced in the early 1950's that have become widely used in the treatment of mental illness. These drugs are popularly known as tranquilizing drugs. These drugs and their derivatives are often effective in relieving anxiety, tension, apprehension, agitation, and hyperactivity without at the same time causing the patient to suffer from a loss of mental alertness. Although the tranquilizing drugs do not remove the underlying causes of emotional disturbance, they do make it possible for many emotionally ill people to remain in the community rather than being hospitalized. Thus it has become necessary for

communities across the nation to become much more concerned with the problem of rehabilitation of the mentally ill person than they were before 1950. Professional workers are trying to develop a program of rehabilitation that will make it possible for a patient to remain in the community after he has been discharged from a psychiatric hospital, since unfortunately, the readmission rate of these discharged patients has been very high. To be successful, such a community program must include the following features: (1) improvement of the treatment approach made by the community agencies that treat patients who are mentally ill; (2) improvement of the social climate and attitudes of acceptance in the community to which the patient returns; (3) education and orientation of the family members to the needs of the recuperating patient; (4) provision for professional supervision of the patient who is living in the community; (5) provision of professional consultation services for the patient's family and for his employer; and (6) provision of compatible employment opportunities in the community.

Contribution of psychiatric hospitals to rehabilitation

The aim of the total treatment program that has been developed in psychiatric hospitals is the ultimate restoration of mentally ill persons to an acceptable level of social and economic responsibility in the community. Even when this goal is not accomplished, the fact still remains that rehabilitation of patients is the objective toward which the hospital staff works.

Hospitalization for mental illness is usually sought only after the patient has become seriously handicapped by emotional problems and can no longer achieve an acceptable social and work adjustment. Inability to maintain an acceptable adjustment may be the result of a profound personality disorder and may involve every aspect of realistic living, or it may involve only certain aspects of life.

The hospital staff begins immediately to help the patient accept the realities of living. To this end, he is encouraged to dress appropriately, to maintain an acceptable level of personal cleanliness, to sleep and eat at regular intervals and in adequate amounts, and to participate in activities designed to help him resume social and occupational activities. The social worker and the psychiatrist work with the family and the patient in an attempt to develop an understanding of him as a unique person with emotional problems and needs. The psychologist carries out a testing program, the results of which help the treatment team in understanding the factors in the patient's emotional life that produce his psychiatric problems. The nurse works toward developing a therapeutic ward environment that will contribute toward his total rehabilitation.

When some understanding of the patient as an individual has been gained, some type of treatment is initiated by the psychiatrist in an attempt to help the patient cope with his emotional problems. Special occupational therapy activities are made available in the hope of maintaining the patient's interest in accomplishing something positive with his talents or creating an interest in new activities.

As soon as the patient is well enough,

if his relationships with his family are at all positive, he is encouraged to spend a few hours at home. As the patient improves, the time spent away from the hospital is lengthened. If family relationships are such that they contribute to the patient's emotional welfare, the family is encouraged to visit the patient, to take him home for holidays and weekends, and to plan for his ultimate homecoming. If possible, the patient's interests and ties with his family and community are encouraged and strengthened.

Before the patient leaves the hospital, plans are usually made for his reemployment in his original job, if this is practical and emotionally acceptable to the patient. If returning to his old job is not possible, then he is encouraged to participate in a program of vocational guidance and training so that he can find suitable employment.

Plans for living away from the hospital are made with the patient by the hospital staff. Sometimes the patient does not feel able to return to the old living situation, which may have been a contributing factor in causing his emotional illness. The appropriate members of the hospital staff work with the patient in an attempt to help him come to some acceptable decisions about the social and personal problems that may have been operating to produce his illness. Plans made for living away from the hospital have as their objective assisting the patient to establish a more emotionally mature and satisfying life.

When the mentally ill patient is well enough to be discharged from the hospital, the professional staff will have tried and had some degree of success in helping him to recognize his emotional problems and find acceptable solutions for those that have been most upsetting. They will have attempted to help him find solutions to, or acceptable substitutes for, his social problems. They will have usually planned with him concerning his future work activities and frequently will have made some provision for the future, in terms of his receiving emotional support through a sustained relationship with some member of the treatment team at the hospital or in an aftercare clinic. Thus the patient is usually well along the road toward being rehabilitated by the time he leaves the modern, well-staffed psychiatric hospital.

Rehabilitation through hospitalization
Case report

Helen was a beautiful, petite, blonde, 17-year-old adolescent when she was admitted to a psychiatric hospital. Her parents had sought admission for their youngest and most beautiful child because she was completely incorrigible. They were chiefly concerned about her sexual behavior, which they feared would bring disgrace upon the entire family, who were very religious and highly thought of in the community. In addition, the parents complained about Helen's excessive drinking, her failing grades in high school, and the exorbitant amounts of money she spent on clothes. She seemed to be entirely self-centered and to care nothing about the effect of her behavior upon her family.

Helen came to the hospital with thirty pairs of shoes, twenty blouses, seventeen skirts, a suitcase full of lovely underwear, and several coats, suits, hats, and purses. Although she was allowed to wear her own clothing in the hospital, there was not room enough for a patient to keep so much. Because of the lack of closet space, the admitting nurse asked Helen to keep several outfits she liked most and to send the rest of the things home with her parents. Although this was a reasonable request, Helen showed her disapproval by reacting with a temper tantrum. She screamed at the nurse, threw things about the room, and refused to give up any of her possessions.

In the hospital, Helen spent hours primping and making herself more beautiful. She wore her lovely blonde hair long and loose about her shoulders and spent much time combing and brushing it. She accepted directions and suggestions from the younger nurses but was sarcastic and hostile toward the more mature and motherly nurses. Toward the psychiatrist to whom she was assigned, Helen was coy and seductive and told everyone that she was going to marry him. At first Helen was somewhat aloof and condescending toward the other patients, but eventually she became the leader of a group of young women who sat together comparing their experiences with young men and discussing their doctors. Helen was always able to tell the most startling story of the evening and was respected by the clique because of her vast amount of experience.

At hospital parties and dances, Helen was so seductive that many of the men were reluctant to dance with her, although she was usually the prettiest girl at the party and the best dancer. Some of the young men were heard to say that they hated her. During refreshment period she liked to sit on the floor at the feet of some young man with her head resting on his knee. She would often look up at him and say, "I'm in love with you. What are you going to do about it?"

The social worker and psychiatrist began a systematic search for the factors in Helen's life that would explain the behavior with which they were trying to deal.

They found, through interviews with members of her family, that she came from a long line of orthodox ministers. In fact, her grandfather and great-grandfather had been leaders of their religious groups in Europe. Her father, born and well-educated in Europe, was the religious leader of a church community in a large eastern city. Her mother, born and educated in Europe, was the daughter of a minister. Helen was the youngest of a family of six children, all of whom were many years older than she. Two of her brothers were ministers in the same eastern city where her father lived. Two sisters were married to ministers.

Helen did not look like any member of her family. Her parents often told her that the way she acted and looked made them wonder if she was really their child. From Helen's earliest memory she was constantly reminded of the fact that she did not look like the rest of the family. Sometimes the family joked about where she could have come from. Helen was required to behave perfectly because she was setting an example for the other little girls in her father's congregation. Consequently, she was always dressed conservatively and was not allowed to do many of the things that her playmates did because her parents felt that it was not becoming for a minister's daughter to act like other children.

Helen was expected to be an excellent student because she came from a family all of whom traditionally achieved honors in academic pursuits. Her psychological tests revealed the fact that she was very bright, but that she did not utilize her intellectual endowments fully. The psychologists also reported that she was a person who did a great deal of phantasizing about running away and setting up her own home in a distant city.

It was obvious that Helen was in a complete state of rebellion against all the members of her family except one unmarried sister was had alway been sympathetic toward her. Consequently, the psychiatrist and the social worker decided to try to help Helen by working with this sister. They asked the other members of the family not to visit Helen be-

cause her symptoms seemed to be exaggerated by their visits.

As the psychiatrist learned to know Helen better, he found that almost all her behavior was designed to embarrass and punish her family. Since she could not control her family in any other way, she sought to do it by acting out her anger against them. Therefore she drank excessively, spent their money recklessly, deliberately failed at school, and dressed seductively. She had almost a compulsive desire to date men who would be particularly distasteful to her parents. Consequently, she picked up poorly dressed boys on the street. One of Helen's greatest problems was her fear of not belonging to her family. She felt that she was not loved because she did not really belong to them.

Helen's rehabilitation began as soon as she reached the hospital because all the family pressures were removed. She no longer contacted her parents and was visited only by a sister. When she began to spend weekends away from the hospital, she stayed with friends or her single sister.

The psychiatrist encouraged Helen to attend school very soon after she came to the hospital. At first she went to the special school held in the hospital, but as soon as possible she was enrolled in a nearby public high school.

The psychiatrist worked with Helen in an attempt to help her understand why she needed to behave in such socially unacceptable ways and to help her see how much more acceptable she would be to people if she behaved in ways more easily understood by them. He explored with her the reasons for her sexual promiscuity and found that unconsciously Helen felt that a woman could get approval and love from men only through seductive behavior. The psychiatrist worked constantly to help Helen feel that he accepted her and cared about her, even though he could not always accept her behavior.

The nurses refrained from censoring Helen

no matter how much makeup she used or how frequently she exhibited temper tantrums. They gave her as many choices as possible in her daily living activities and praised her when she looked especially attractive or was helpful about the ward. Eventually, Helen was able to accept one older, motherly nurse. She began to talk in a straightforward manner to her psychiatrist about her poblems and was able to give up her seductive behavior toward him.

Helen graduated from high school while living at the hospital and, through the help and guidance of the vocational rehabilitation center in the city, decided that her abilities could best be used in the capacity of a stenographer. While living at the hospital, she completed a nine-month course in secretarial training and was able to find a job as an office manager. This job required a great deal of Helen. She frequently returned to the hospital in a state of panic. She confided her fears to the nurse on duty. She often said, "I can't do this job. It is too hard for me. I am a sick girl. How can they expect me to earn my own living?"

With the support of the nurse, the psychiatrist, and the social worker, Helen was able to hold her job, although she frequently said in the evening that she could not go back the next day. During this period of stress, the psychiatrist prescribed one of the tranquilizing drugs for her and talked with her almost every evening.

During the period of adjusting to the job, Helen became involved with a young man she met on the street and began to fear that she was pregnant. Some days she refused to go to work and lay on her bed and screamed and cried. When her fears were proved to be false, the psychiatrist helped her to see that this was an unconscious attempt to remain within the protective environment of the hospital. He then began to suggest that she needed to think about finding a place to live outside the hospital. This was a very threatening idea to Helen. She was more upset than ever when she returned from work in the evening. Helen sometimes stood at the door of the nurse's station trembling and pleading for a sedative. Once or twice she collapsed on the floor to demonstrate how weak and sick she was. She said repeatedly, "How can they ask someone who is so sick to live by herself away from the hospital?"

After a few weeks the social worker located a room in the city in a girls' club where Helen might live away from the hospital but still be in a relatively protected environment. At first Helen refused to go with the social worker to look at the room, but after a few days she made the necessary trip. Helen wept every evening for a week, but she was finally able to accept the idea of living away from the hospital. When the social worker helped her into the taxi with her bags, Helen was able to tell her hospital friends good-bye without tears. She had been in the hospital almost two years.

Her doctor continued to see her twice a week for almost a year after she went to live in the girls' club. Eventually Helen married a young man of her family's religion and racial heritage.

Helen's rehabilitation was a long and difficult one for her, and for the hospital staff. Her future mental health depends to a great extent upon the maturity of the man she married and the insight and understanding she gained while being treated in the hospital.

Influence of community attitudes on rehabilitation

The most important factors confronting a convalescing psychiatric patient who seeks to reestablish himself as a contributing member of the community are the attitudes with which his family, friends, and former employer greet him. If the family considers the discharged patient a burden, a disgrace, and a liability, his adjustment to the community is likely to be seriously jeopardized. If employment is denied him on the basis of his previous mental illness, his chances for remaining in the community as a contributing citizen are very limited. If his friends shun him and if he feels unwanted, his return to the accepting care of the psychiatric hospital is practically assured. Therefore it is essential that members of the staffs of psychiatric hospitals work closely with families, employers, and staffs of other community agencies in planning for the patient's return to the community.

Altering community attitudes toward persons who have been psychiatric casualties or who have received psychiatric help requires a vigorous and continuous educational campaign on the part of every agency that is interested in human welfare. Recently a good deal of national effort has been directed toward changing attitudes in the direction of more acceptance for people who find themselves in need of psychiatric help. Some evidence of positive change is apparent, but changing of attitudes is probably the most difficult part of our national effort to help mentally ill persons.

Role of the public health nurse in rehabilitating the patient

The public health nurse has become increasingly involved in the rehabilitation of psychiatric patients since the introduction of the tranquilizing drugs and the resulting discharge of hundreds of patients who continue to require professional supervision. The public health nurse is frequently the key professional person who helps the family develop an understanding and acceptance of the patient so that the postdischarge period will be a constructive part of the entire rehabilitation process. Families may be afraid to accept the hospitalized member back in the home because they remember how difficult his sick behavior was for them to handle. They may feel guilty and ashamed because they placed the patient in the hospital. Some families have utilized the patient's living space for some other individual and may require help in finding enough room for him. The public health nurse can be of inestimable assistance to a family group who are anticipating the return of a discharged member. She can assist the family to make realistic plans for the future. After the patient resumes his place in the home, her visits provide an opportunity for the family to ventilate their concerns about new problems the patient's behavior may precipitate and new needs they have identified.

As the public health nurse visits the family, she will be able to evaluate the adjustment the patient is making and will report her findings to the appropriate physician or clinic. She can encourage the patient to continue taking the medication prescribed by the hospital physician or encourage the patient to visit the clinic if a reevaluation of the effectiveness of the prescribed drug appears indicated. She will also offer valuable assistance in supporting the family and helping them to recognize the progress the returning member is making. If the patient is having a difficult time in adjusting to his family and the community, the public health nurse can help him and his family make the decision that he should reenter the hospital if such a step is indicated. Today, public health nurses need to be as skilled in meeting the needs of the psychiatric patient and his family as they are in meeting the needs of other patients who require assistance with health problems.

The public health nurse is usually aware of the agencies in the community that offer help to families and can assist them in contacting appropriate agencies when additional services are required.

Need of families for help in understanding their role in rehabilitation

One of the frequent fears from which mentally ill patients suffer is a feeling of not belonging and of not being wanted. Unfortunately, in some family situations very little love and acceptance have been available, and patients may actually not be wanted by their families. Some people who suffer from such negative family relationships have been able to find the love they need in various ways, such as by establishing families of their own or through cultivating friends. A few individuals are never able to find a way to fill this human need. These lonely, unloved people frequently find adjustment to life situations difficult and sometimes impossible. Such poorly adjusted individuals may become psychiatric casualties if the pressures of life become severe. One of the approaches a psychiatric treatment situation seeks to make in helping such a person is to offer him warmth, acceptance, and friendship. It is obvious that it would be a serious mistake for a person to leave the psychiatric hospital and return

to a rejecting, hostile, unloving family.

Families that are able to provide an atmosphere of warmth, love, and acceptance are a significant factor in supporting a convalescing mentally ill patient through the trying period of rehabilitation. These positive attitudes may need to be encouraged and developed in the family before the convalescing patient returns to the family situation.

Families need help in understanding and accepting an emotionally ill member who is returning after an experience in a psychiatric treatment center. Families need help in learning what to say, how to act, and what to avoid when dealing with the emotionally ill or convalescing member. Families need reassurance and guidance. They need an objective, professional person with whom they can discuss the many fancied or real problems a mentally ill member presents. Some family situations are in such turmoil and filled with so many problems that the convalescing member would not be helped by returning to the home. If the patient is to be helped to accept the role of a self-directing, contributing member of a community, his family frequently needs almost as much help as he does.

Because families are so important in supporting the patient during the period of rehabilitation and because families need so much help, there is need for psychiatric social workers or public health nurses with psychiatric preparation to work continuously over a period of time with families. These workers can help the family to prepare the way so that the homecoming will be a therapeutic experience rather than a traumatizing one. Sometimes social workers may need to help the patient avoid a traumatizing family situation by planning with him and his physician for a substitute living arrangement. Such arrangements may be a foster home or a room in a club or some other suitable place. Communities need to provide a variety of substitute homes for mentally ill patients who are ready to return to the community but who for a variety of reasons cannot live with their families.

Contribution of aftercare clinics to rehabilitation

Support and guidance may be provided for the newly discharged patient by some type of aftercare clinic that he may attend whenever he feels the need for help. In such a clinic the patient may see the same physician with whom he was acquainted in the hospital. This carry-over of professional help is in itself a reassuring experience.

In rehabilitating a mentally ill patient, some type of follow-up care after hospitalization is usually essential. Clinic care usually becomes less necessary as time goes on and the recovering patient is able to make an increasingly effective adjustment. The patient feels reassured when he realizes that the security of the clinic is always available to him and that the greater security of the hospital is available if the pressures of living become too great.

Contribution of day care hospitals and comprehensive community mental health centers to rehabilitation

This discussion of the rehabilitation of patients suffering from mental illness has until now been focused upon the patient who has been discharged from a psychiatric treatment hospital. There are probably more individuals living in the community who are in need of psychiatric help than there are patients in the psychiatric hospitals which serve that community. Until recently, most communities made no medical provision for the individual who was in need of psychiatric help but who did not require hospital admission. Sometimes a community may have been fortunate enough to have a few private psychiatrists to whom such emotionally ill persons might turn for help. However, private psychiatric help has always been so expensive that many citizens could not afford it, and many communities have had no psychiatric help available.

Today, the comprehensive community mental health center is becoming a well-accepted part of many community health programs. These centers offer treatment services to individuals who are able to live at home and receive the help they require. Such agencies are usually staffed with psychiatrists, psychiatric social workers, nurses, and psychologists. Group therapy is available for patients needing this type of treatment. Help for families who need assistance in understanding and accepting their emotionally ill member is available through the services of psychiatric social workers. Marriage counseling and help in understanding and handling family problems may be a part of the service. Such community mental health centers make it possible for families to remain intact while one member receives treatment for an emotional problem. The comprehensive community mental health center has become an essential part of

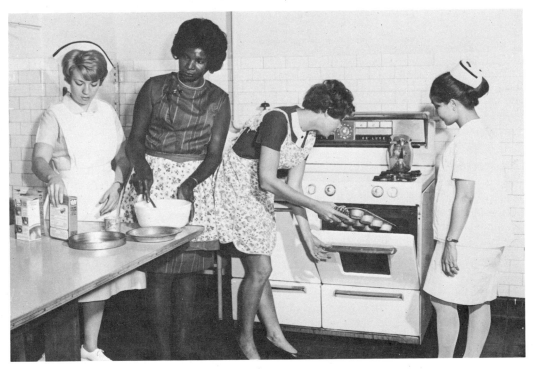

FIG. 20. *Rehabilitation for emotionally ill women includes helping them accept the role of homemaker.*

adequate community health services. The vocational rehabilitation center usually works closely with the comprehensive mental health center in offering professional assistance to members of the community who need help in making a more adequate work adjustment.

Another relatively new approach to the rehabilitation of mentally ill persons is the day care hospital. Such an institution treats mentally ill patients during the day. It opens about 9 A.M., closes late in the afternoon, and offers patients all the treatments and therapies available in any psychiatric hospital. Thus patients may receive electric shock, drug therapy, individual psychotherapy, or group therapy. They may participate in occupational and recreational therapy. In a day care hospital the patient usually takes the evening meal with his family and spends the night at home. This plan serves to keep the family intact, capitalizes upon the therapeutic aspects of family living, and avoids the stigma of hospitalization. Social workers are available to help the families accept their role in helping the patient. Not all mentally ill patients can profit from an experience in a day care hospital. Not all home situations have a therapeutic potential. Day care hospitals can be of real service to some patients and can make it possible for some patients to avoid the traumatic experience of breaking completely with family and community life. Day care hospitals are much less costly than the traditional psychiatric hospital and are becoming increasingly popular.

There have been many variations of the day care hospital as communities have sought to meet the unique needs of individuals. Some day care hospitals have a census of patients who spend 8 hours in the hospital from nine in the morning until five in the evening and a different census of patients who spend the late evening and night hours at the hospital. This arrangement meets the needs of a group of patients who are usually able to cope with a job situation and perhaps to spend part of the evening at home. However, they may be too emotionally fragile to completely bridge the gap between the relatively protective climate of the psychiatric hospital and the emotionally demanding life in the community. They still need the security that comes from spending the late evening and night in a protected environment.

Contribution of social clubs to rehabilitation

Patients may sucessfully achieve discharge from the psychiatric hospital and gain some measure of success in a job without making a satisfactory social adjustment. Many people who have found it necessary to seek psychiatric help have been characteristically shy and ill at ease in social situations throughout their entire lives and continue to make this kind of adjustment after discharge from the hospital. Other patients make a marginal adjustment at home and at work but spend their evenings in solitary activity. Many of these discharged patients struggle to interact socially with others and sometimes express feelings of loneliness and defeat when they are not socially successful. Because of these realistic social needs of psychiatric patients, social clubs composed of these patients have sprung up in several of the major cities in the United States. It is understandable that many of these people can feel comfortable

and accepted only by other discharged patients. It is not unusual for patients to make close friends among fellow patients while in the hospital and to comment that they have never been able to make friends before. It appears to be logical and often therapeutic for groups of patients who have been congenial and mutually supportive while in the hospital to seek to continue this relationship after discharge.

Authorities disagree as to the value of social clubs formed entirely of discharged psychiatric patients. Some psychiatrists take the position that such social groups are natural and meet a specific unmet need. Others believe that discharged patients should be assisted and required to seek social activities among groups of people who have not necessarily shared a psychiatric hospitalization. Because of these divergent views, all social clubs formed by discharged patients have not gained official sanction. However, their existence probably suggests that families and communities need to be aware of the unmet social needs of discharged psychiatric patients and should make some provision to meet these needs. Certainly the postdischarge period in the patient's life is crucial and should receive much more consideration and thoughtful planning than it has had to date.

Vocational guidance centers aid in rehabilitation

Many communities now provide vocational rehabilitation centers that offer guidance to individuals who are returning to the community from an experience as a patient. Some persons who have been emotionally ill are able to make a marginal adjustment in the community by living at home, if they are not required to take on the additional pressures of a job. Most people, however, become discouraged if they are not able to find work. Performing successfully in a work situation is an ego-strengthening experience.

Because rehabilitation experts have recognized the therapeutic aspects of performing successfully in a work situation and the emotional significance of being able to earn a living, vocational guidance centers have been established to help handicapped persons achieve success in some kind of work.

Vocational guidance centers usually offer a testing service to help the individual identify the areas of his highest aptitudes and greatest abilities. They frequently provide an opportunity for convalescing patients to receive training to equip them to perform the specific work for which they seem best fitted. In addition, these centers usually help their clients find jobs after their period of training has been completed. Staffs from psychiatric hospitals need to work closely with vocational rehabilitation centers to provide discharged patients with the help they may need in becoming economically independent members of the community.

From the standpoint of job placement, one of the most serious problems facing the vocational guidance center is the community attitude toward the former psychiatric patient. Although attitudes vary from community to community, it is safe to say that many employers are reluctant to accept discharged psychiatric patients as employees. For many years the Veterans Administration has been actively working on developing more acceptance of dis-

charged veterans as employees and has achieved some success. The problem requires persistent, intelligent, and long-term community education on the part of skillful professional workers. Even today, in many sections of this country it is not wise for discharged psychiatric patients to divulge information concerning their emotional health record to potential employers if they hope to be considered for a position. This situation is unfortunate because such withholding of information has implications concerning the patient's emotional security as well as his future job security.

The sheltered workshop

Some persons who have been emotionally ill are able and willing to work but are not stable enough to withstand the pressures and competition of the usual job. For such individuals, the sheltered workshop may be the answer. Such a work situation pays slightly less than the same position in general industry, but less pressure is placed upon the worker and more understanding and acceptance of him as an individual is offered. Sheltered workshops are an essential part of a community program of rehabilitation for mentally ill persons. If such sheltered working situations are available, many convalescing patients who have been mentally ill can have the therapeutic experience of being economically independent.

The role of religion in rehabilitation

Today, clergy representing all faiths in this country have developed an awareness of the need of many emotionally ill persons for spiritual help and guidance. More and more frequently pastoral counseling is being included as a part of the preparation with which a young clergyman is equipped before he leaves the theological seminary.

Ministers, priests, and rabbis are striving to develop an understanding of the manifestations of emotional illness and to learn how they may increase their effectiveness in helping emotionally disturbed persons who seek their help.

The weekly programs of most modern churches offer many favorable circumstances for lonely persons to find companionship and the opportunities for socialization so essential to good mental health. This is an especially important factor in large modern urban areas where family ties may be tenuous and often nonexistent. Church groups sometimes offer the individual who is convalescing from an emotional illness the only real warmth and acceptance he finds in the community.

A renewal or strengthening of religious faith may be the ingredient in life that enables the convalescing psychiatric patient to find the courage to face the reality of problems of living and to work toward solving these problems. Because of the significance of a religious faith in restoring mental health there has been a renewed emphasis upon religion in the lives of hospitalized patients during the last decade. Modern psychiatric hospitals now make available to all patients the services of rabbis, ministers, and priests. Church services are now included in the activities of all modern psychiatric hospitals. Community churches are frequently utilized as an integral part of the community resources for the rehabilitation of emotion-ally ill persons. Some research concerning the role of religion in the maintenance of mental health and the prevention and treatment of emotional illness has been carried on. Many psychiatrists and members of the clergy of various faiths are working together in a team relationship, recognizing that each group can profit from the knowledge and skills of the other and that humanity will be significantly benefited by this collaborative effort. This trend toward coordination of efforts by the clergy and by psychiatrists is one of the many hopeful signs in the attack that this nation is making upon mental illness, which is presently its largest health problem.

• • •

Many communities are only beginning to develop facilities for rehabilitating patients who have experienced mental illness. More study and research are required in this area of human need to improve these services and to discover better and more effective ways of accomplishing the goals of rehabilitation.

IMPORTANT CONCEPTS

1. The objective of hospitalization is to restore the patient to the fullest possible level of normal living within the limitations of his emotional handicaps.
2. Hospitalization can be a positive learning experience in human relations.
3. Successful rehabilitation of the mentally ill patient is a matter of teamwork on the part of many professional persons.

4. The public health nurse is frequently the key professional person who helps the family develop an understanding and acceptance of the patient so that the postdischarge period will be a constructive part of the entire rehabilitation process.
5. A successful community program for rehabilitating mentally ill patients requires the following:
   a. Improvement of the treatment agencies
   b. Improvement of the social climate and attitudes of acceptance toward discharged patients
   c. Education and orientation of family members to the needs of the recuperating patient
   d. Provision of professional consultation services for the patient's family and his employer
   e. Provision of professional supervision for the discharged patient
   f. Provision of compatible employment opportunities
6. The mentally ill patient is usually well along the road toward being rehabilitated by the time he leaves the modern well-staffed psychiatric hospital.

7. Attitudes of his family, friends, and former employer are some of the most important factors with which the convalescing psychiatric patient is confronted when he attempts to reestablish himself as a contributing member of the community.
8. Communities need to provide a variety of substitute homes for mentally ill patients who are ready to return to the community but who for a variety of reasons cannot return to their own family.
9. Because of the therapeutic significance of successful performance in a work situation, vocational guidance centers have been established in many communities to help handicapped persons achieve success in some type of work.
10. During the last decade there has been a renewed emphasis upon religion in helping to rehabilitate psychiatrically ill patients.
11. The rehabilitation of any individual depends on finding answers to these three fundamental human needs: (a) somewhere to live, (b) some work to do, and (c) someone to care.

SUGGESTED SOURCES OF ADDITIONAL INFORMATION

Burling, Temple: The vocational rehabilitation of the mentally handicapped, Amer. J. Orthopsychiat. 20:202-207, 1950.

Davis, John E.: An introduction to the problems of rehabilitation, Ment. Hyg. 29:217-230, 1945.

Davis, John E.: Rehabilitation, its principles and practice, New York, 1946, A. S. Barnes & Co., Inc.

Fisher, Saul H.: The recovered patient returns to the community, Ment. Hyg. 42:463-473, 1958.

Hartigan, Helen: Nursing responsibilities in rehabilitation, Nurs. Outlook 2:649-651, Dec., 1954.

Hunt, Robert C.: Ingredients of a rehabilitation program. In Proceedings of the Thirty-Fourth Annual Conference of the Milbank Memorial Fund, part I, New York, 1958, The Milbank Memorial Fund.

Jones, Maxwell: The therapeutic community—a new treatment in psychiatry, New York, 1953, Basic Books, Inc., Publishers.

Mandelbrote, Bertram: Development of a comprehensive psychiatric community service around the mental hospital, Ment. Hyg. 43:368-377, 1959.

Noble, Douglas: The use of therapeutic activities in psychiatry, Amer. J. Occup. Therapy 3:62-68, 1949.

Palmer, Mary B.: Social rehabilitation for mental patients, Ment. Hyg. 42:24-28, 1958.

Rennie, Thomas A. C.: Psychiatric rehabilitation therapy, Amer. J. Psychiat. 101:476-485, 1945.

Rosner, S. Steven: After care services for the mental hospital patient, Ment. Hyg. 44:417-425, 1960.

Stevenson, George S.: Dynamic considerations in community functions, Ment. Hyg. 34:531-546, 1950.

Switzer, Mary E.: Rehabilitation and mental handicaps, Ment. Hyg. 30:390-396, 1946.

The psychiatric nurse in the mental hospital, report of the Committee on Psychiatric Nursing and the Committee on Hospitals of the Group for the Advancement of Psychiatry, Topeka, Kansas, May, 1952.

CHAPTER TWENTY-TWO

Community mental health— a new concept

Community psychiatry is a relatively new and rapidly expanding development in the field of mental health. The basic principles underlying this concept are being put into practical use in centers called comprehensive community mental health centers. Currently, great variations exist among these centers as each one attempts to define the unique needs of its clientele and to develop methods for meeting these needs.

Community psychiatry is said to be one of the three or four revolutionary developments in the field of psychiatry. The first of these was achieved by Pinel in 1793 when he struck off the chains of mentally ill patients who were confined in Bicêtre outside of Paris. The second was the development of the psychoanalytic method of treatment by Freud about a hundred years later. The third is said by some to be the development in the early 1950's of the tranquilizing drugs.

The concept of community psychiatry is not new in the sense that the basic services are new, but it is new in the way these services are being organized and delivered to the people of the community. It requires a total realignment of the roles of the professional workers involved in these centers and a change in their philosophical approach to the prevention of mental illness and the treatment of people in need of emotional and psychological help. The comprehensive community mental health center is organized around a demographic unit with a population small enough to permit the development of comprehensive mental health services. It seeks to serve the people who reside in a specific geographic area of a city or a locality that is referred to as a *catchment* area. The workers in the center attempt to assist individuals who have become mentally ill to maintain their ties with the community and when hospitalization is necessary, to return to community living as soon as possible.

Community psychiatry has developed in response to the realization that much of the effort expended in the past as treatment for mentally ill patients encouraged chronicity rather than a return to the community. Thus the current trend is to treat the patient immediately in his community, no matter what his mental problem may be. In this way it is hoped that the development of chronic symptomatology and the rupturing of community ties through institutionalization can be avoided.

Even when patients require hospitalization, the staff of the comprehensive community mental health center expects the period of institutionalization to be as short as possible, with the patient returning to his home and community during the first two or three weeks for visits. The patient will be treated as an outpatient as soon as possible and will be encouraged to accept a reasonable number of his former responsibilities, including a return to work. Thus the depersonalization effect upon the individual of a large institution will be avoided.

The early return of patients to their homes and to the community makes it essential that all helping agencies share information freely and cooperate effectively.

When fully developed, a comprehensive community mental health center will include inpatient services, outpatient services, and services to make partial hospitalization possible. These partial hospitalization services include facilities for day, night, and weekend care. In addition, the community mental health center is expected to offer services to the community that include consultation to community agencies and professional personnel, diagnostic services, and rehabilitative services including vocational and educational programs. Precare and aftercare community services will also be a part of the program of a comprehensive community mental health center. Precare and aftercare services will include foster home placement, home visiting, and halfway houses. Finally, the community mental health center will provide training for professional and paraprofessional workers, carry on research into the prevention, cause, and treatment of mental illness, and evaluate the effectiveness of the program being carried forward.

Like all other significant changes, the concept of community psychiatry did not spring into being without many smaller changes first contributing to the improvement of the situation for the mentally ill in the United States and Canada.

DEVELOPMENT OF THE COMMUNITY MENTAL HEALTH MOVEMENT

Knowledge of the historical background of the community mental health movement helps us to understand and appreciate it. Some authorities place its earliest beginnings in 1908 when Clifford Beers, a psychiatric patient who was hospitalized several times during an otherwise productive life, published a book entitled *A Mind That Found Itself*. This book about his experiences as a mentally

ill patient provided the impetus for the beginning of the mental health movement in the United States. Child guidance clinics developed and flourished from the early 1920's through the 1930's. A heritage from this era is the staffing pattern of the traditional clinic team, which included a psychiatrist, a psychologist, and a social worker. The nurse was omitted. This oversight probably grew out of the belief that the expertise of the nurse lay solely in caring for the physically ill. Since most children who required help from child guidance clinics were not physically ill, the usefulness of the nurse in such clinics was thought to be limited or nonexistent.

Schools of nursing did not traditionally include mental health or psychiatric nursing in the curriculum until the late 1930's. Thus most physicians and social workers thought of the nurse's work as dealing almost entirely with physical problems. Unfortunately, this attitude continues today to be the firm position of many professional people who represent the three professions traditionally staffing the child guidance clinics.

One of the greatest forward looking actions the nation has ever taken in relation to mental illness was achieved when the National Mental Health Act was passed in 1946. Among other accomplishments it established the National Institute of Mental Health within the Public Health Service of the Department of Health, Education and Welfare. An act was passed about the same time in Canada. It was similar to the National Mental Health Act enacted in the United States and has had a similar effect in moving Canada into the forefront in the field of mental health. Both these acts provided for the financing of research and training programs. Through their enactment the governments expressed their belief that it was necessary to acquire more knowledge concerning the cause, prevention, and treatment of mental illness and that more professionally trained workers were needed to improve the care and treatment of the mentally ill. Financial support for the education of psychologists, psychiatric social workers, psychiatrists, and psychiatric nurses is still available in the United States through the National Mental Health Act.

The National Mental Health Act grew out of the experiences the nation had during World War II when more men in the armed forces were disabled by mental illness than by all actual military action. The hundreds of soldiers who were incapacitated by acute and chronic mental illness alerted the nation to the need for many more trained professional workers in the field, for greater knowledge about the problem, and for greatly improved treatment techniques.

During World War II the psychiatrists in the medical corps, led by Dr. William Menninger, learned the importance of early recognition of psychiatric problems and the significance of initiating treatment rapidly and close to the place where the difficulty occurred. They developed a method of crisis-oriented treatment, which promoted adaptation and an early return to duty. To individuals in decision-making positions, they demonstrated the usefulness of consultation where issues that affected the mental well-being of soldiers were concerned. This knowledge and skill, which was developed

pragmatically in the armed forces, has been incorporated today into the principles of the community mental health movement.

The tranquilizing or ataractic drugs played a large role in the development of community psychiatry. They were first used experimentally in 1953. By 1956 the populations of the state mental hospitals were reported to have fallen slightly, instead of increasing as they had done for decades. This development was largely due to the fact that with the help of the drugs, patients could control their behavior and thus could spend time outside the hospital in the community. Had it not been for these drugs, many patients would never have been able to control their unusual behavior sufficiently to remain at home and thus be available for help away from an institution.

In the late 1940's and the early 1950's, the large public institutions for the care of psychiatric patients began to change significantly through the development of new methods for approaching and understanding patients. Some of these new methods included family diagnosis, the introduction of short- and long-term treatment programs, and the advent of crisis-oriented therapy. At about the same time, several new ideas were introduced into public psychiatric hospitals. Such developments as the therapeutic community concept, which attempted to alter certain segments of larger psychiatric institutions in order to provide patients with an opportunity for achieving a more constructive social adjustment, the concept described as milieu therapy, and the approach known as the open door hospital were introduced and refined. Some of these ideas, especially the open-door hospital and the therapeutic community, came to the United States directly from experimentation carried on in England.

In 1955 the Congress of the United States passed the Mental Health Study Act. This Act provided money for a five-year study of the problem of mental illness in the United States. As a result of the Act, the Joint Commission on Mental Illness was established. On December 31, 1960, this commission submitted its final report to the Congress, to the Surgeon General of the Public Health Service, and to the governors of the fifty states. The published report was entitled *Action for Mental Health* and was available to the public in 1961. It was widely read and provided an impetus for developing more effective services for people in need of psychiatric help and was the basis for additional legislation. Because of its statements concerning the need to develop and utilize the potential therapeutic abilities of all other professional workers in psychiatric settings, in addition to psychiatrists, it added strength to the position that had already been taken by professional nurses who were working in psychiatric situations. Many of these nurses had maintained for several years that the nurse had a legitimate and specific role in providing therapy for patients.

A milestone in the nation's developing awareness of the need for an improved approach to the problems of mental health and illness was reached when on February 5, 1963, President Kennedy delivered his special message to the Congress on mental illness and mental retardation. In this speech he mentioned a few goals: "Central to a new mental health program is comprehensive community care . . . . The mentally ill can achieve . . . a constructive social adjustment . . . . The centers will focus on community resources . . . . Prevention as well as treatment will be a major activity."* In that same year, 1963, the Community Mental Health Centers Construction Act was passed, followed in 1965 by the Staffing Act for the Community Mental Health Centers. These acts made money available to build and staff the centers and were the impetus for the rapid development of many centers in a relatively short period of time.

PHILOSOPHICAL ASSUMPTIONS UNDERLYING THE CONCEPT OF COMMUNITY MENTAL HEALTH

The basic assumption underlying the community mental health movement is that behavior is a function of two sets of variables—the person and the situation. That is, behavior is related both to attributes of the behaving individual and attributes of his environment. Thus the term community mental health has come to represent all mental health activities carried out in a community, and the theoretical formulation has evolved as an alternative to the medical model.†

The medical model successfully used

---

*From Ozarin, Lucy D.: The community mental health center: concept and commitment, Ment. Hyg. **52**:78, 1968.
†Blackman, Sheldon, and Goldstein, Kenneth M.: Some aspects of a theory of community mental health, Community Mental Health J. **4**:86, 1968.

by physicians to identify and treat physically ill individuals was employed for many years by psychiatrists because they were trained as physicians and until recently as neurologists. In dealing with a mentally ill individual, the psychiatrist frequently removed him from the community and prescribed a treatment program designed to correct the sickness that lay within the patient's personality. Even the treatment technique known as psychoanalysis was developed out of Freud's experiences, some of which he had as a neurologist. Psychoanalysis seeks to help the patient to identify his own interpersonal or intrapsychic problems and to make appropriate changes through developing self-understanding and insight.

As social science research has developed and grown in importance, it has become increasingly evident that mental health problems are intimately related to the environment and that there are many environmental factors that may contribute to the mental health or mental illness of an individual. Thus there has been a growing dissatisfaction with the medical model or the idea that mental illness is inherent within the personality of the individual. As dissatisfactions grew, attempts have been made to develop a theoretical model to replace the medical model that has been in use so long.

Thus the theoretical formulations underlying the current movement in community psychiatry were developed. They deal with the belief that much deviant behavior is learned behavior and develops in response to a negative environmental situation that reinforces and encourages the development of deviance. It follows that if a type of behavior is learned it can be unlearned or that a more socially acceptable type of behavior can be substituted. It also follows that if deviant behavior develops in relation to environmental influences, as much social science research has demonstrated, the environment should be the focus of the attention of professional workers who seek to alter the situation in a positive direction. Social scientists have come to recognize that inadequate, overcrowded housing, poor or nonexistent community recreation facilities, unemployment, poverty, broken homes, and poor schools are all factors that contribute to high rates of mental illness among the population in some communities. One approach to preventing mental illness in individuals living in a community is to improve the conditions existing in the community. Thus community psychiatry not only focuses upon the individual and his family but upon the community itself.

CHARACTERISTICS OF A COMPREHENSIVE COMMUNITY MENTAL HEALTH CENTER

Specific requirements for a fully developed comprehensive community mental health center have been identified in the law that makes government funding available. These requirements have been recorded in an earlier portion of this chapter. Although inpatient services, outpatient services, and partial hospitalization must be made available, the government expects individual communities to identify which services will be developed first, which will be emphasized most, and what the specific focus of the clinic will be.

The need for suicide prevention and

crisis clinics was identified early in the development of some mental health services in some communities, whereas other communities concentrated on the development of day care and night care centers. Thus each comprehensive community mental health center developed differently, depending upon the needs of the community it served, the philosophy of the professionals involved in the development of the services, and the relationship the community had with the center.

In spite of many differences there are some significant similarities in comprehensive community mental health centers. There are also departures from the more traditional approach to the treatment of psychiatric problems. Some of these departures from the traditional psychiatric treatment approach include the following:

1. The treatment modality is focused upon helping the patient through the use of groups of which he is a member rather than by relying therapeutically upon the use of the individual one-to-one relationship. Thus the treatment focus is upon family therapy, group therapy, the therapeutic community, and crisis intervention. The development of knowledge and skill in the use of the group process is essential for all professional workers who hope to be involved in working therapeutically with comprehensive community mental health centers.

2. The services of individuals who are already working with the larger population of the catchment area are utilized. These individuals may include welfare workers, police, clergy, teachers, public health nurses, and other community leaders. Some community mental health centers have involved individuals identified as indigenous workers. These are people who may lack formal education but who have lived in the community and understand the unofficial community organization. They are aware of the real hopes, interests, and concerns of the people. In addition, they speak and understand the language commonly used by the people being served. With professional guidance the indigenous workers have been surprisingly successful in some community mental health centers because of their ability to understand the people seeking help and to offer it to them on a level that is acceptable and useful.

3. Role definitions are becoming blurred as the various representatives of the professional disciplines work in the interdisciplinary climate of the comprehensive community mental health centers. All disciplines share treatment responsibilities in these centers. The leadership of the clinic team may be held by any one of the members of the team, depending upon the background, experience, interests, and abilities of the individual team members. Group or family therapy may be carried on by the nurse as a therapist or as a cotherapist with some other member of the professional team. Thus the nurse who looks forward to working in a comprehensive community mental health center needs to think in terms of seeking additional preparation in individual and group therapy before undertaking such responsibility.

4. Prevention is a major focus in the new mental health centers. Thus consultation and educational activities become as important in the centers as treatment.

Many of the professional workers spend more time in the consultation and educational aspects of their work than in the treatment aspects. They seek to help mothers of children, school teachers, public health nurses, workers in the juvenile courts, and individuals employed in social agencies to understand the concepts of mental health and the contribution they can make in the areas of prevention of mental illness and the promotion of mental health among the groups with whom they deal.

5. Planned social change is another focus of the comprehensive community mental health centers. Professional workers are concerned not only with the individuals who seek help but also with the community itself, which is the incubator, in a sense of the word, of the mental health problems from which the population suffers. Thus the professional staff of the community mental health center works to improve the social systems that serve the population within the community, that is, the family, the churches, the schools, the hospitals, recreational facilities, the court system, housing, local government, industry, and so on.

6. Comprehensive and continuous service to the patient is emphasized in the community mental health centers. The patient is seen immediately when he feels that he is in need of help. No longer are individuals asked to wait for weeks or months for an appointment. Some clinics are called crisis clinics. Others are referred to as trouble clinics to emphasize the fact that they are available to anyone who feels that he is in some kind of urgent difficulty or trouble. Many of these clinics have a psychiatrist available

around the clock. Cooperation among agencies is basic if these centers are to offer a comprehensive program that can deal with the range of mental problems that arise in any community.

7. Research into the cause and treatment of mental illness is a part of every well-developed community mental health center.

ROLE OF THE NURSE IN THE COMPREHENSIVE COMMUNITY MENTAL HEALTH CENTERS

As has been stated, the role definitions of the professional workers in the community mental health centers are becoming blurred as each worker is free to utilize the knowledge and skill that he brings to the situation or that he has developed in the course of his experience at the center.

Many nurses who work in community mental health centers are involved in carrying on a variety of therapeutic activities that focus upon group and family therapy and mental health consultation. Because nurses have had more experience with home visiting than many other professional workers, there are some activities through which the nurse can make a unique contribution. One of these is helping the patient's family as they prepare to welcome him back into the home after a period of hospitalization in a psychiatric facility. Another contribution is working with the family and the patient after his return in order to assist with the adjustment period. This work might involve the supervision of the patient in the continuation of his medications, assisting the patient in his adjustment to the family, and helping to prevent his return to the hospital. Another type of home visiting that the nurse has done and that has been beneficial is the initial visit to the family after the patient has been referred to the center for help. Through this visit the nurse is able to evaluate the situation, relay this information to the treatment team, and initiate whatever therapeutic intervention is indicated in relation to the social situation.

The community mental health center provides the professionally prepared nurse with an unusual opportunity to fill an expanding therapeutic role. In no other clinical situation does the nurse have so many opportunities to utilize her professional potential to achieve the maximum therapeutic benefit for the patient, his family, and the community.

IMPORTANT CONCEPTS

1. The basic principles underlying the concept of community psychiatry are being utilized in comprehensive community mental health centers.
2. Community psychiatry requires a total realignment of the roles of the professional workers who are involved and a change in their philosophical approach to the prevention of mental illness and the treatment of mentally ill people.
3. The comprehensive community mental health center attempts to treat mentally ill patients while helping them to maintain their ties with the community.
4. The comprehensive community mental health center hopes to avoid the depersonalization effect that a large

institution has upon an individual.
5. When fully developed, a comprehensive community mental health center will include inpatient services, outpatient services, facilities for partial hospitalization, consultation services, diagnostic services, rehabilitation services, training for professional and paraprofessional workers, and a research program.
6. The National Mental Health Act was passed by the U. S. Congress in 1946 and made it possible for the nation to begin its attack on the problem of mental illness through the financing of research and training programs.
7. The tranquilizing or ataractic drugs, first used experimentally in 1953, played a large role in the development of community psychiatry by helping mentally disturbed patients control their behavior and remain in the community.
8. The final published report of the Joint Commission on Mental Illness was entitled *Action for Mental Health* and was issued in 1961.
9. The term community mental health has come to represent all mental health activities carried on in a community, and the theoretical formulation basic to their functioning has evolved as an alternative to the medical model.
10. It has become increasingly evident that mental health problems are intimately related to the environment and that many environmental factors contribute to the individual's mental health or illness.
11. The theoretical formulations underlying community psychiatry deal with

the belief that much deviant behavior is learned behavior in response to a negative environmental situation.

12. One approach to preventing mental illness and improving the mental health of individuals in a community is to improve the social conditions that exist in the community.

13. Each comprehensive community mental health center developed differently depending upon the needs of the community it served, the philosophy of the professional workers involved, and the relationship of the community to the center.

14. The treatment modality in the comprehensive community mental health center is focused upon helping the patient through the use of group techniques.

15. Role definitions are becoming blurred as the representatives of several professional disciplines work together in an interdisciplinary climate.

16. The major focuses of the comprehensive community mental health centers include: (a) prevention, (b) planned social change, (c) comprehensive and continuous service to the patient, and (d) research into the cause and treatment of mental illness.

SUGGESTED SOURCES OF ADDITIONAL INFORMATION

Blackman, Sheldon, and Goldstein, Kenneth M.: Some aspects of a theory of community mental health, Community Mental Health J. 4:85-90, Feb., 1968.

Bulbulyan, Ann, Davidites, Rose Marie, and Williams, Florence: Nurses in a community mental health center, Amer. J. Nurs. 69:328-331, Feb., 1969.

Caplan, Gerald: An approach to community mental health, New York, 1966, Grune & Stratton, Inc.

Daniels, Robert S.: Community psychiatry—a new profession, a developing sub specialty, or effective clinical psychiatry, Community Mental Health J. 2:47-54, Spring, 1966.

DePaul, Alice V.: The nurse as a central figure in a mental health center, Perspect. Psychiat. Care 6:17-24, 1968.

DeYoung, Carol D.: Nursing's contribution in family crisis treatment, Nurs. Outlook 16:60-62, Feb., 1968.

Evans, Frances M. C.: The role of the nurse in community mental health, New York, 1966, The Macmillan Co.

Joint Commission on Mental Illness and Health: Action for mental health, New York, 1961, Basic Books, Inc., Publishers.

Kardiner, Sheldon H.: The family: structure, patterns, and therapy, Ment. Hyg. 52:524-531, 1968.

LaFave, Hugh G.: Community care of the mentally ill: implementation of the Saskatchewan plan, Community Mental Health J. 4:37-45, Feb., 1968.

Leininger, Madeleine M.: Community psychiatric nursing: trends, issues, and problems, Perspect. Psychiat. Care 7:10-20, 1969.

Lief, Victor F., and Brotman, Richard: The psychiatrist and community mental health practice, Community Mental Health J. 4:134-143, April, 1968.

Margolin, Reuben J.: A concept of mental illness: a new look at some old assumptions, Community Mental Health J. 4:417-424, Oct., 1968.

McGee, Richard K.: Community mental health concepts as demonstrated by suicide prevention programs in Florida, Community Mental Health J. 4:144-152, April, 1968.

Mereness, Dorothy: The potential significant role in community mental health services, Perspect. Psychiat. Care 1:34-39, 1963.

Mistr, Virginia R.: Community nursing service for psychiatric patients, Perspect. Psychiat. Care 6:36-41, 1968.

Ozarin, Lucy D.: The community mental health

center: concept and commitment, Ment. Hyg. **52**:76-80, 1968.

Report of Work Conference in Graduate Education, Psychiatric Mental Health Nursing sponsored by the School of Nursing of the University of Maryland and National Institute of Mental Health, Baltimore, April 24-28, 1967.

Rosenblum, Gershen, and Hassol, Leonard: Training for new mental health roles, Ment. Hyg. **52**:81-85, 1968.

Saper, Bernard: Current trends in comprehensive mental health services, Ment. Hyg. **51**:100-107, 1967.

Scarpitti, Frank R., Albini, Joseph, Baker, E., and others: Public health nurses in a community care program for the mentally ill, Amer. J. Nurs. **65**:89-95, June, 1965.

Sheldon, Alan, and Hope, Penelope: The developing role of the nurse in a community mental health program, Perspect. Psychiat. Care **5**:272-279, 1967.

Stretch, John J.: Community mental health: the evolution of a concept in social policy, Community Mental Health J. **3**:5-12, Spring, 1967.

Stueks, Alice M.: Working together collaboratively with other professions, Community Mental Health J. **1**:316-319, Winter, 1965.

Ujhely, Gertrud B.: The nurse in community psychiatry, Amer. J. Nurs. **69**:1001-1005, May, 1969.

CHAPTER TWENTY-THREE

Making use of psychiatric nursing principles in improving nursing care for the physically ill

The knowledge and skills used by the psychiatric nurse in the care of mentally ill patients are applicable and necessary in providing comprehensive nursing care for patients who are physically ill. Differentiation between the emotional needs of mentally ill patients and those of patients who are physically ill is artificial and unrealistic. Physically ill patients have feelings of intense anxiety, hostility, depression, elation, fear, anger, and sorrow. These are the same feelings expressed by mentally ill patients. Perhaps one of the few differentiations that can be made between the reactions of these two groups of patients is the presumed ability of the physically ill to maintain conscious control of behavior and to utilize better judgment than do patients who are mentally ill. However, even these expected differences are not always observed.

Placing psychiatric units in general hospitals has been one attempt to eradicate the traditionally artificial boundaries between the needs of patients who are mentally ill and those who are physically ill. Use of the psychosomatic concept in medicine is another attempt to encourage professional workers to recognize the interrelationship between the body and the mind.

There is growing dissatisfaction with the nursing care received by patients in general hospitals in the United States. Studies of these dissatisfactions point up the fact that only a few of them are related to the physical care given. The large majority of complaints have to do with failure of professional nurses to establish satisfying interpersonal relationships with patients. The nurse is frequently said to lack warmth in her attitude toward patients, to fail to give patients a feeling of being important human beings, to fail to listen sympathetically to the concerns of the patients, or to fail to ask enough questions to gather the necessary data from patients to make wise decisions about their needs.

Listening to patients, helping patients feel that they are important, and demonstrating that she cares about the patients and their problems does make some demands on the professional nurse's already limited time. However, the understanding and emotional support that physically ill patients deserve and are demanding is omitted more often because the nurse does not understand the character of the emotional needs of patients and how to provide the help they require than because she lacks the time to give this type of care.

It is often more difficult and more challenging to recognize and cope with the emotional needs of physically ill patients than it is to work effectively with the emotional needs of mentally ill patients. Because part of a mentally ill patient's problem is his lack of emotional control, he sometimes expresses his needs openly and directly. The emotionally ill patient's needs may be difficult to understand, but their existence is obvious. Because he is said to be mentally ill, the nurse realizes that part of her task is to help the patient with his emotional problems. In contrast, the physically ill patient usually tries to control his feelings and to solve his own problems. Nurses frequently expect the patient to handle his own emotional problems. They sometimes fail to recognize that in addition to their responsibility for his physical care they are also responsible for dealing with his emotional needs.

Any physical illness for which hospitalization is necessary forces the patient to assume a dependent role that may be disturbing to the individual. This is especially true for men, who may see physical illness as an expression of weakness. In our culture, physical illness does not coincide with our concept of the strong, masculine role expected of men. Inability to accept the forced dependency required in many hospitals is one reason for the uncooperative behavior of some patients.

The modern hospital is a highly organized creation of our mechanized world. The patient is expected to submit to a variety of procedures without always understanding what they are for or why they are being done. He often believes that they are being performed without his consent or without his having been given any explanation about them. Although the patient may have signed an operative permit, he is not likely to realize that this may cover a variety of tests and procedures before the actual operation is undertaken. The physician may have explained the preoperative tests, but the anxiety level of many patients is so high that they are unable to hear what the doctor is saying. Even when patients are able to concentrate upon the doctor's words, they do not always understand the full meaning of them, and the preoperative procedures may still come as a shocking surprise. It is not difficult to understand that a newly admitted surgical patient may be frightened and feel that he has lost his identity. Such a situation could be eased if nurses understood the importance of giving reassurance, if they could identify the patient's need, and if they were skillful in giving emotional support. Sometimes reassurance requires only a few minutes of time spent listening to the patient, answering questions, and recognizing him as a unique human being who is reaching out for understanding and help.

Some of the results of hospital procedures, especially surgical procedures, precipitate an emotional crisis for some patients. Such a crisis is overwhelming for a patient who has already developed the feeling that he is lost, forgotten, and reduced to a childlike state of dependence in the hospital. These feelings may actually impede his recovery and may cause him to view his hospitalization as an extremely traumatizing experience.

EMOTIONAL PROBLEMS PRECIPITATED BY SURGICAL PROCEDURES

Every person has a mental picture of his own body that is sometimes called the body image. This body image may be realistic, or it may be part of the individual's wish-fulfilling phantasy about himself. To a large extent an individual functions within the boundaries of this unconscious image. A patient once said in a hopeless voice, "I can never marry. What woman would want a man with one short leg?" This man's body image was so misshapen and ugly that he could not accept it. Because he could not accept his own body, he was convinced that no one else could. He was especially convinced that no woman could want him as a marriage partner. His reaction to all aspects of life was in keeping with this attitude of being worthless and of having an unacceptable body.

In contrast, some women maintain an unrealistic image of themselves, which they developed early in their lives. It is not uncommon to hear a large, matronly woman ask a saleswoman in a dress shop for a size 12 dress. Without making a comment the understanding clerk brings out the required large size and helps her try on the garment. When this same woman, who still sees herself as beautiful, desirable, and attractive, requires the surgical removal of a breast or of the uterus, it is understandable that she is emotionally devastated by the procedure.

Surgical removal of a breast or the uterus is among the most emotionally disturbing surgical procedures that women must face. It is unfortunate that more nurses have not been helped to understand the meaning these experiences have for many women and have not been assisted in helping these patients with the feelings precipitated by surgery.

Although people respond in highly individual and unique ways to the same surgical procedures, almost all women unconsciously feel that they have been mutilated by a breast amputation or the removal of the uterus. If given an opportunity after such a surgical procedure they will express feelings about not being a whole woman or about being of less value to the world than they were before the operation. Such patients may express fears about losing the acceptance of their marital partners.

Most women pass through a period of mourning for the lost part of the body. Nurses need to understand the realistic reasons that underlie the frequent tears in a gynecological section of the hospital and should accept this as an expression of a normal emotional response about an extremely upsetting experience. Crying is probably one of the most helpful ways of expressing grief. Unfortunately, some women cannot cry about this kind of problem. Instead, they repress their feelings of despair and sadness and respond in other ways that may be more difficult for the nurse to understand and cope with. After breast surgery one patient turned her face to the wall, refused to see any visitors, and requested that even her husband be excluded from the room.

Sadness and mourning may be expressed in a reaction that appears to an observer as an outburst of anger. The patient may respond as does a child when something of value is taken away. This response may be an expression of underlying depression, but the external reaction is one of anger at having lost a valued part of the body. Another frequent response to surgical loss is an unconscious feeling on the part of the patient that she is being punished for some real or phantasized transgression that may have occurred years before. This feeling may lead the patient to respond as if she were unworthy of attention from friends or relatives.

The possible reasons for the many emotional reactions to breast amputation and hysterectomy are as varied as the patients who submit to these procedures. The important thing for the nurse to remember is that these experiences are difficult for women to accept, that patients respond to them in highly individual ways, depending on their life situation and personality, and that the nurse needs to demonstrate that she cares about the patient and her feelings. Good physical care is always the first place to start in meeting the emotional needs of physically ill patients. Ways in which the nurse can demonstrate that she really cares about the patient include an unhurried approach, attentive, perceptive listening to the patient, and anticipation of the patient's physical needs before it is necessary for the patient to ask for care.

Women are not the only patients who are unable to accept an altered body image. All patients who submit to disfiguring surgery of any type have a variety of fears, which focus upon their concern about being acceptable to other people, especially to their marital partners. Operations involving amputations of a leg or disfiguring facial surgery are especially difficult for patients to accept. However, it has been noted that patients are able to accept body mutilation more readily when the location is such that it is evident to everyone. This phenomenon may be due to the fact that something that is obvious must be recognized and talked about. Some patients refrain from mentioning a problem that is hidden under clothing. They are therefore burdened with a tremendous amount of unresolved sensitivity for years. Perhaps the much joked about American habit of discussing one's operation and exhibiting the surgical scar at social gatherings has some psychologically healing attributes. The nurse is being more therapeutic than she sometimes realizes when she is able to help patients discuss the way they feel about the surgical procedure they have experienced.

Nurses should avoid censoring patients who blame the surgeon for their disfigured bodies. It is a natural human response to relieve anxiety by blaming someone else for an unhappy situation that the individual cannot control with his usual defenses. One example of this kind of reaction

was a man who was hospitalized for plastic reconstruction of a thumb that was lost in an accident involving high voltage electricity. After several skin grafts and months of hospitalization, the patient was disturbed when he saw the reconstructed thumb. It was many times larger than a normal thumb and was covered with short hair because the skin graft had been taken from the patient's thigh. He had expected a normal-looking thumb and had looked forward to having a functioning hand as a reward for the long period of boring hospitalization. He was bitterly disappointed and disgusted at the appearance of the thumb. The patient remarked to the nurse, "Look at that! It's obscene! I am going to sign myself out of this hospital and have my own doctor cut this thing off." The nurse reported this reaction to the head nurse who said, "He should be ashamed of himself for criticizing his doctor, who is the best plastic surgeon in this part of the country. The doctor has worked terribly hard on that thumb."

The patient did leave the hospital against medical advice. He was angry and disappointed. If someone had explained to this patient that the surgeon planned to shape the thumb to normal proportions after the body had established effective circulation to the new tissues, he might have been helped to wait for a few more weeks for the surgeon to complete the delicate and tedious work. Unfortunately, the nurse with whom the patient had developed a positive relationship did not know enough about plastic surgery to use the opportunity to be helpful to the patient at the time when he needed reassurance.

A colostomy is another emotionally disturbing experience for patients. In our culture the emphasis placed on cleanliness and fastidiousness in personal hygiene creates a serious conflict for patients who find it medically necessary to resort to a colostomy. Cultural attitudes toward toileting, which are taught early in a child's life, sometimes cause the adult patient to rebel at the thought of caring for a colostomy. Probably no surgical procedure presents patients with more emotional and social problems than does a colostomy. Although hundreds of patients have been able to adjust successfully to a colostomy, the nurse should not forget that the patient who is just beginning to cope with the problems presented by the loss of normal bowel function has many hurdles ahead of him. The following clinical report points up the effect that a colostomy can have on some fastidious people.

A fastidious man who understood English poorly entered the hospital with a diagnosis of far-advanced carcinoma of the rectum. He had suffered a great deal before coming to the hospital and was grateful when surgery relieved the pain. A colostomy opening was established. His physical recovery was rapid. When he was discharged he left many gifts for the hospital staff. In every way he appeared to be a happy and a grateful patient. The surgeon had attempted to explain the seriousness of the problem to the patient before surgery. The hospital staff believed that the patient understood the nature of his operation and the need for a permanent colostomy. One week after discharge he returned to the surgical clinic and requested admission to the hospital in order to have the colostomy opening closed. Again the surgeon explained the nature of the operation and the perma-nent character of the surgery. The patient left the clinic without appearing to be upset. The next day the newspapers carried a notice of the patient's suicide. This problem undoubtedly grew out of this individual's language handicap and his attitude toward importance of physical cleanliness. Although this response to the colostomy was unusual, many patients will admit that in the beginning of their experience with a colostomy they occasionally wondered if life was worthwhile under such circumstances. Colostomy patients worry about their acceptability to their friends and their marital partners. Unfortunately, many colostomy patients find that after a few months it is impossible to carry on marital relations. It would be helpful if patients could be encouraged to express their feelings, attitudes, and questions about their condition. Patients are not helped by nurses who insist upon the light, gay approach and refuse to involve themselves in serious conversation about these problems. The patient with a colostomy deserves a nurse who will give his situation thoughtful, sympathetic, realistic consideration.

Such procedures as the colostomy operations are performed only when they are necessary to save the life of a patient. The nurse cannot alter the problems that patients who need the operation must solve, but she can help the patient to talk about the problem, to begin to accept the reality of the situation, and to begin to learn all he can about his condition so that he can handle it as effectively as possible.

Surgical operations on the male genitourinary tract sometimes present patients with disturbing emotional conflicts. Occasionally such an operation precipitates a psychotic reaction. The following clinical report presents an example of such a situation.

A middle-aged gentleman who was a devoted church member was admitted to a surgical unit because of symptoms of prostatic hypertrophy. A successful operation was performed to relieve the distressing symptoms. Within a day or two the patient was complaining of the suggestive pictures on the walls of his room, which he said the hospital authorities had placed there for the purpose of tormenting him. The nurses were confused by these complaints because no pictures were hanging in his room. The psychiatrist who was called to talk with the patient reported that the annoying pictures were of young, nude women. The patient stated that a man of his principles should not be surrounded by such lewd art. The psychiatrist concluded that the patient was not able to accept the fact that a man of his social standing would indulge in such an active, unconscious phantasy life dealing with sexual material. To relieve his own anxiety about his unconscious sexual longings, which were dramatically brought to light by his complaint about the nude pictures, the patient utilized the mechanism of projection. It was much more acceptable to him and safer from the standpoint of his self-esteem to blame the hospital for hanging nude pictures around the room than to accept the explanation that the pictures represented his own phantasies.

This unusual reaction was undoubtedly precipitated by the surgical procedure, but it would not be accurate to say that the procedure caused the response. During most of this patient's life he probably exerted a great deal of emotional energy to repress unacceptable sexual thoughts. The emotional crisis presented by the surgical experience was apparently enough to make it impossible for this patient to continue to keep his unacceptable thoughts repressed.

EMOTIONAL PROBLEMS AMONG OBSTETRICAL PATIENTS

Many nurses choose to work with obstetrical patients because the obstetrical unit is such a happy place to work. In talking about their work, obstetrical nurses frequently emphasize the great happiness of mothers and fathers when a new baby arrives. It is true that there is much happiness among obstetrical patients, but nurses should not overlook the fact that there are a few new mothers who are emotionally distressed and in great need of understanding and reassurance because they have delivered imperfect babies. Young mothers who deliver imperfect babies are apt to be more troubled than mothers whose babies are stillborn. Death is an accomplished, final fact that can be accepted and explained to some extent. Death of a new baby will undoubtedly precipitate sadness and grief. However, our culture has provided some ways of helping people handle these feelings. Funeral services provide culturally sanctioned opportunities for the expression of grief. Families offer much emotional support at such a time. Many mothers can console themselves by looking forward to a second child.

On the other hand, mothers of imperfectly formed babies or premature infants are distressed by doubts concerning their own adequacy as mothers and by guilt about their responsibility for the existence of the problem. It may surprise some nurses to learn that almost all mothers whose babies are born prematurely or congenitally imperfect respond with questions about their abilities as mothers. They ask themselves questions such as, "What did I do to cause this?" or "Why has this happened to me?" Sometimes a scientific explanation does little to remove a young mother's sense of failure as a woman. Production of perfect babies is one of the most important tasks performed by the woman in our culture. When a woman fails in this effort, she sometimes wonders about her effectiveness and her intrinsic value. Some women who have set high achievement goals for themselves find it difficult to accept an imperfect product. The following clinical report demonstrates this point.

An English professor from a large midwestern university found that she was pregnant for the first time at the age of 40. She and her husband were moderately happy about this new development in their lives. However, they were sorry to have to give up their plans for a sabbatical leave and a trip abroad. When the baby boy was born, he had a bilateral harelip and a cleft palate. When the nurse brought the baby to the mother, she looked at him and said, "That can't possibly be my child." The nurse assured the mother that it was her little boy. She said to the nurse, "Don't bring that baby in here again. I won't have a baby that looks like that!" In five days the mother left the hospital without asking to see her baby again. The father arranged for a nurse to help him take his son to a distant city where a famous surgeon specialized in repairing harelips.

This story suggests something of the difficulty that some women have in accepting an imperfect product, even when it is a living child.

Guilt causes people to feel uncomfortable. When a mother feels guilty about her baby's imperfections she may reject it outright or may spend the rest of her life punishing herself for failing to give

her child a perfect body. This punishment may take the form of slavishly serving the child in an attempt to make up in every possible way for the child's poor start in life. This reaction is one of the disguised forms that rejection may take.

As in many other situations, the nurse cannot alter the reality of the difficult situation, but she can encourage the mother to talk about her feelings. If the mother can be helped to discuss some of these feelings, she may come to feel less guilty and may be able to clear away some of the emotion about the problem so that constructive steps can be taken and solutions can be planned.

Many other problems of patients in general hospitals could be discussed from the standpoint of the emotional needs of the patient and the role that a warm, supportive, caring nurse can take in helping these patients cope with their anxieties, fears, guilt, and repressed feelings. It is hoped that this discussion has underscored our original contention regarding the enormous need of all physically ill patients for nurses who make use of psychiatric nursing skills.

IMPORTANT CONCEPTS

1. The knowledge and skills used by the psychiatric nurse in the care of mentally ill patients are applicable and necessary in providing comprehensive nursing care for patients who are physically ill.
2. Differentiation between the emotional needs of mentally ill patients and those of patients who are physically ill is artificial and unrealistic.
3. The large majority of complaints

made by patients concerning their hospital care have to do with the failure of professional nurses to establish satisfying interpersonal relationships with patients.

4. The understanding and emotional support that physically ill patients deserve and are demanding is omitted more often because the nurse does not understand the character of the emotional needs and how to cope with them than because she lacks the time to give this type of help.

5. Any physical illness for which hospitalization is necessary forces the patient to partially assume a dependent role that may be disturbing to the individual and may cause him to react with what is sometimes called uncooperative behavior.

6. Newly admitted patients in general hospitals may feel frightened and may develop a sense of having lost their identity.

7. Every person has a mental picture of his body, which is sometimes called the body image and which may be realistic or part of the individual's wish-fulfilling phantasy about himself.

8. Surgical removal of a breast or the uterus is among the most emotionally disturbing surgical procedures that human beings are called upon to accept.

9. Although people respond in highly individual and unique ways to the same surgical procedures, almost all women unconsciously feel that they have been multilated by amputation of a breast or the removal of the uterus.

10. All patients who submit to disfiguring surgery of any type have a variety of fears that focus upon their concern about being acceptable to other people, especially their marital partners.

11. The nurse is being more therapeutic than she sometimes realizes when she is able to help patients talk about the way they feel regarding the surgical procedure that they have experienced.

12. In our culture the emphasis placed on cleanliness and fastidiousness in personal hygiene creates a serious conflict for patients who find it medically necessary to resort to a colostomy.

13. Mothers of imperfectly formed babies and premature babies are distressed by doubts concerning their own adequacy and are guilt ridden concerning their own responsibility for the existence of the problem.

14. As in many other situations, the nurse cannot alter the reality of the difficult situation for the new mother with an imperfect baby, but she can encourage her to talk about her feelings and lessen her guilt. This may make it possible for her to view the problem realistically and to plan solutions.

SUGGESTED SOURCES OF ADDITIONAL INFORMATION

Aronson, Morton J.: Emotional aspects of nursing the cancer patient, Ment. Hyg. **42**:267-273, 1958.

Bird, Brian: Psychological aspects of preoperative and postoperative care, Amer. J. Nurs. **55**:685-687, June, 1955.

Bojar, Samuel: The psychotherapeutic function of the general nurse, Nurs. Outlook 6:151-153, March, 1958.

Cohen, Sidney, and Klein, Hazel K.: The delirious patient, Amer. J. Nurs. 58:685-687, May, 1958.

Crate, Marjorie: Nursing functions in adaptation to chronic illness, Amer. J. Nurs. 65:72-76, Oct., 1965.

Gelb, Lester A.: Personality disorganization camoflaged by physical handicaps, Ment. Hyg. 45:207-215, 1961.

Gregg, Dorothy: Reassurance, Amer. J. Nurs. 55:171-174, Feb., 1955.

Ingals, Thelma: Do patients feel lost in a general hospital? Amer. J. Nurs. 60:648-651, May, 1960.

Jensen, Hellene N., and Tillotson, Gene: Dependency in nurse-patient relationships, Amer. J. Nurs. 61:81-84, Feb., 1961.

Jourard, Sidney M.: To whom can a nurse give personalized care? Amer. J. Nurs. 61:86-88, March, 1961.

Jourard, Sidney M.: The bedside manner, Amer. J. Nurs. 60:63-66, Jan., 1960.

Kaufmann, Margaret A., and Brown, Dorothy E.:

Pain wears many faces, Amer. J. Nurs. 61:48-51, Jan., 1961.

Larsen, Virginia A.: What hospitalization means to patients, Amer. J. Nurs. 61:44-47, May, 1961.

Martin, Harry W., and Prange, Arthur J.: The stages of illness—psychosocial approach, Nurs. Outlook 10:168-171, March, 1962.

Mead, Margaret: Understanding cultural patterns, Nurs. Outlook 4:260-262, May, 1956.

Neylan, Margaret Prowse: The depressed patient, Amer. J. Nurs. 61:77-78, July, 1961.

Oliva, Anthony T.: Personality factors in human relations, Nurs. Outlook 2:578-579, Nov., 1954.

Skipper, James K., Tagliacozzo, Daisey L., and Mauksch, Hans O.: What communication means to patients, Amer. J. Nurs. 64:101-103, April, 1964.

Tarnower, William: Psychological needs of the hospitalized patient, Nurs. Outlook 13:28-30, July, 1965.

Thomas, Betty J.: Clues to patient's behavior, Amer. J. Nurs. 63:100-102, July, 1963.

Wesseling, Elizabeth: The adolescent facing amputation, Amer. J. Nurs. 65:90-94, Jan., 1965.

CHAPTER TWENTY-FOUR

Psychiatry and the law

Neither physician nor nurse should be unaware of the rudimentary principles of law that concern the mental patient and his legal status. A psychiatric nurse should be sufficiently acquainted with the legal aspects of psychiatry so that she can avoid giving poor advice or innocently involving herself in a legal entanglement.

The legal significance of psychiatry is of special concern because mental illness affects the behavior of the individual and his reaction to others. If behavior varies considerably from those standards established by society the person is considered either a criminal or insane. It should be emphasized that the term insanity is a legal rather than a medical one. According to Singer and Krohn, the *definition for legal insanity* is as follows: "An insane person or lunatic is one in whom there exists, due to disease, a more or less prolonged deviation from his normal method of behavior and who is, therefore, incapable of managing his affairs or transacting ordinary business, who is dangerous to himself, to others, or to property, or who interferes with the peace of society." The definition does not include the idiot or imbecile. The determination of insanity in a legal sense is based upon the particular act or misbehavior in each case, and in each case must therefore be tried on its own merits.

If an individual is guilty of a crime by reason of insanity, he is committed to an institution, not so much to protect society as to allow him to receive the benefits of treatment. This is a step in a more humane and rational direction, since it implies that the wrongdoer is not a criminal but is mentally ill.

Every state has made some sort of provision for the care and treatment of the mentally ill persons. In most instances this consists of a state hospital system consisting of one or more institutions. In a few states the actual care is left in the hands of county authorities, but is under close inspection by state officials. This system is changing rapidly in many states with comprehensive community mental health centers providing treatment in the patient's community. More and more often the patient is being treated while remaining at home.

METHODS OF COMMITMENT

There is no uniformity of commitment methods in the several states, but no one can be deprived of his liberty without due process of law. In a few parts of this country the commitment proceedings still imply that the mentally ill person is a criminal in that he must be tried by jury. A jury is not always competent to decide on such complicated and technical matters as whether a person is mentally ill, and the entire ordeal is such that it may often act as a great psychological shock to the patient.

It is much better to simplify the legal side of commitment and to reduce it to a simple and very informal procedure while at the same time protecting the individual's legal and constitutional rights. In general the commitment proceedings consist of three parts: (1) the application, (2) the examination, and (3) detention in some type of institution.

The action is initiated generally by relatives or friends who have become aware of the mental abnormality. Any legally appointed officer of the law, a policeman, a sheriff or his deputies, members of charitable organizations, a public health official, or any private citizen may make the application, which will bring the matter to the attention of the proper court. In most states the court that settles matters of insanity is the common pleas court or the probate court. Here the application is submitted; statements by interested parties are heard under oath; and all available information about the patient and his behavior is recorded.

Frequently the application must be accompanied by the certificates of one or more physicians. The judge may, however, appoint one or two physicians to conduct the psychiatric examination. Specially certified physicians who make medicolegal examinations and submit their opinions to the court are known as alienists. Each alienist must satisfy himself that mental disease exists before he can lawfully certify the patient for commitment. The testimony of lay witnesses and of the examining physicians must be sufficient to convince a judge or jury that the person in question is a social menace and needs to be restrained and treated.

If the court finds that the need exists for institutionalization, the patient is generally committed to a state hospital. In some localities provision is made for temporary commitment in a detention hospital. This observation period is usually from five to thirty days, and during this interval additional data are obtained to determine whether or not final action is justified.

LEGAL RIGHTS OF THE CONFINED MENTAL PATIENT

Every nurse who has charge of mental patients in an institution should be ac-quainted with the legal status of such patients. Statutes provide for maintaining certain rights of citizenship, even though the patient be already certified as insane. A patient may be allowed to have visitors, may send unopened letters to judges and hospital staff members, and may make contact with attorneys. However, both nurse and doctor may exercise a reasonable control over the matter of the patient's correspondence. If by reason of his psychosis a patient is dangerously paranoid or maniacal and may take to writing threatening, abusive, or obscene letters to strangers or public officials, it is better to distract the individual by encouraging other activities or to turn over such correspondence to relatives, who can dispose of them without causing undue concern or worry to others.

Many people still believe that a large number of patients are confined in mental hospitals without good reason or justification. Actually, under the present methods of commitment such a miscarriage of justice is rare or next to impossible. If illegal detention is suspected, any individual is free to force court action through *habeas corpus* proceedings. By this means the patient can be brought to court for a hearing and the cause for confinement must be clearly shown by those who detain him.

Patients in state hospitals cannot, under ordinary circumstances, be treated by their own personal physicians, and the latter do not usually care to assume such responsibilities. The directing head of the hospital usually decides the question of medical consultation but may, as a matter of pure courtesy, allow the family physician to visit the patient.

A patient who has been judged to be legally insane may lose certain rights, and these cannot be regained until such time as he recovers full mental capacity. A certified patient cannot, for instance, enter into a valid contract unless it can be proved that such contract was made during a lucid interval. Even the simple endorsement of a check can be questioned as to its legality if the patient has been committed and confined for mental illness.

GUARDIANSHIP

To protect the patient's rights and property, a guardian is appointed either by the court that commits him or by the state authorities. If the amount of property warrants the expense of guardianship or if necessary business involving such property is transacted, the guardian's responsibilities are not trivial. In some states this property guardian is called a conservator. A guardian is one who has direct responsibility for the patient's personal welfare. He is generally a near relative. He cannot confine the patient in an institution without permission or approval of the court but can dictate, within certain limits, the nature of the patient's treatment, and he can sign a permit for a major operation. He may also have custody of the minor children of the patient if the mother is incapable of this herself.

The wife or husband of a patient, rather than the parents, is regarded as the natural guardian. Every guardian must give bond for the proper performance of his duties. At regular intervals he is required to make an accounting of expenses and income. His first consideration must be the comfort of the patient. The guardian is required to guard the patient's welfare judiciously.

LEAVE OF
ABSENCE AND DISCHARGE

In most states at the discretion of the directing physician, committed patients may be permitted to return to their homes on trial visit for a period of a few days, a few weeks, or even a year. This plan provides for a "trying-out" period, during which the patient can demonstrate the degree of recovery as measured by his capacity to cope with normal social situations. The patient, however, remains under the supervision of the hospital and must continue to visit regularly with the psychiatrist or social worker assigned to him. If the trial visit progresses satisfactorily, the patient may then be legally discharged.

Usually the legal discharge of a mental patient is not as formal a procedure as is the commitment. The hospital physicians in a staff meeting make a final examination, and the superintendent merely issues the order for release. The patient may be discharged because he has recovered or is greatly improved or because his relatives have made satisfactory arrangements for treatment in a private institution. This does not, however, apply to the patient who is criminally insane, since he is subject to the orders of a regular criminal court.

In all instances in which a patient has been legally discharged, the hospital authorities notify the court responsible for the commitment.

VOLUNTARY COMMITMENT

The most desirable manner of obtaining treatment for mental illness is voluntary commitment. Unfortunately this is not always done because many mentally ill individuals have limited insight concerning their own behavior, and the average patient will not of his own volition go to a hospital. Under voluntary commitment the patient need not undergo a court action, but simply signs an application and agrees to submit himself for treatment and to abide by the rules of the hospital. By doing this, he will neither lose his rights as a citizen nor commit himself for an indefinite period. Upon giving three days' notice he is entitled to leave the hospital. If in the judgment of the physician in charge, however, his discharge constitutes a menace to the community, relatives can be quickly notified, a legal commitment can be arranged, and further detention assured. Otherwise the patient under voluntary commitment is free to go, with no other formality.

MENTAL CAPACITY IN MAKING A WILL

The question as to the mental qualifications of an elderly person making a will is often an important problem in legal psychiatry. A nurse who is in charge of an aging patient may frequently be called upon for testimony as to his testamentary capacity; she may be asked to witness the signature to a will or even to draw up a will. It is important for her to be aware of the important considerations necessary to establish or to recognize whether a patient can make or sign a will.

As a rule, a patient who is able to carry on his ordinary business is qualified. If, however, an individual has been an invalid for some length of time and has not clearly demonstrated this capacity, it should be ascertained whether he has an understanding and knowledge of his business or vocation, whether his memory is such that he knows what property he possesses, whether he has a knowledge of the persons or organizations to whom he desires to will his property, and whether he shows reasonably good judgment pertaining to the disposal of his property.

Senile individuals may have periods of mental clouding and confusion, but they may also have lucid intervals. A will is legal if it is made during a lucid period as long as it can be proved that such a period of mental clarity existed at the time.

The question of testamentary capacity in the mental patient, particularly in the elderly person, is always a trying one, as indicated by the frequent legal controversies that arise between beneficiaries and nonbeneficiaries when considerable property is involved.

The wise nurse will avoid getting involved with the question of whether a patient is capable of making a will by requesting assistance from the legal department of the hospital.

PRIVILEGED COMMUNICATION

Privileged communication is a legal term referring to any matter or information necessarily held in professional confidence, as between a patient and a physician, which is not admissible as evidence in a court. It is an evasion of the law to submit in evidence on the witness stand any facts dealing with methods of treatment. The psychiatric nurse should remember that the medical chart and the data thereon are regarded as privileged communication. It is a part of the nurse's duty to protect this record from scrutiny by unauthorized or curious individuals. If any doubt arises as to rights and privileges in this respect, the matter should be referred to the administrative officers of the hospital or to the physician in charge.

SUGGESTED SOURCES OF ADDITIONAL INFORMATION

Davidson, Henry A.: Forensic psychiatry, New York, 1952, The Ronald Press Co.

Davidson, Henry A.: Civil rights and mental hospitals, Perspect. Psychiat. Care 1:28-33, 1963.

Ginsberg, Leon H.: Civil rights of the mentally ill—a review of the issues, Community Mental Health J. 4:244-250, June, 1968.

Gray, K. G.: Law and the practice of medicine, Toronto, 1955, Ryerson Press.

Guttmacher, M. S., and Weihofen, H.: Psychiatry and the law, New York, 1952, W. W. Norton & Co., Inc.

Hoch, Paul H., and Zubin, Joseph, editors: Psychiatry and the law, vol. 9, New York, 1955, Grune & Stratton, Inc.

Overholser, W.: The psychiatrist and the law, New York, 1953, Harcourt, Brace & World, Inc.

Ostrow, Seymour: The medico-legal conflict, Amer. J. Nurs. 63:67-71, July, 1963.

Ploscowe, Morris: Sex and the law, New York, 1951, Prentice-Hall, Inc.

Sherwin, R. V.: Sex and the statutory law, New York, 1949, Oceana Publications, Inc.

Szasz, Thomas S.: Law, liberty and psychiatry, New York, 1963, The Macmillan Co.

Zilboorg, Gregory: The psychology of the criminal act and punishment, New York, 1954, Harcourt, Brace & World, Inc.

Appendixes

Glossary

The following list of words are those frequently used by the psychiatric nurse. Many of the definitions were taken from *A Psychiatric Glossary.** A larger and equally useful book is the *Psychiatric Dictionary.*†

abulia absence or deficiency in will power.

acting out expression of unconscious emotional conflicts or feelings of hostility or love in actions that the protagonist does not consciously know are related to such conflicts or feelings.

addiction strong emotional and physiological dependence upon alcohol or a drug that has progressed beyond voluntary control.

affect a person's emotional feeling tone; affect and emotional response are commonly used interchangeably.

affective psychosis a psychotic reaction in which the predominant feature is a severe disorder of mood or emotional feelings.

aggression as used in psychiatry, forceful attacking action (physical, verbal, or symbolic).

agitation state of chronic restlessness; psychomotor expression of emotional tension.

ambivalence coexistence of two opposing drives, desires, feelings, or emotions toward the same person, object, or goal; may be conscious or partly conscious.

anxiety apprehension, tension, or uneasiness that stems from the anticipation of danger, the source of which is largely unknown or unrecognized; primarily of intrapsychic origin, in distinction to fear, which is the emotional response to a consciously recognized and usually external threat or danger.

autism (autistic thinking) form of thinking that attempts to gratify unfulfilled desires without due regard for reality; objective facts are distorted, obscured, or excluded in varying degrees.

autoerotism securing or attempting to secure sensual gratification from oneself as in masturbation; a characteristic of an early stage of emotional development.

blocking difficulty in recollection or interruption of a train of thought or speech, due to emotional factors usually unconscious.

brain syndrome a group of symptoms resulting from impaired function of the brain; may be acute (reversible) or chronic (irreversible).

catatonia type of schizophrenia characterized by immobility with muscular rigidity or inflexibity; alternating periods of psysical hyperactivity and excitability may occur; generally there is marked inaccessibility to ordinary methods of communication.

cathexis investment of an object or idea with special significance or value to the individual.

cerea flexibilitas the "waxy flexibility" often present in catatonic schizophrenia in which the patient's arm or leg remain passively in the position in which it is placed.

cognitive refers to mental processes of comprehension, judgment, memory, and reasoning.

compensation (1) mental mechanism, operating unconsciously, by which the individual attempts to make up for real or fancied deficiencies; (2) conscious process by which the individual strives to make up for real or imagined defects in such areas as physique, performance, skills, or psychologic attributes—the two types frequently merge.

complex a group of associated ideas that have a common strong emotional tone; these may be in part unconscious and may significantly influence attitudes and associations.

compulsion insistent, repetitive, intrusive, and unwanted urge to perform an act that is contrary to the person's ordinary conscious wishes or standards; a defensive substitute for hidden and still more unacceptable ideas and wishes (anxiety results from failure to perform the compulsive act).

---

*Committee on Public Information of the American Psychiatric Association: A psychiatric glossary, Washington, D. C., 1957, American Psychiatric Association.

†Hinsie, Leland E., and Campbell, Robert J.: Psychiatric dictionary, ed. 3, New York, 1960, Oxford University Press.

concept mental image.

condensation psychologic process often present in dreams in which two or more concepts are fused so that a single symbol represents the multiple components.

confabulation unconscious, defensive "filling in" of actual memory gaps by imaginary or fantastic experiences, often complex, that are recounted in a detailed and plausible way as though they were factual.

conflict clash, conscious or unconscious, between two opposing emotional forces; if unconscious, an internal (instinctual) wish or striving is opposed by another internal and contradictory wish.

confusion disturbed orientation in respect to time, place, or person; sometimes accompanied by disturbances of consciousness.

consciousness clear awareness of self and the environment.

conversion mental mechanism, operating unconsciously, by which intrapsychic conflicts, which would otherwise give rise to anxiety, are instead given symbolic external expression; the repressed ideas or impulses plus the psychologic defenses against them are converted into a variety of somatic symptoms.

countertransference the psychiatrist's conscious or unconscious emotional reaction to his patient.

delirium disturbance in thinking with disorientation and confusion; illusions, delusions, or hallucinations may be present.

delusion false belief out of keeping with the individual's level of knowledge and his cultural group; the belief is maintained against logical argument and despite objective contradictory evidence.

delusions of grandeur exaggerated unrealistic ideas of one's importance or identity.

delusions of persecution ideas that one has been singled out for persecution.

delusions of reference incorrect assumption that certain casual or unrelated remarks or the behavior of others applies to oneself.

dementia old term denoting madness or insanity; now used entirely to denote organic loss of intellectual function

dementia praecox obsolescent descriptive term for schizophrenia.

denial mental mechanism, operating unconsciously, used to resolve emotional conflict and to allay consequent anxiety by denying some of the important elements; the feelings denied may be thoughts, wishes, needs, or external reality factors; what is consciously intolerable is simply disowned by the protectively automatic and unconscious denial of its existence.

dependency needs vital infantile needs for mothering, love, affection, shelter, protection, security, food, and warmth; these needs may continue beyond infancy in overt or hidden forms, or be increased in the adult as a regressive manifestation.

depersonalization feelings of unreality or strangeness concerning either the environment or the self.

depression used in the psychiatric sense, a morbid sadness, dejection, or melancholy; may vary in depth from neurosis to psychosis; to be differentiated from grief that is realistic and proportionate to what has been lost.

dereistic describes mental activity that is not in accordance with reality, logic, or experience; similar to autistic.

disorientation loss of awareness of the position of self in relation to space, time, or persons.

displacement a mental mechanism, operating unconsciously, by which an emotion is transferred or "displaced" from its original object to a more acceptable substitute object.

dissociation psychologic separation or splitting off; an intrapsychic defensive process, which operates automatically and unconsciously, through which emotional significance and affect are separated and detached from an idea, situation, or object.

dynamic psychiatry psychiatry stressing the existence of mental forces that energetically demand expression; dynamic psychiatry implies the study of the active, energy-laden, and changing factors in human behavior, as opposed to the older, more static, and descriptive study of clinical patterns, symptoms, and classification.

dysarthria impaired, difficult speech, usually due to organic disorders of the nervous system; sometimes applied to emotional speech difficulties such as stammering and stuttering.

ego refers to the conscious self, the "I"; in

Freudian theory, the central part of the personality that deals with reality and is influenced by social forces; the ego modifies behavior by largely unconscious compromise between the primitive instinctual drives (the id) and the conscience (the superego).

ego ideal that part of the personality that comprises the aims and goals of the self; usually refers to the conscious or unconscious emulation of significant persons with whom it has identified.

emotion subjective feeling such as fear, anger, grief, joy, or love.

empathy objective and insightful awareness of the feelings, emotions, and behavior of another person, and their meaning and significance; to be distinguished from sympathy, which is nonobjective and usually noncritical.

euphoria exaggerated feeling of physical and emotional well-being not consonant with apparent stimuli or events; usually of psychologic origin, but also seen in organic brain disease and toxic states.

exhibitionism commonly, showing off; psychiatrically, body exposure, usually of the male genitals to females; sexual stimulation or gratification usually accompanies the act.

extroversion state in which attention and energies are largely directed outward from the self, as opposed to interest primarily directed toward the self as in introversion.

fabrication relating imaginary events as true, not in the sense of lying but to cover up gaps in memory.

fixation arrest of psychosexual maturation at an immature level; depending on degree, may be either normal or pathological.

flight of ideas verbal skipping from one idea to another before the preceding one has been concluded; the ideas appear to be continuous but are fragmentary and determined by chance associations.

free association in psychoanalytic therapy, unselected verbalization by the patient of whatever comes to mind.

free-floating anxiety pervasive anxiety that the patient cannot explain to his own satisfaction.

functional mental illness illness of emotional origin in which organic or structural changes are either absent or are developed secondarily to prolonged emotional stress.

general paresis a psychosis associated with organic disease of the central nervous system resulting from chronic syphilitic infection.

globus hystericus sensation of having a ball in the throat; a hysterical spasm of the esophagus.

grandiose in psychiatry, refers to delusions of great wealth, power, fame.

hallucination false sensory perception in the absence of an actual external stimulus; may be of emotional or chemical (drugs, alcohol, etc.) origin and may occur in any of the five senses.

homosexual panic acute and severe attack of anxiety based upon unconscious conflicts involving homosexuality.

homosexuality sexual attraction or relationship between members of the same sex; active homosexuality is marked by overt activity, whereas latent homosexuality is marked by unconscious homosexual desires or conscious desires consistently denied expression.

hypnosis altered state of conscious awareness induced in a suggestible subject; under hypnosis a person manifests increased receptivity to suggestion and direction.

hysteria illness resulting from emotional conflict and generally characterized by immaturity, impulsiveness, attention-seeking, dependency, and use of the mental mechanisms of conversion and dissociation.

id in Freudian theory, that part of the personality structure which harbors the unconscious instinctive desires and strivings of the individual.

ideas of reference incorrect interpretation of casual incidents and external events as having direct reference to oneself. May reach sufficient intensity to constitute delusions.

identification mental mechanism, operating unconsciously, by which an individual endeavors to pattern himself after another; plays a major role in the development of one's personality and specifically of one's superego (conscience).

idiopathic term applied to diseases of unknown cause, for example, idiopathic epilepsy.

illusion misinterpretation of a real external sensory experience.

incorporation primitive mental mechanism, operating unconsciously, by which a person, or parts of another person, are symbolically ingested and assimilated; for example, infantile fantasy that the mother's breast has been ingested and is a part of oneself.

infantilism applied to adults who are childish or mentally or physically immature.

inhibition unconscious interference with or restriction of instinctual drives.

insight self-understanding; a major goal of psychotherapy; the extent of the individual's understanding of the origin, nature, and mechanisms of his attitudes and behavior.

instinct inborn drive; human instincts include those of self-preservation, sexuality, and (according to some authorities) the *ego instincts* and the herd or social instincts.

integration useful organization of both new and old data, experience, and emotional capacities into the personality; also refers to the organization and amalgamation of functions at various levels of psychosexual development.

introjection mental mechanism, operating unconsciously, whereby loved or hated external objects are taken within oneself symbolically; the converse of *projection;* may serve as a defense against conscious recognition of intolerable hostile impulses, for example, in severe depression the individual may unconsciously direct unacceptable hatred or aggression toward himself, that is, toward the introjected object within himself; related to the more primitive mechanism of *incorporation.*

introversion preoccupation with oneself, with accompanying reduction of interest in the outside world; roughly the reverse of extroversion.

involutional psychosis psychotic reaction taking place during the involutional period, climacteric or menopause, characterized most commonly by depression, and occasionally by paranoid thinking; the course tends to be prolonged, and the condition may be manifested by feelings of guilt, anxiety, agitation, delusional ideas, insomnia, and somatic preoccupation.

kleptomania compulsive stealing, largely without regard to any apparent material need for the stolen objects.

Korsakoff's psychosis (Korsakoff's syndrome) disorder marked by disturbance of attention and memory, as evidenced by confabulation and by involvement of the peripheral nerves; may

be due to alcohol, certain poisons, or infections.

labile rapidly shifting emotions.

latency period in psychoanalysis, a phase between the oedipal (or phallic) and adolescent periods of psychosexual development; characterized by a marked decrease of sexual behavior and interest in sex.

libido psychic drive or energy usually associated with the sexual instinct (sexual is used here in the broad sense to include pleasure and love-object seeking); also used broadly to connote the psychic energy associated with instincts in general.

lucid interval period during which there is a remission of symptoms in a psychosis.

malingerer conscious simulation of illness used to avoid a personally unpleasant or intolerable alternative.

manic-depressive psychosis major emotional illness marked by severe mood swings alternating from elation to depression and a tendency to remission and recurrence; depressed type is characterized by depression of mood with retardation and inhibition of thinking and physical activity; manic type is characterized by elation, overtalkativeness, extremely rapid ideation, and increased motor activity.

megalomania syndrome marked by delusions of great self-importance, wealth, or power.

melancholia pathologic dejection, usually of psychotic depth.

mental mechanisms also called defense mechanisms and mental dynamisms; specific intrapsychic defensive processes, operating unconsciously, which are employed to seek resolution of emotional conflict and freedom from anxiety; conscious efforts are frequently made for the same reasons, but true mental mechanisms are out of awareness (unconscious).

milieu the environment, the people and objects with which the individual deals.

mysophobia morbid fear of dirt, germs, or contamination.

narcissism self-love; in a broader sense indicates a degree of self-interest normal in early childhood but pathologic when seen in similar degree in adulthood.

narcolepsy condition in which the individual is overcome by short irresistible periods of sleep.

negative feelings as used in psychiatry, refers to hostile, unfriendly feelings.

negativism perverse opposition and resistance to suggestions or advice; often observed in people who subjectively feel "pushed around."

neologism in psychiatry, new word or condensed combination of several words coined by a patient to express a highly complex meaning related to his conflicts; not readily understood by others; common in schizophrenia.

neuroses emotional maladaptations due to unresolved unconscious conflicts; one of the two major categories of emotional illness, the other being the psychoses; usually less severe than a psychosis, with minimal loss of contact with reality; thinking and judgment may be impaired; a neurotic illness represents the attempted resolution of unconscious emotional conflicts; types of neuroses are usually classified according to the particular predominate symptoms.

nihilism as used in psychiatry, refers to the delusion of nonexistence of the self or part of self.

obsession persistent, unwanted idea or impulse that cannot be eliminated by usual logic or reasoning.

oral erotism pleasurable sensation obtained from the mouth; first experienced in suckling at the breast; later modified and sublimated but still persisting as in kissing.

oral stage includes both the oral-erotic and oral-sadistic phases of infantile psychosexual development, lasting from birth to 12 months or longer; oral-erotic phase is the initial pleasurable experience of nursing; oral-sadistic phase is the subsequent aggressive (biting) phase; both erotism and sadism normally continue in later life in disguised and sublimated forms.

orientation awareness of oneself in relation to time, place, and person.

orthopsychiatry psychiatry concerned with the study of children; emphasis is placed on preventive techniques to promote normal, healthy emotional growth and development.

overcompensation conscious or unconscious process by which a real or fancied physical or psychologic deficit inspires exaggerated correction.

panic as used in psychiatry, refers to an attack of acute, intense, and overwhelming anxiety, accompanied by a considerable degree of personality disorganization.

paranoia rare psychotic disorder that develops slowly and becomes chronic; characterized by an intricate and internally logical system of persecutory or grandiose delusions, or both; stands by itself and does not interfere with the remainder of the personality, which continues essentially normal and apparently intact; to be distinguished from paranoid schizophrenic reactions and paranoid states.

penis envy literally, envy by the female of the penis of the male; more generally, the female's wish for male attributes, position, or advantages; believed by many to be a significant factor in female character development.

perversion substitution of another aim for the usual aim in any activity; usually related to sexual activity when a component of sex or an earlier stage of sexual development is substituted for normal coitus.

phallic stage period of psychosexual development from the age of about 2½ to 6 years during which sexual interest, curiosity, and pleasurable experience center about the penis and in girls, to a lesser extent, the clitoris.

phobia obsessive, persistent, unrealistic fear of an external object or situation such as heights, open spaces, dirt, and animals; fear believed to arise through a process of displacing an internal (unconscious) conflict to an external object symbolically related to the conflict.

pleasure principle basic psychoanalytic concept that man instinctually seeks to avoid pain and discomfort and strives for gratification and pleasure; in personality development theories, the pleasure principle antedates and subsequently comes in conflict with the *reality principle*.

preconscious referring to thoughts that are not in immediate awareness but that can be recalled by conscious effort.

projection mental mechanism, operating unconsciously, whereby that which is emotionally unacceptable in the self is unconsciously rejected and attributed (projected) to others; attributes so assigned to another are real to the self and the self reacts accordingly.

psyche the mind, in distinction to the soma, or body.

psychodynamic the systematized knowledge and theory of human behavior and its motivation, the study of which depends largely upon the functional significance of emotion; psychodynamics recognizes the role of the unconscious motivation in human behavior; a predictive science, based on the assumption that a person's total makeup and probable reactions at any given moment are the product of past interactions between his specific genetic endowment and the environment in which he has lived from conception onward.

psychogenesis production or causation of a symptom or illness by mental or psychic factors as opposed to organic ones.

psychosexual development the changes and stages that characterize the development of the psychological aspect of sexuality during the period from birth to adult life.

pyromania morbid compulsion to set fires.

rapport confidential relationships between the patient and the professional person who is in a helping relationship with the patient.

rationalization mental mechanism, operating unconsciously, by which the individual attempts to justify or make consciously tolerable, by plausible means, feelings, behavior, and motives that would otherwise be intolerable (not to be confused with conscious evasion or dissimulation).

reaction formation mental mechanism, operating unconsciously, wherein attitudes and behavior are adopted that are the opposites of impulses the individual disowns either consciously or unconsciously—for example, excessive moral zeal may be the product of strong but repressed antisocial impulses.

reality principle in Freudian theory, the concept that the *pleasure principle* in personality development in infancy is normally modified by the inescapable demands and requirements of external reality; the process by which this compromise is effected is technically known as "reality testing," both in normal growth and in psychiatric treatment.

regression partial or symbolic return to more infantile ways of gratification; most clearly seen in severe psychoses.

repression mental mechanism, operating unconsciously; the common denominator and unconscious precursor of all mental mechanisms in which there is involuntary relegation of unbearable ideas and impulses into the unconscious from whence they are not ordinarily subject to voluntary recall but may emerge in disguised form through utilization of one of the various mental mechanisms; particularly operative in early years.

resistance in psychiatry, an individual's massive psychologic defense against bringing repressed (unconscious) thoughts or impulses into awareness, thus avoiding anxiety.

Rorschach test psychologic test developed by the Swiss psychiatrist Hermann Rorschach (1884-1922), which seeks to disclose conscious and unconscious personality traits and emotional conflicts through eliciting the patient's associations to a standard set of inkblots.

sadism pleasure derived from inflicting physical or psychological pain on others; the sexual significance of sadistic wishes or behavior may be conscious or unconscious; the reverse of masochism.

schizoid adjective describing traits of shyness, introspection, and introversion.

schizophrenia severe emotional disorder of psychotic depth characteristically marked by a retreat from reality with delusion formations, hallucinations, emotional disharmony, and regressive behavior; formerly called dementia praecox.

sensorium roughly approximates consciousness; includes the special sensory perceptive powers and their central correlation and integration in the brain; a clear sensorium conveys the presence of a reasonably accurate memory together with a correct orientation for time, place, and person.

soma the body, the physical aspect of man as distinguished from the psyche.

somatic bodily, having reference to the body or its organs.

stereotypy persistent, mechanical repetition of an activity, common in schizophrenia.

subconscious psychiatrically obsolescent; refers in general to both that which is not subject to recall and to that which may, with independent effort, be recalled.

sublimation mental mechanism, operating unconsciously, through which consciously unacceptable instinctual drives are diverted into personally and socially acceptable channels.

substitution mental mechanism, operating unconsciously, by which an unattainable or unacceptable goal, emotion, or object is replaced by one that is more attainable or acceptable.

suggestibility referring to a person's susceptibility to having his ideas or actions changed by the influence of others.

superego in Freudian theory, that part of the mind that has unconsciously identified itself with important and esteemed persons from early life, particularly parents; the supposed or actual wishes of these significant persons are taken over as part of one's own personal standards to help form the "conscience." These standards may remain anachronistic and overpunitive, especially in psychoneurotic patients.

suppression conscious effort to overcome unacceptable thoughts or desires.

symbolization mental mechanism, operating unconsciously, in which a person forms an abstract representation of a particular object, idea, or constellation thereof. The symbol carries, in more or less disguised form, the emotional feelings vested in the initial object or ideas.

toxic psychosis psychosis resulting from the toxic effect of chemicals and drugs, including those produced in the body.

transference unconscious attachment to others of feelings and attitudes that were originally associated with important figures (parents, siblings, etc.) in one's early life. The transference relationship follows roughly the pattern of its prototype; the psychiatrist utilizes the phenomenon as a therapeutic tool to help the patient understand his emotional problems and their origin; in the patient-physician relationship the transference may be negative (hostile) or positive (affectionate).

transvestism sexual pleasure derived from dressing or masquerading in the clothing of the opposite sex; the sexual origins of transvestism may be unconscious.

unconscious in Freudian theory, that part of the mind or mental functioning the content of which is only rarely subject to awareness; a repository for data that has never been conscious (primary repression) or that may have become conscious briefly and was then repressed (secondary repression).

undoing primitive defense mechanism, operating unconsciously, by which something unacceptable and already done is symbolically acted out in reverse, usually repetitiously, in the hope of "undoing" it and thus relieving anxiety.

verbigeration stereotyped and seemingly meaningless verbal responses without relevance to the attempt of another to converse.

volition the will.

word salad voluble speech in which words and phrases have no logical connection or meaning.

zones, erotic regions such as the lips, breasts, genitoanal area, etc., stimulation of which causes erotic excitement.

Tranquilizers and antidepressants*

TABLE 1. *Tranquilizers*

| Drug | Dosage | | Use | Side effects and precautions |
	Minimum	Maximum		
Chlorpromazine (Thorazine)	10 to 25 mg. t.i.d. *Children:* ¼ mg. per pound to 100 mg. per day	1,500 to 2,000 mg. per day	Agitation, hyperactivity, and anxiety in psychoses (schizophrenia, manic-depressive states, and organic psychoses)	Incidence of various side effects varies widely (from 0 to 50%), depending upon drug used, size of dose, and individual sensitivity of patient *Hypotension, convulsive seizures, and blood dyscrasias (leukopenia and agranulocytosis) more common with these diethylamine phenothiazines*
Promazine (Sparine)	25 to 200 mg. t.i.d. *Children:* Over 12 years 10 to 25 mg. t.i.d.	1,000 mg. per day	Psychoneurosis, behavior disorders, and alcoholism	Nurse also to be on alert for following: jaundice, liver damage, urticaria, contact dermatitis, photosensitivity, gastrointestinal syndrome, parkinsonism, blurry vision, depression, constipation, urinary difficulties, vomiting, drowsiness, fatigue, cataleptic seizures, impairment of power of voluntary motion, and excessive lactation These drugs also potentiate CNS depressants (alcohol, barbiturates, etc.)

*Adapted from Ulett, George A., and Goodrich, D. Wells: A synopsis of contemporary psychiatry, ed. 4, St. Louis, 1969, The C. V. Mosby Co.

Continued.

TABLE 1. *Tranquilizers—cont'd*

| Drug | Dosage | | Use | Side effects and precautions |
	Minimum	*Maximum*		
Prochlorperazine (Compazine)	15 to 20 mg. per day *Children:* 5 to 25 mg. per day	75 to 150 mg. per day	Agitation, hyperactivity, and anxiety in psychoses (schizophrenia, manic-depressive states, and organic psychoses) Psychoneurosis, behavior disorders, and alcoholism	Incidence of various side effects varies widely (from 0% to 50%), depending upon drug used, size of dose, and individual sensitivity of patient *Dystonic reactions (parkinsonism, cataleptic seizures) seen commonly with the piperazinyl phenothiazines* Nurse also to be on alert for following: jaundice, liver damage, leukopenia, agranulocytosis, urticaria, contact dermatitis, photosensitivity, gastrointestinal syndrome, blurry vision, convulsive seizures, hypotension, depression, constipation, urinary difficulty, vomiting, drowsiness, fatigue, and excessive lactation This drug also potentiates CNS depressants (alcohol, barbiturates, etc.)

TABLE 1. *Tranquilizers—cont'd*

| Drug | Dosage | | Use | Side effects and precautions |
	Minimum	Maximum		
Perphenazine (Trilafon)	2 mg. t.i.d.	64 mg. per day	Agitation, hyperactivity, and anxiety in psychoses (schizophrenia, manic-depressive states, and organic psychoses)	Incidence of various side effects varies widely (from 0 to 50%), depending upon drug used, size of dose, and individual sensitivity of patient
				Dystonic reactions (parkinsonism, cataleptic seizures) seen commonly with the piperazinyl phenothiazines
Trifluoperazine (Stelazine)	2 mg. t.i.d.	80 mg. per day	Psychoneurosis, behavior disorders, and alcoholism	Nurse also to be on alert for following: jaundice, liver damage, leukopenia, agranulocytosis, urticaria, contact dermatitis, photosensitivity, gastrointestinal syndrome, blurry vision, convulsive seizures, hypotension, depression, constipation, urinary difficulty, vomiting, drowsiness, fatigue, and excessive lactation
				These drugs also potentiate CNS depressants (alcohol, barbiturates, etc.)

Continued.

TABLE 1. *Tranquilizers—cont'd*

Drug	Dosage		Use	Side effects and precautions
	Minimum	*Maximum*		
Thioridazine hydrochloride (Mellaril)	10 mg. t.i.d. *Children:* 10 mg. t.i.d.	800 mg. per day	Agitation, hyperactivity, and anxiety in psychoses (schizophrenia, manic-depressive states, and organic psychoses) Psychoneurosis, behavior disorders, and alcoholism	Incidence of various side effects varies widely (from 0 to 50%), depending upon drug used, size of dose, and individual sensitivity of patient Nurse to be on alert for following: jaundice, liver damage, leukopenia, agranulocytosis, urticaria, contact dermatitis, photosensitivity, gastrointestinal syndrome, parkinsonism, blurry vision, convulsive seizures, hypotension, depression, constipation, urinary difficulty, vomiting, drowsiness, fatigue, cataleptic seizures, impairment of power of voluntary motion, and excessive lactation This drug also potentiates CNS depressants (alcohol, barbiturates, etc.)

TABLE 2. *Tranquilizers—Rauwolfia alkaloids*

Source	Drug	Dosage	Use	Side effects and precautions
Rauwolfia ser-pentina, Benth (shrub of Apocynaceae family indigenous to India); powdered whole root	Raudixin	200 mg. initially; after 10 days adjust maintenance dose to 50 to 300 mg.	Sedation and tranquilization in anxiety and agitation of psychoses and psychoneuroses	*Include:* Adverse behavioral effects (fatigue, listlessness, somnolence, weakness), Parkinson's syndrome (5%), dystonic syndrome, seizures, hypotension, edema, mental depression, activation of peptic ulcer
Purified alkaloid reserpine	Serpasil	0.25 mg. b.i.d. starting dose; maintenance, 0.25 mg. per day for hypertension and mild emotional disturbances 3 to 20 mg. per day for psychotics	Potentiates action of barbiturates and other sedatives Hypertension	*Less severe:* Nasal congestion, excess salivation, bradycardia, flushing, vomiting, diarrhea Initial sedation may give way to period of restlessness and to occurrence of mild side reactions, which disappear as favorable response begins in second or third week

315

TABLE 3. *Tranquilizers—glycol, glycol derivatives, and others*

Drug	Dosage		Use	Side effects and precautions
	Adults	*Children*		
Meprobamate (Equanil) (Miltown)	400 mg. b.i.d. to q.i.d.	100 mg. t.i.d. 200 mg. 3 years and over	Tranquilization Antianxiety and muscle relaxation	Produces addiction and withdrawal syndrome with convulsions Allergic reactions: rash, drowsiness
Oxanamide (Quiactin)	400 mg. q.i.d.		Anxiety and tension	
Chlordiaze-poxide (Librium)	10 mg. b.i.d. to 25 mg. q.i.d.	5 mg. t.i.d.	Anxiety and tension, especially psychoneuroses, and behavioral disorders of children	Observe caution in patients with renal or hepatic insufficiency

TABLE 4. *Antidepressants (psychic energizers): nonhydrazine monoamino oxidase inhibitors (MAO)*

Drug	Dosage			Use	Side effects	Precautions
	Start	*Treatment*	*Maintenance*			
Isocarbox-azid (analog of iproni-azid) (Marplan)	10 mg. t.i.d.	Same	10 mg. b.i.d. or t.i.d.	Depression of all types, including both psychotic and psycho-neurotic; also depression with chronic illness	Hypertensive crises (hypertensive reaction with headache, nausea and vomiting, palpitations, and rarely intracranial bleeding) presumably a result of sympatho-mimetic actions of phenelzine and tranylcypromine, have been reported immediately following administration of amphetamine or ingestion of certain foods	Observe for effects of over-stimulation
Phenelzine dihydrogen sulfate (Nardil)	15 mg. t.i.d.	Improvement seen in 7 to 14 days; reduce to 15 mg. per day	Continue 2 to 5 weeks			Suicide always a danger during recovery from depressions
				Angina pectoris		Contraindicated in patients with cerebrovascular and cardiovascular disorders
Nialamide (Niamid)	25 mg. t.i.d. or q.i.d.	Increase to 200 mg. if no response within a few days	Reduce to meet individual requirements			
					Constipation and delayed micturition	
					Edema	
					Blurred vision, dry mouth	
					Sweating	
					Occasional weakness, lethargy, headaches	
					Occasional skin rash	
					Occasional nausea	

Continued.

317

TABLE 4. *Antidepressants (psychic energizers): nonhydrazine monoamino oxidase inhibitors (MAO)—cont'd*

Drug	Dosage			Use	Side effects	Precautions
	Start	*Treatment*	*Maintenance*			
Tranylcypromine (Parnate)	10 mg. b.i.d. for 2 to 3 weeks	Same	10 to 30 mg.; above 60 mg. not advised	Severe depression in patients under 60 and under supervision in hospital	Postural hypotension, constipation, urinary hesitancy, blurring of vision, vertigo, nausea, and anorexia; severe hypertensive reactions have occurred following ingestion of cheese	Contraindicated in patients with cerebrovascular or cardiovascular disease
		Intensive: Intensive: 20 mg. A.M. 10 mg. P.M.				Do not give in conjunction with other amino oxidase inhibitors or with Tofranil or Elavil
						Observe for effects of overstimulation
						Not to be given in combination with amphetamines, alcohol, or with diuretic, antihistaminic, or sedative drugs
						Cheese must be withheld from diet
						Frequent blood pressure readings are essential

TABLE 5. *Antidepressants (psychic energizers); Dibenzazepine derivatives* (not MAO inhibitors)*

Drug	Dosage			Use	Side effects	Precautions
	Start	Treat-ment	Mainte-nance			
Imipramine hydrochloride (Tofranil)	26 mg. t.i.d.	Increase to 150 mg. per day if necessary	Reduce gradually to 50 mg. per day if possible	Depression, anxiety, tension, psychosomatic disorders, alcohol intoxication; used in combination with phenothiazines for psychoses, mental deficiency, schizophrenia, etc.	Dry mouth, blurred vision, insomnia, dizziness, headache, nausea, skin rash, tremor, occasionally drowsiness, constipation, or G. I. disturbances	Do not give with monoamine oxidase inhibitor and give with care in patients with convulsive disorder; use with caution in glaucoma or patients with a propensity to urinary retention. Observe for effects of overstimulation. Suicide always a danger during recovery from depressions

*These drugs should never be administered concurrently with any monoamino oxidase inhibitors

TABLE 6. *Antidepressants—the stimulants*

Drug	Dosage	Use	Side effects and precautions
Dextroamphetamine (Dexedrine)	Up to 30 mg. per day Spansule capsule gives 10 to 12 hour therapeutic effect	Mild depression; and lethargy; hyperactive children, behavior disorders	
Methamphetamine (Desoxyn)	2.5 mg., b.i.d. or t.i.d. before breakfast and at noon Long-release tablets given once daily in morning	Mild stimulant and antidepressant; stimulates freer verbalization Neurotic and psychotic depression, drug induced depressions	Sympathomimetic effects; may potentiate epinephrine; check blood pressure with repeated doses
Methylphenidate (Ritalin)	Oral: 10 to 20 mg. t.i.d. Injectable (I.V., I.M., or subcutaneously): 10 to 50 mg. q.½h. or as indicated		

Classification of mental illnesses

The following is a classification of mental illnesses that has been prepared by the committee on Nomenclature and Statistics of the American Psychiatric Association. The classification was published in the *Diagnostic and Statistical Manual of Mental Disorders*, Washington, D. C., in 1968 by the American Psychiatric Association Mental Hospital Service.

LIST OF DSM-II
DIAGNOSES AND CODE NUMBERS†

I MENTAL RETARDATION

310	Borderline
311	Mild
312	Moderate
313	Severe
314	Profound
315	Unspecified

With each: Following or associated with

.0	Infection or intoxication
.1	Trauma or physical agent
.2	Disorders of metabolism, growth, or nutrition
.3	Gross brain disease (postnatal)
.4	Unknown prenatal influence
.5	Chromosomal abnormality
.6	Prematurity
+ .7	Major psychiatric disorder
+ .8	Psychosocial (environmental) deprivation
.9	Other condition

II ORGANIC BRAIN SYNDROMES (OBS)
A PSYCHOSES
Senile and presenile dementia

290.0	Senile dementia
290.1	Presenile dementia

Alcoholic psychosis

+ 291.0	Delirium tremens
+ 291.1	Korsakov's psychosis
+ 291.2	Other alcoholic hallucinosis
+ 291.3	Alcohol paranoid state
+ 291.4*	Acute alcohol intoxication*
+ 291.5*	Alcoholic deterioration*
+ 291.6*	Pathological intoxication*
291.9	Other alcoholic psychosis

Psychosis associated with intracranial infection

292.0	General paralysis
292.1	Syphilis of CNS
292.2	Epidemic encephalitis
292.3	Other and unspecified encephalitis
292.9	Other intracranial infection

Psychosis associated with other cerebral condition

293.0	Cerebral arteriosclerosis
293.1	Other cerebrovascular disturbance
293.2	Epilepsy
293.3	Intracranial neoplasm
293.4	Degenerative disease of the CNS
293.5	Brain trauma
293.9	Other cerebral condition

Psychosis associated with other physical condition

294.0	Endocrine disorder
294.1	Metabolic and nutritional disorder
294.2	Systemic infection
294.3	Drug or poison intoxication (other than alcohol)
+ 294.4	Childbirth
294.8	Other and unspecified physical condition

B NONPSYCHOTIC OBS

309.0	Intracranial infection
+ 309.13*	Alcohol* (simple drunkenness)
+ 309.14*	Other drug, poison or systemic intoxication*
309.2	Brain trauma
309.3	Circulatory disturbance
309.4	Epilepsy
309.5	Disturbance of metabolism, growth, or nutrition
309.6	Senile or presenile brain disease

†Many of the titles here are listed in abbreviated form.
+These are new diagnoses that do not appear in DSM-1.
*These diagnoses are for use in the United States only and do not appear in ICD-8.

309.7 Intracranial neoplasm
309.8 Degenerative disease of the CNS
309.9 Other physical condition

III PSYCHOSES NOT ATTRIBUTED TO PHYSICAL CONDITIONS LISTED PREVIOUSLY

Schizophrenia

	295.0	Simple
	295.1	Hebephrenic
	295.2	Catatonic
+	295.23*	Catatonic type, excited*
+	295.24*	Catatonic type, withdrawn*
	295.3	Paranoid
+	295.4	Acute schizophrenic episode
+	295.5	Latent
	295.6	Residual
	295.7	Schizo-affective
+	295.73*	Schizo-affective, excited*
+	295.74*	Schizo-affective, depressed*
	295.8*	Childhood*
	295.90*	Chronic undifferentiated*
	295.99*	Other schizophrenia*

Major affective disorders

	296.0	Involutional melancholia
	296.1	Manic-depressive illness, manic
	296.2	Manic-depressive illness, depressed
	296.3	Manic-depressive illness, circular
+	296.33*	Manic-depressive, circular, manic*
+	296.34*	Manic-depressive, circular, depressed*
	296.8	Other major affective disorder

Paranoid states

	297.0	Paranoia
+	297.1	Involutional paranoid state
	297.9	Other paranoid state

Other psychoses

298.0 Psychotic depressive reaction

IV NEUROSES

	300.0	Anxiety
	300.1	Hysterical
+	300.13*	Hysterical, conversion type*
+	300.14*	Hysterical, dissociative type*
	300.2	Phobic
	300.3	Obsessive, compulsive
	300.4	Depressive
+	300.5	Neurasthenic

+	300.6	Depersonalization
+	300.7	Hypochondriacal
	300.8	Other neurosis

V PERSONALITY DISORDERS AND CERTAIN OTHER NONPSYCHOTIC MENTAL DISORDERS

Personality disorders

	301.0	Paranoid
	301.1	Cyclothymic
	301.2	Schizoid
+	301.3	Explosive
	301.4	Obsessive compulsive
+	301.5	Hysterical
+	301.6	Asthenic
	301.7	Antisocial
	301.81*	Passive-aggressive*
	301.82*	Inadequate*
	301.89*	Other specified types*

Sexual deviation

+	302.0	Homosexuality
+	302.1	Fetishism
+	302.2	Pedophilia
+	302.3	Transvestitism
+	302.4	Exhibitionism
+	302.5*	Voyeurism*
+	302.6*	Sadism*
+	302.7*	Masochism*
	302.8	Other sexual deviation

Alcoholism

+	303.0	Episodic excessive drinking
+	303.1	Habitual excessive drinking
+	303.2	Alcohol addiction
	303.9	Other alcoholism

Drug dependence

+	304.0	Opium, opium alkaloids and their derivatives
+	304.1	Synthetic analgesics with morphine-like effects
+	304.2	Barbiturates
+	304.3	Other hypnotics and sedatives or "tranquilizers"
+	304.4	Cocaine
+	304.5	Cannabis sativa (hashish, marihuana)
+	304.6	Other psychostimulants
+	304.7	Hallucinogens
	304.8	Other drug dependence

VI PSYCHOPHYSIOLOGIC DISORDERS

  305.0   Skin
  305.1   Musculoskeletal
  305.2   Respiratory
  305.3   Cardiovascular
  305.4   Hemic and lymphatic
  305.5   Gastrointestinal
  305.6   Genitourinary
  305.7   Endocrine
  305.8   Organ of special sense
  305.9   Other type

VII SPECIAL SYMPTOMS

    306.0   Speech disturbance
    306.1   Specific learning disturbance
+ 306.2   Tic
+ 306.3   Other psychomotor disorder
+ 306.4   Disorders of sleep
+ 306.5   Feeding disturbance
    306.6   Enuresis
+ 306.7   Encopresis
+ 306.8   Cephalalgia
    306.9   Other special symptom

VIII TRANSIENT SITUATIONAL DISTURBANCES

  307.0*   Adjustment reaction of infancy*
  307.1*   Adjustment reaction of childhood*
  307.2*   Adjustment reaction of adolescence*
  307.3*   Adjustment reaction of adult life*
  307.4*   Adjustment reaction of late life*

IX BEHAVIOR DISORDERS OF CHILDHOOD AND ADOLESCENCE

+ 308.0*   Hyperkinetic reaction*
+ 308.1*   Withdrawing reaction*
+ 308.2*   Overanxious reaction*
+ 308.3*   Runaway reaction*
+ 308.4*   Unsocialized aggressive reaction*
+ 308.5*   Group delinquent reaction*
    308.9*   Other reaction*

X CONDITIONS WITHOUT MANIFEST PSYCHIATRIC DISORDER AND NONSPECIFIC CONDITIONS

Social maladjustment without manifest psychiatric disorder

+ 316.0*   Marital maladjustment*
+ 316.1*   Social maladjustment*
+ 316.2*   Occupational maladjustment*
    316.3*   Dyssocial behavior*
+ 316.9*   Other social maladjustment*

Nonspecific conditions

+ 317*   Nonspecific conditions*

No mental disorder

+ 318*   No mental disorder*

XI NONDIAGNOSTIC TERMS FOR ADMINISTRATIVE USE

  319.0   Diagnosis deferred*
  319.1*   Boarder*
  319.2*   Experiment only*
  319.3*   Other*

Index